Neurosurgical Treatments for Psychiatric Disorders

Bomin Sun · Antonio De Salles
Editors

Neurosurgical Treatments for Psychiatric Disorders

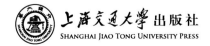 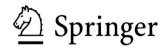

Editors
Bomin Sun
Ruijin Hospital, Center for Functional
 Neurosurgery
Shanghai Jiao Tong University
Shanghai
China

Antonio De Salles
Neurosurgery
University of California
Los Angeles
USA

and

HCor Neuroscience
Sao Paulo
Brazil

ISBN 978-94-017-9575-3   ISBN 978-94-017-9576-0   (eBook)
DOI 10.1007/978-94-017-9576-0
Springer Dordrecht Heidelberg New York London

Library of Congress Control Number: 2014953249

Jointly published with Shanghai Jiao Tong University Press

© Shanghai Jiao Tong University Press, Shanghai and Springer Science+Business Media
Dordrecht 2015
This work is subject to copyright. All rights are reserved by the Publishers, whether the whole
or part of the material is concerned, specifically the rights of translation, reprinting, reuse of
illustrations, recitation, broadcasting, reproduction on microfilms or in any other physical way,
and transmission or information storage and retrieval, electronic adaptation, computer software,
or by similar or dissimilar methodology now known or hereafter developed. Exempted from this
legal reservation are brief excerpts in connection with reviews or scholarly analysis or material
supplied specifically for the purpose of being entered and executed on a computer system, for
exclusive use by the purchaser of the work. Duplication of this publication or parts thereof is
permitted only under the provisions of the Copyright Law of the Publishers' locations, in its
current version, and permission for use must always be obtained from Springer. Permissions for
use may be obtained through RightsLink at the Copyright Clearance Center. Violations are
liable to prosecution under the respective Copyright Law.
The use of general descriptive names, registered names, trademarks, service marks, etc. in this
publication does not imply, even in the absence of a specific statement, that such names are
exempt from the relevant protective laws and regulations and therefore free for general use.
While the advice and information in this book are believed to be true and accurate at the date of
publication, neither the authors nor the editors nor the publishers can accept any legal
responsibility for any errors or omissions that may be made. The publishers make no warranty,
express or implied, with respect to the material contained herein.

Printed on acid-free paper

Springer is part of Springer Science+Business Media (www.springer.com)

Foreword I

Modern Psychiatric Surgery and Old Fears

Although it is acceptable to prescribe medication to patients, damping brain circuitry, to a point that the patients' cognition, sexual function, balance, and motor function are impaired, surgical procedures to improve brain function, guided to a specific disturbance detected by functional imaging are still in their infancy, chiefly for established psychiatric diseases. It is important that the specificity of these procedures bypass at large the systemic side effects related to medications. The effectiveness, safety, and reversibility of novel surgical procedures directed to psychiatric symptoms, for example, continuous electrical stimulation, or nonreversible novel lesion-making techniques, such as high frequency ultrasound and gamma knife surgery, which does not even violate the skull, are attractive for highly suffering patients.

Functional imaging is bringing to light previous studies of neurosurgeons, psychiatrists, and neurologists working together to understand brain circuitry and the consequences of structural modification of this circuitry, either secondary to structural diseases or iatrogenic. While at the birth of behavioral surgery the procedures were massively aggressive to the brain and practiced indiscriminately, now the multidisciplinary approach, institutional review boards, and improved methods of diagnosis of psychiatric disorders make the possibility of poor practice of behavioral surgery very remote. Moreover, some of the current procedures are reversible, such as deep brain stimulation.

The association of functional imaging to structural imaging based on robust software for imaging analysis and device development to influence brain function is the center of the novel "Why Fly Over the Cuckoo's Nest, Psychosurgery in My Brain Please," by Antonio De Salles (Ref. [28] of the Chap. 19), challenging the outdated control by civil authorities of the so-called "psychosurgery." To what degree are civil authorities and the general public aware of the important differences between current behavioral/psychiatry neurosurgery, psychiatry and neuroscience, and the stereotypes evoked by the controversial figures of the past exemplified by Dr. William Friedman, who performed lobotomies indiscriminately and without respect to event the most basic surgical practices of asepsis and hemostasis?

While tight control of surgical procedures modifying the human brain for therapeutic reasons seems to be outdated, the hideous use of such practices to change the individual minds due to disagreement of political and cultural views has fortunately been abolished from "medical" practice. The confusion between patient's need for surgery and the malpractice of medicine for profit in disregard to patient's interest is still a matter of worry though. On the other hand, thousands of helpless patients with intractable psychiatric symptoms (by currently available noninvasive treatments) remain without access to surgical procedures that have been proven to be both safe and effective. To what degree is the psychosurgery stigma guarding us from old fears or merely precluding the access of needy patients to treatment?

Lincoln Frias
Ricardo de Oliveira
Jorge Moll
D'Or Institute for Research and Education (IDOR)
Rio de Janeiro
Brazil

Foreword II

Functional Imaging and developments in pacemakers for the brain, as well as the acceptance of the psychiatric community of medical therapy's failure to help a substantial number of patients with psychiatric diseases has brought back the interest in Psychiatric Surgery.

"Surgical Treatment for Psychiatric Disorders": Is there a chance to have society broadly agreeing to the renaissance of what was in the past called "Psychosurgery," the terrible invasion of the human mind? Are we prepared to undertake this controversial field ahead and avoid the terrible wounds of the past from being reopened, as described by a lobotomized patient in 1960?

"I am a bus driver. I am a survivor: In 1960, when I was twelve years old, I was given a transorbital, or "ice pick" lobotomy. My stepmother arranged it. My father agreed to it. Dr. Walter Freeman, the father of American lobotomy, told me he was going to do some "tests." It took ten minutes and cost two hundred dollars. The surgery damaged me in many ways. But it didn't "fix" me, or turn me into a robot. So my family put me into an institution. I spent the next four decades in and out of insane asylums, jails, and halfway houses. I was homeless, alcoholic, and drug-addicted. I was lost, I knew I wasn't crazy. But I knew something was wrong with me. Was it the lobotomy? Was it something else? I hadn't been a bad kid. I hadn't ever hurt anyone. Or had I? Was there something I had done, and forgotten – something so horrible that I deserved a lobotomy? I asked myself that question for more than forty years. I thought about my lobotomy all the time, but I never talked about it. It was my terrible secret. What had been so wrong with me?"

My Lobotomy
Howard Dully

Preface

This now over 50 year-old man was hurt for life by the abuse of a Psychiatrist, a luminary of the "Surgical Treatment of Psychiatric Disorder" field at that time.

While these kinds of stories are examples that come from that dark past, patients were also helped by surgery, otherwise it would not have arrived as far as it did during those years, when it was even a reason for a Nobel prize, at a time when the psychiatrists did not see the brain structure and function in a living patient as we can see today. Therefore, surgery was performed based on the subjective decision of a doctor, influenced by the desire of mal-intentioned people (this 12-year-old boy's story exemplifies this influence), by doctors' vanity and greediness, and by the financial pressure of public administrators dealing with the burden of overcrowded psychiatric hospitals. Unfortunately, the field was victim of the later reasons, since the most important tool supporting a surgical indication and precision was not available at that time, i.e., the visualization of the diseased brain and its functioning.

Presented in the pages of this textbook, written by specialists in Psychiatry, Neurosurgery, Neurology, Neuroanatomy, Neuroradiology, and Ethics, the reader will decide by himself if he is prepared to assume the heavy responsibility to help patients suffering from the most terrible suffering that a human can suffer, the suffering of the mind. They are not understood by their family members and society, and are therefore discriminated and doped so they do not participate and do not disturb normal lives. They become depressed to a point of not having the drive to work, date, and enjoy life. This leads to a very high addiction and suicidal rate, so high that it accounts as one of the diseases that kills most humans, close to the death rate of cancer, stroke, or heart disease. It also represents a terrible economical burden to society on jobs loss, absenteeism, and expenses with the care for these patients.

The first three chapters of the book bring the reader updated with the neuroanatomy and pathophysiology of the Psychiatric Disorders based on modern imaging, including connectivity and functional changes in specific areas of the brain. Following, come three chapters bringing lessons learned from the past, when the poor practice of this important field reigned and no rules existed. The ways lesions were made in the brain and the consequences of these lesions are stressed. These historical lessons are employed to discuss the ethical meanders of the Psychiatric Surgery practice. Once these issues are settled, the patients are prepared for surgery in a chapter dedicated to preoperative issues. At this point the reader is ready to learn and judge applications of novel techniques for modifying brain function, comparing them to the older approaches used for specific diseases. Further, applications in development, expanding the horizons of the field, are presented in the last six chapters.

This book is to be seen as an update of anatomical, ethical, and indications of "Surgery for Psychiatric Disease," opening the mind of the reader to the future of this promising field. It is expected that the reader acquire understanding of the surgical anatomy, the surgical techniques at hand, and ethical judgment of the power of this field, with the knowledge that this practice is in frank evolution and therefore controversial.

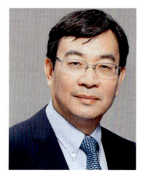

Bomin Sun

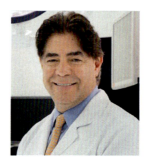

Antonio De Salles

Acknowledgments

After I graduated from medical school, I trained in Psychiatry. There, I understood that there were so many psychiatric patients who did not respond to psychological therapy and neuroleptics. There was really a need for an alternative treatment for these refractory patients. In 1986, by chance, I had been involved in a group performing stereotactic surgical treatment for mental disorders; at that time we only used ventriculography-guided surgery. Since then, I became very interested in surgical treatment for psychiatric disorders and I started training in neurosurgery including stereotactic and functional neurosurgery.

At UCLA medical center, I trained with Prof. Antonio De Salles as a fellow in stereotactic and functional neurosurgery and learned many basic knowledge and skills. During that period, I had the chance to meet many world class experts and discussed with them surgical treatment for psychiatric disorders. I remember that during a meeting of the ASSFN in 1999, Dr. Marwan Hariz taught me how to do capsulotomy in a swimming pool in Salt Lake city.

Since there are too many debates and misunderstandings on surgical treatment for psychiatric disorders, I was thinking that we needed a book that systematically and comprehensively discusses surgical treatment for mental disorders. My friend Prof. Keith Matthews, Psychiatrist from Dundee, Scotland provided many suggestions. Dr. Ree Cosgrove in Boston also provided detailed and constructive help toward this book.

I would like to express a special word of gratitude to my two great mentors. Dr. Jian-ping Xu, a pioneer of surgical treatment for psychiatric disorders in China, who triggered and stimulated my interest in stereotactic and functional neurosurgery while I was a resident in psychiatry. And to Prof. Antonio De Salles, who taught me advanced stereotactic and functional neurosurgery and opened my view to worldwide functional neurosurgery. Furthermore, he encouraged me to go back to China to establish a functional neurosurgery center after my training in UCLA, so that I had my platform to make effort toward stereotactic and functional neurosurgery.

Finally, I would also like to express a special word of gratitude to my colleagues, residents and fellows who over the years have contributed so much to the development of neurosurgical treatment for psychiatric disorders and their contributed to this book.

Bomin Sun

Contents

1 Related Circuitry and Synaptic Connectivity in Psychiatric Disorders 1
Jean-Jacques Lemaire

2 High-angular diffusion MRI in reward-based psychiatric disorders 21
Wenwen Yu, Qiming Lv, Chencheng Zhang, Zhuangming Shen, Bomin Sun and Zheng Wang

3 Neuroimaging in Psychiatry 35
Chuantao Zuo and Huiwei Zhang

4 DBS in Psychiatry and the Pendulum of History 47
Marwan I. Hariz

5 Ablative Surgery for Neuropsychiatric Disorders: Past, Present, Future 53
Yosef Chodakiewitz, John Williams, Jacob Chodakiewitz and Garth Rees Cosgrove

6 Legal Issues in Behavioral Surgery 69
Sam Eljamel

7 Preoperative Evaluation and Postoperative Follow-up of Deep Brain Stimulation for Psychiatric Disorders 77
Loes Gabriëls, Hemmings Wu and Bart Nuttin

8 Ablative Surgery for Depression 87
Sam Eljamel

9 Deep Brain Stimulation for the Management of Treatment-Refractory Major Depressive Disorder 95
Nir Lipsman, Peter Giacobbe and Andres M. Lozano

10 Ablative Surgery for Obsessive-Compulsive Disorders 105
Roberto Martinez-Alvarez

| 11 | **DBS for Obsessive-Compulsive Disorder** | 113 |

11 **DBS for Obsessive-Compulsive Disorder** 113
Mayur Sharma, Emam Saleh, Milind Deogaonkar
and Ali Rezai

12 **Focused Ultrasound for the Treatment
of Obsessive-Compulsive Disorder** 125
Young Cheol Na, Hyun Ho Jung and Jin Woo Chang

13 **Deep Brain Stimulation for Tourette Syndrome** 143
Jianuo Zhang, Yan Ge and Fangang Meng

14 **Stereotactic Neurosurgery for Drug Addiction** 161
Guodong Gao and Xuelian Wang

15 **Surgical Treatments for Anorexia Nervosa**............. 175
Bomin Sun, Dianyou Li, Wei Liu, Shikun Zhan,
Yixin Pan and Xiaoxiao Zhang

16 **Neurosurgery for the Treatment of Refractory
Schizophrenia**.................................. 189
Bomin Sun, Wei Liu, Shikun Zhan, Qianqian Hao,
Dianyou Li, Yixin Pan, Yongchao Li and Guozhen Lin

17 **Surgical Management for Aggressive Behavior**.......... 203
Wei Wang and Peng Li

18 **Deep Brain Stimulation in Aggressive Behavior** 211
Giuseppe Messina, Giovanni Broggi, Roberto Cordella
and Angelo Franzini

19 **Radiosurgery for Psychiatric Disorders** 217
Antônio De Salles and Alessandra A. Gorgulho

Index 227

Related Circuitry and Synaptic Connectivity in Psychiatric Disorders

1

Jean-Jacques Lemaire

Abstract

Deciphering the connectivity supporting brain function in psychiatric disorders is one of the major challenges in clinical neurosciences. Neural correlates of psychiatric disorders are not well-known because experimental research is extremely difficult to carry on facing the complexity of biological, medical and socio-psychological concepts. Although far from an extensive knowledge of such complex issue, one can summarize most main macroscopic or microscopic circuits known in human and higher species, but also in rodents. After a reminder of scales and functionality of neurobiological circuits, anatomo-functional correlates of the executive-behavioral system and psychiatric disorders are exposed, focusing on most frequent domains of psychiatry, anxiety, mood, substance disorders and memory.

1.1 Network Scales and Functionality of Neurobiological Circuits

The functionality of circuits involved in psychiatric disorders can be described from the molecular to the connectomics scales. The molecular scale is the neuronal transmission of information, still not extensively mastered, which can be split into two main types [2]: wiring transmission relying on synapses, neurotransmitters, excitatory such as the glutamate or inhibitory such as the gamma-amino-butyric acid (GABA), and gated ion channels; volume transmission relying on neuromodulators within the extracellular space and cerebrospinal fluid, such as dopamine and serotonin monoamine circuits, affecting large population of neurons through G protein-coupled receptors. Neurons can release several neurotransmitters, fast such as the glutamate and GABA, and modulatory, such as the dopamine [9]; typically within the striatum, medium-sized spiny neurons contain GABA and either substance P or enkephalin (see [32, 65]). Within the cortex, the complex distribution of neuromodulator and neurotransmitter receptors makes difficult the analysis of functionality of circuitries accounting molecular transmission of information, in particular in the context of psychiatric disorders (see e.g. [86]). At microscopic level, the study of structural microanatomy still relies

---

J.-J. Lemaire (✉)
Image-Guided Clinical Neuroscience and Connectomics, Auvergne University, Clermont-Ferrand, France
e-mail: jjlemaire@chu-clermontferrand.fr

J.-J. Lemaire
Service of Neurosurgery, University Hospital of Clermont-Ferrand, Clermont-Ferrand, France

---

B. Sun and A. De Salles (eds.), *Neurosurgical Treatments for Psychiatric Disorders*,
DOI 10.1007/978-94-017-9576-0_1
© Shanghai Jiao Tong University Press, Shanghai and Springer Science+Business Media Dordrecht 2015

on ex vivo histologic sampling; axonal tracing having harvested a lot of data on micro connectivity in humans and other species, however still complex to extrapolate at large scale. Molecular imaging using Petscan could explore in vivo components of neuronal signaling process, such as dopaminergic neurotransmission [105]. Nano circuitry of inter and intra cellular signaling (see e.g. [74]) is beyond the purpose of chapter, limited to microcircuits, i.e. inter neuronal connectivity. Ongoing researches tackling the challenge of mastering brain function based on bio-molecular controls should help in the near future [12, 14, 63, 111]. On the other hand, the connectomics scale, meso-macroscopic or millimetric, relies on segregation of brain function and parcellation of gray matter (GM); it is very close to the size of circuit elements described at the functional anatomy scale currently used in clinics for reasoning, and should likely be suitable for deciphering, at least partially, psychiatric disorder pathophysiology. Recent advances in optogenetic [75] rise hopes that future technologies mix electrical and pharmacological modulation, tuning finely neuromodulation at the core of neural circuits. Diffusion tensor imaging (DTI) fiber tracking (FT) enables in vivo analysis of the macroscopic connectivity of brain, probing white matter (WM) structures connecting cortical areas and deep GM regions. DTI is a fast magnetic resonance imaging (MRI) sequence exploring water molecule movements sequentially in several directions, usually from 6 to 20. The main orientation of water motion is resolved within each MRI voxel, resulting, after fiber tracking computational post processing, in colored fibers displayed in 3D within the whole MRI voxel data set. It is assumed that the anisotropic organization of WM due to nerve fiber (or axon) bundles explains the fibers resulting of DTI FT analysis. WM organization was explored by pioneering neuro-anatomists using brain hardening techniques of anatomic specimen [16, 50], introducing the term WM fascicle, later defined as microscopically delimited bundle of nerve fibers [89]. Tractus and pathways referred to bundles of nerve fibers subserving functions and

systems [89]: tractus or tract defined groups of fibers, such as the cortico-spinal tract subserving the motor system; pathway or path define chains of neurons, such as the visual pathway. Practically the macroscopic WM bundles, as those displayed by DTI FT, are structural, whereas tractus or pathways are related to known function; however the terms are often mixed up. With recent advances of functional connectivity and connectomics in vivo analysis, these differences could be of importance, connectomics referring to structure and functional connectivity to function, which are still not explored at the same time, at least with the same technique: functional MRI (fMRI; at rest and activation), 3D electroencephalography, molecular imaging, and magneto encephalography explore function; structural MRI is the most precise in vivo imaging technique to explore the brain meso- and macroarchitecture. Exploration of macro connectivity of psychiatric disorders using DTI could facilitate the understanding of abnormalities [41].

Fill the gap between micro and meso-macro connectivity is of upmost importance, and challenging, in psychosurgery, as we do not master the full functionality of the executive-behavioral system. Consequently we must deal with macro and micro approaches of pathologies and related circuits: topography of anatomo-functional elements of macro circuits, and molecular functionality of micro circuits. The tremendous knowledge of biochemical neuromodulation and transmission within the executive-behavioral system, enables the integration of micro and macro connectivity, which is however far to be extensively mastered. Among the circuits of the executive-behavioral system, the mesocorticolimbic circuitry, involved in reward [44] and mood disorder [86], is emblematic of the long way covered and also the considerable distance still to cover. Schematically the mesocorticolimbic system corresponds to the efferent connection of the ventral tegmental area (VTA) with neo and transitional cortices, such as the sensorimotor cortex, medial prefrontal cortices and the insula, and with limbic structures, such as the accumbens nucleus, the septal region, the cingulate and the hippocampus-amygdala complex [76]. VTA projects to the striatum together with the SN compacta, forming the VTA-nigral complex. The mesocorticolimbic system is often called reward system because most neurons, dopaminergic (VTA A10 neurons) or GABA, modify their activity when signaling salient events. Glutamate neurons activate VTA dopaminergic neurons [44], which target modulatory interneurons, under the control of inhibitory gabaergic neurons [13]. Dopaminergic neurons project to the pallidum and striatum, and control the direct and indirect pathways using specific dopamine receptors. GABA medium spiny neurons of striatum project to the lateral and the internal pallidum, and evoke potentials through co-transmission of information, respectively with enkephalin and substance P: (i) the direct pathway reinforces positively behavior, inhibiting the internal pallidum, hence provokes thalamus activation; (ii) the indirect pathway reinforces negatively behavior, inhibiting the external pallidum, hence activates the subthalamic nucleus (STN) and consequently inhibits the thalamus (for a review see [37]) (Fig. 1.1). Cholinergic modulatory interneurons are present within the striatum [78], and in large numbers within the basal forebrain, such as the pallidum, the substantia innominata, the septum, the diagonal band of Broca, the lateral hypothalamus, and particularly the nucleus of Meynert 90 % cholinergic [40] and the nucleus ansa lenticularis 50 % cholinergic in rodents [49].

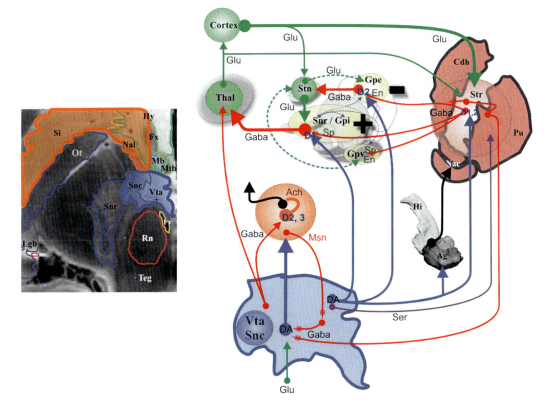

Fig. 1.1 Mesocorticolimbic system. *Left* axial high field MRI slice overlaid with anatomical structures of the executive-behavioral system, containing predominantly, dopamine (*blue*) or acetylcholine (*orange*) neurons. *Right* mesocorticolimbic system

1.2 Anatomo-Functional Correlates of the Executive-Behavioral System

The frontal, the temporal and the limbic lobes, coupled with basal ganglia, thalamus, hypothalamus, and upper midbrain nuclei are the main structures modulating behavioral phenotypes, and are all or part linked with psychiatric disorders. The cerebellum could be involved in psychiatric symptoms, through the cerebello-thalamo-cortico-pontine loop, in the posterior a fossa, and the cerebellar cognitive affective syndromes and others cognitive and affective disorders [15, 69].

The core system supporting neural correlates of psychiatric disorders is the executive-behavioral system involving the prefrontal and the cingulate cortices, and the rest of the limbic system, which includes the limbic lobe (Fig. 1.2). From the clinical experience, the whole frontal lobe could be involved in the executive-behavioral system, however this has to be interpreted cautiously [4], even though recent data shows that the supplementary motor area of medial motor cortex could participate to action-monitoring system, adjusting behavior according to the result of action [8]. Functional imaging should help to segregate functionalities supporting executive-behavior functions within the frontal lobe [102].

The executive-behavioral system supports the so-called "emotional brain" and "social brain" [24, 52], coming from pioneering works of Broca introducing the term "grand lobe limbique" [11], Papez [79] proposing the concept of corticothalamic correlate of emotions, and MacLean [58] extending Papez's work with the visceral brain (Fig. 1.3). A lot of connections between these structures are known, although the functionality, physiologic and pathophysiologic, of circuits is not fully mastered.

Broadly elements of executive-behavioral system are pushed aside by WM fascicles of the internal capsule, separating two groups: (i) the medial group, hypothalamus, subthalamus, thalamus, head of caudate nucleus, accumbens nucleus; (ii) the lateral group, hippocampus-amygdala complex, lateral striatum (putamen and

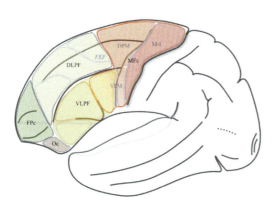 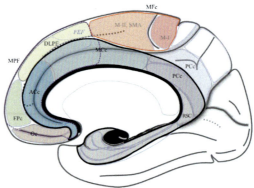

Fig. 1.2 Frontal and cingulate functional territories, and the limbic lobe. Segregation of frontal and cingulate cortices into functional territories [30, 82, 107], semi-schematic drawing; the frontal cortex is subdivided into motor and prefrontal regions. The motor cortex is made up of the primary motor (M-I; B4), dorsal premotor (DPM; B6), ventral premotor (VPM; B6, 44 and 45) and medial premotor (or supplementary motor area; MII-SMA; B6) cortices. The prefrontal cortex is made up of the ventrolateral prefrontal, the dorsolateral prefrontal (DLPF), the frontopolar (FPc), the orbitofrontal and the medial prefrontal cortex, which involves, (1) the medial part of the DLPF and the FPc cortex, and (2) the anterior cingulate cortex (ACc) and the rostral part of midcingulate cortex. The cingulate cortex is made up of ACc, MCc, posterior cingulate and retrosplenial cingulate cortices. The limbic lobe [19] is made up of the limbic (B27, 51 and 34) and paralimbic cortices (*grey*), the subcallosal and cingulate gyri, the isthmus and the parahippocampal gyrus, and the intralimbic gyrus (*black*), with 3 segments, anterior, superior and inferior or hypocampus (*fine white line*)

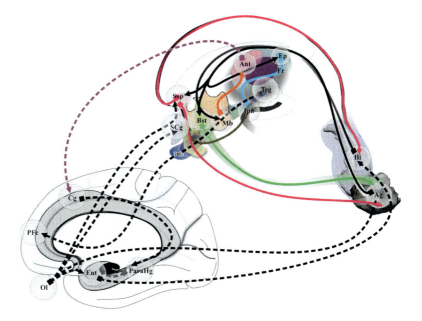

Fig. 1.3 Broca's, Papez's and Maclean's contributions to the emotional, social and limbic brain

tale of caudate nucleus), pallidal complex, substantia innominata, claustrum and insula. GM territories lined by arched fascicles connect the medial and lateral groups: superior (dorsal) system, cingulum with the cingulate, hippocampal, para hippocampal (including the entorhinal area), subcallosal and anterior intralimbic gyrii, olfactive fascicle, stria terminalis, fornix, and body of caudate; inferior (ventral) system, nucleus of ansa lenticularis and ansa lenticularis, extended amygdala, diagonal band of Broca and ventral pallidum. Commissural structures linked right and left elements of the executive-behavioral system, such as the corpus callosum, the fornix and the anterior commissure. The Fig. 1.4 summarizes anatomic elements of the executive-behavioral system.

The cingulum (Fig. 1.5) is made up of three fascicles [89]: anterior connecting the anterior perforate substantia with the frontal lobe, the horizontal connecting frontal, limbic and parietal gyrii; the posterior connects medial and lateral

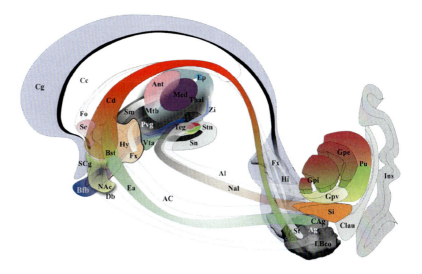

Fig. 1.4 Anatomic elements of the executive-behavioral system

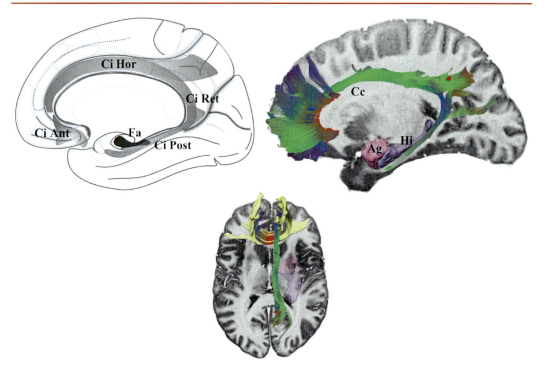

Fig. 1.5 Cingulum. *Left* fascicles of the cingulum. *Right* DTI tractography of the cingulum showing different components; note that anterior commissural fibers of the beak of callosum (*yellow*) merge with anterior fibers of the cingulum

occipito-temporal gyrii with the temporal gyrus. Recent advances have added new insights into the cingulum bundle, showing the multiple connection fibers merged [46]. In monkeys the cingulum also contains fibers connecting the prefrontal dorsolateral cortex and the hippocampal formation [31]. The distal, rostral, anterior cingulate is a part of the sub cingulo-callosal region that includes also the subcallosal (or subcallosal cingulate) gyrus and the carrefour olfactif of Broca (paraolfactory area). The gyrus rectus merges with the anterior cingulate and the subcallosal gyrus within the carrefour olfactif [89]. The organization of the WM of the sub cingulo-callosal region illustrates the complexity of connections, allowing the prefrontal cortex to connect with the lateral and the medial groups of elements of the executive-behavioral system (Fig. 1.6). The fornix connects the hypothalamus (mammillary and tubero mammillaris), the septum, and the habenula, with the Amon horn (alveus; medial) and the gyrus dentatus (fimbria; lateral). The olfactive fascicle connects the posterior septum and cingulate through the corpus callosum, with the anterior septal nuclei and the anterior perforate area, and continues to the amygdala, the substantia innominata and the uncus, through the diagonal band of Broca [89]. The stria terminalis connects the septal and paraseptal region (or bed of the stria terminalis) with the amygdala; the extended amygdala, a network of sparse cells and connections within the rostral mediobasal forebrain, located laterally to the hypothalamus and below the lenticular nucleus, bridges the bed nucleus of stria terminalis and the centromedial amygdala [27, 26]. The hypothalamus, made of 11 nuclei, had a large connectivity with the cortex and the deep brain [55] (Fig. 1.7), some features seems specific: dorsomedial nucleus mostly connected with the medial thalamus and the midline gray substance; ventromedial area (ventromedial nucleus and the adjacent tuberomamillaris nucleus) strongly connected with the prefrontal cortex; preoptic

1 Related Circuitry and Synaptic Connectivity in Psychiatric Disorders

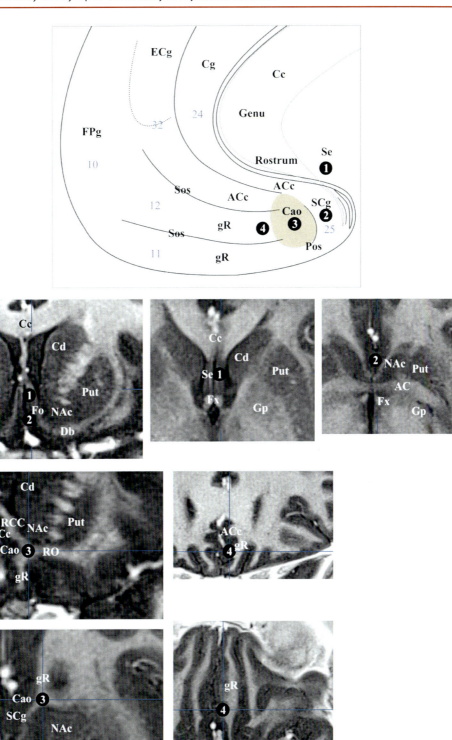

Fig. 1.6 Sub cingulo-callosal region. *Top* semi-schematic drawing, medial view, *bottom* MRI slices going through 1 and 2 (top row; left, coronal, intermediate and right axial), 3 (left column; top, coronal, and, bottom, axial) and 4 (right column; top, coronal, and, bottom, axial). Brodmann's areas are specified (*light gray* numbers)

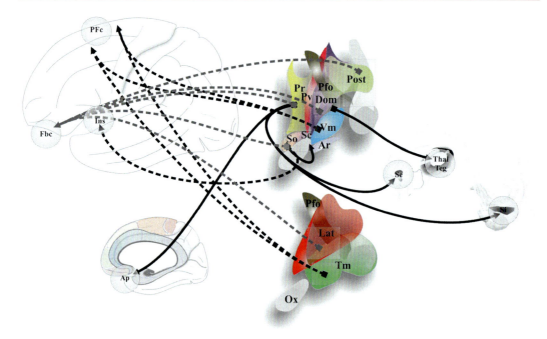

Fig. 1.7 Hypothalamus connections. Cortical and deep brain connections

region predominantly connected with the septal region, the substantia innominata of Reichert and the anterior perforate region. The posterior part of hypothalamus belongs to the ventral tegmental area (see [23]), which is closely related functionally with the substantia nigra compacta and the retrorubral nucleus (or retrorubral field), so called VTA-nigral complex in rodents [22]. The VTA is subdivided into centromedial and lateral parts, which project respectively to the core and shell of accumbens nucleus; VTA also projects to the dorsal striatum, the septum, the lateral habenula and the amygdala, and has reciprocal connections with cortices in particular the pre frontal [22, 76, 104]. The thalamus is made of numerous nuclei, which can be labelled in a simplified way according to the human brain orientation and segregated into 9 groups: anterior or oral, dorsal, intermediate, ventral, medial, laminar, posterior or caudal, superficial and related nuclei [54] (Fig. 1.8). The functional limbic territory of the striato-pallidal system is rostro-ventral and is called the ventral pallidum, internal and external, and the ventral striatum [34, 47]. The internal ventral pallidum is well-defined below the anterior commissure, although laterally it overlaps with the globus pallidum external and internal, and the substantia innominata. The accumbens nucleus, also called ventral striatum [43], can be separated into two functional territories, the core, dorsal and the shell, ventral [108] (Fig. 1.9). The ventral striatum also includes the olfactory region of the anterior perforate substantia [104]. The claustrum origins from the cortex [85, 89] and is connected ventrally with fibers of the anterior commissure and the olfactive fascicle [89]. The insula is, *inter alia*, limbic [68]. The striato-limbic substantia innominata of Reichert has numerous connections (Fig. 1.10) and contains the nucleus basal of Meynert (medial) merging with the nucleus ansa lenticularis [39, 72, 81, 89, 94]. The thalamo-tegmental reticular system makes the link between sensori-motor inputs and executive-behavioral system. It is made up notably of the centromedian-parafascicular complex and the reticular formation of the brain stem, and has numerous connections with the cortico-striato-pallido-subthalamo-thalamo-cortical loop (see e.g. [93]). The effectiveness of vagus nerve

1 Related Circuitry and Synaptic Connectivity in Psychiatric Disorders

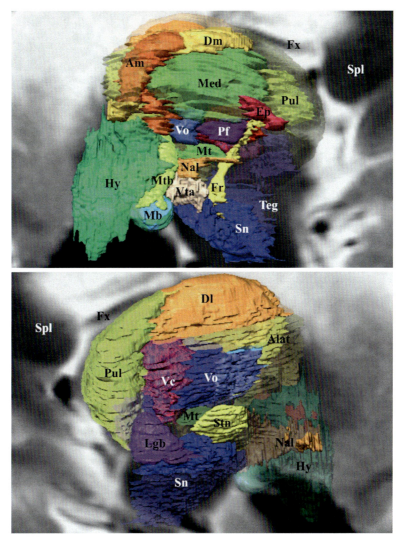

Fig. 1.8 Thalamus, hypothalamus and subthalamus. Medial (*top*) and lateral (*bottom*) views of reconstructed anatomical structures from high-field MRI of human brain (background, sagittal MRI slices)

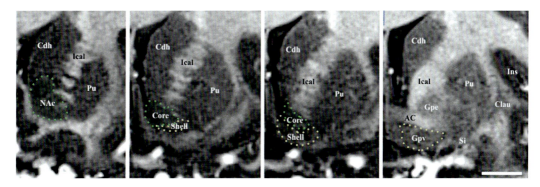

Fig. 1.9 Accumbens nucleus. Coronal MRI sections of the nucleus accumbens (from *left* to *right*, from rostral to caudal). Delineation of core and shell (*dotted lines*) is done according to [108]; note that the caudal shell is mixed up with the ventral pallidum. White bar = 10 mm

Fig. 1.10 Substantia innominata. *Top* connections; *bottom* MRI topography (coronal slice)

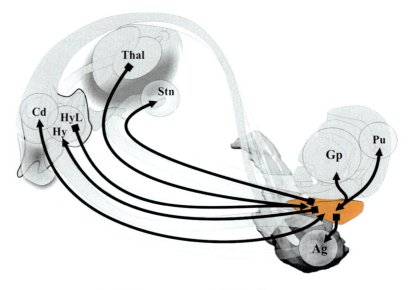
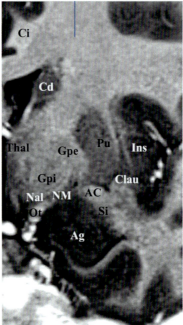

stimulation alleviating symptoms of drug-refractory depression could be explain by the role of thalamo-tegmental reticular system [71]. The gabaergic reticular nucleus of the thalamus, placed between cortices and thalamic nuclei, could participate to the pathophysiology of schizophrenia [21].

1.3 Anatomo-Functional Correlates of Psychiatric Disorders

The concept of emotional brain had progressively involved all deep brain structures, in particular the sensorimotor's and notably their limbic part.

The importance of interactions between the cortex and deep GM nuclei in psychiatric disorders is highlighted through the so-called cortico-basal circuitry. Compulsive and repetitive behavior observed in obsessive compulsive disorder (OCD) and autism spectrum disorders, are the most emblematic symptoms linked with the cortico-striato-pallido-subthalamo-thalamo-cortical loop [101]. The dorso-ventral segregation of basal ganglia circuits into limbic-emotional, ventral, associative-cognitive, intermediate, and sensory-motor, dorsal, systems exemplifies the interrelations of basal ganglia and thalamus with the frontal cortex during behavior control, notably emotional [34, 35, 38]. For instance, the sensation of pleasure, emotional, would be mediated by a ventral striato-pallidal circuit, while motivation ("wanting") used a dorsal striato-GPi/SNr circuit [62]. The sensory-motor circuitry, especially the hyper direct pathway between cortex and STN [73] (Fig. 1.11a), plays a role within the cortico-sub-cortical circuitry involving a lot of ventral connections (Fig. 1.11b). Clinical reports of chronic electric stimulation (DBS) illustrate the involvement of basal ganglia into the executive-behavioral system, and in particular the STN concentrating the three functional territories within a very limited volume. DBS of the anterior and medial part improves compulsive behavior in OCD patients [60], and DBS of the sensori-motor part can provoke symptoms of depression in severe Parkinson's disease [99]. In severe Parkinson's disease, stimulo-induced hypomania was reported with stimulation of the limbic part of STN [59], but also when contacts are within the substantia nigra [103]. Pallidal DBS can also provokes hypomania in parkinsonians [70].

Known and hypothetical neural correlates of emotional states of mood, such as depression and anxiety (negative valence) and mania and hypomania (positive valence), serve as models of circuitry of mood-affective disorders, e.g. in depression, OCD and bipolar disorders. Depressive mood disorders are associated with chronic stress, supported by the hypothalamic–pituitary–adrenal axis (paraventricular nucleus) [57, 96]. Chronic stress is also linked with obesity, thus metabolism control and mood interacts [42]

notably through the leptin pathway in the hypothalamus (paraventricular and arcuate nuclei) and the hippocampus [29]. Hypothalamus is a key actor of regulation of food intake (see neuro-modulation examples [67, 110]) controlling metabolism and behavior. Effects of STN and internal pallidum DBS also show the involvement of basal ganglia in food intake; weight gain is explained, *inter alia*, by modifications of metabolism and eating behavior [88]. Anxiety and fear fall when pathologic in anxiety disorders, such as the generalized anxiety disorder. Substance disorders, abuse and dependence refer to persistent, compulsive and repetitive behaviors, and associated harm, thus consequently to rewarding. Mood and reward are not independent as inferred from food intake behavior [109].

Emotion perception could be supported by two systems [83]: ventral, amygdala, insula, ventral striatum and ventral anterior cingulate and prefrontal cortices; dorsal, hippocampus, dorsal anterior cingulate and prefrontal cortices. Processes of emotion regulation could support models of bipolar disorder [84] (Fig. 1.12). Prefrontal cortex participates differently according to the type of regulation: automatic emotion regulation by medial prefrontal along with hippocampus and para hippocampus cortices; voluntary emotion regulation by lateral prefrontal cortex [90]. The sub cingulo-callosal prefrontal region, modulating mood, is atrophied at the expense of glia in major depressive disorder and bipolar disorder, and the metabolic activity increased in major depressive disorders diminishes after treatments [17, 18, 64]. DBS within the sub cingulo-callosal region modulates mood and anxiety, but also anorexia nervosa-related OCD [56]. More globally the emotional-limbic brain, including medial thalamic and sub-ventricular relays, modulates mood and related disorders [87], involving most basal ganglia circuitry [62], up to the insula [5]. In the core of the executive-behavioral system, is the hippocampus-amygdala complex. The hippocampus mediates temporo-spatial encoding and recalling of events, and is co-activated with the amygdala during fear conditions; short connections link functionally amygdala and hippocampus [27]. The amygdala participates to a variety of emotion

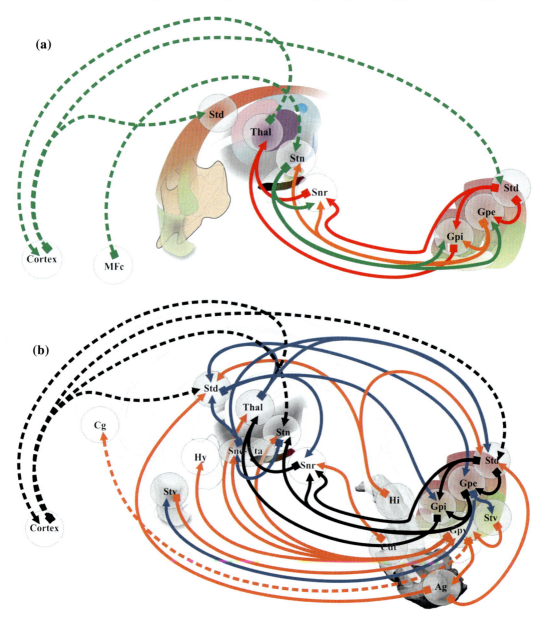

Fig. 1.11 Cortico-sub-cortical circuitry. **a** motor loop; **b** cortico-subcortical circuitry; according to Alexander et al. [3], Marchand [62], Nambu et al. [73], Parent and Hazrati [80]

processes, during fear, reward, attention, perception and explicit memory; it is connected to hippocampus, cortex, thalamus, hypothalamus, ventral striatum, periaqueductal gray and neurovegetative systems [53]. It has been proposed that the bed nucleus of the stria terminalis participates to alcohol abuse disorder [48, 97]. Finally the amygdala should play a role in psychosis, in particular though dopamine inputs [25]; most basal forebrain structures could be involved. Reward is a positive emotional stimuli, such as food, sex and social interaction [91], reinforcing behavior, leading to conditioned behavior [45]. The reward circuit encompasses a lot of mediobasal structures

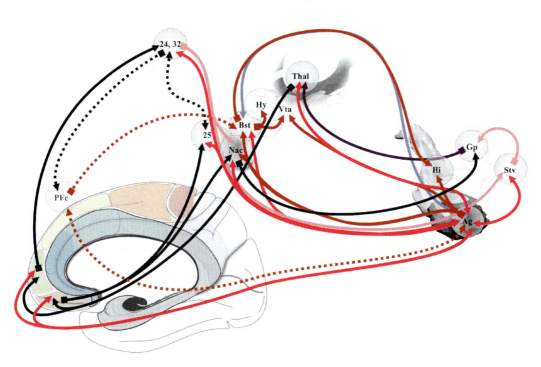

Fig. 1.12 Neural correlates of bipolar disorder. According to Strakowsky et al. [98]. Numbers specify Brodmann's areas

[45, 91], such as VTA, hypothalamus, ventral striatum and medial prefrontal cortex, modulated in particular by dopamine release in the ventral striatum, the amygdala, and the prefrontal cortex [10, 25, 97] (Fig. 1.13). The insula is also involved in addiction [28, 95]. DBS of the anterior limb of the internal capsule, in the vicinity of ventral striatum and pallidum, accumbens nucleus and lateral hypothalamus improves OCD patients and treatment-resistant depression, on both compulsive activity and depression [33, 61]. Right hemisphere dominance of mood and reward controls could exist [55, 92]. Stimulo-induced, fear, panic and smile were observed when contact are positioned in the ventral part of the anterior limb—accumbens nucleus region [77]. DBS of the accumbens nucleus in OCD alleviates symptoms of depression, anxiety and anhedonia [7].

Neural correlates of memory (Fig. 1.14) were first described at the beginning of the 20th century when memory defects were analyzed in clinics (see [6] for a review); they involved the mammillary bodies, the fornix and the hippocampus, often called Papez's circuit. Recent clinical studies have shown memory enhancement when stimulating entorhinal cortex [100] and fornical area [51]. The nucleus ventral tegmental of Gudden would participate to memory processing [106]; the anterior thalamus could be an integrative relay from hypothalamus and hippocampus [1]. The memory circuit is at the core of the executive-behavioral system where two structures are particularly involved in memory process: the medial prefrontal cortex [20] and the amygdala for emotional dimension [66].

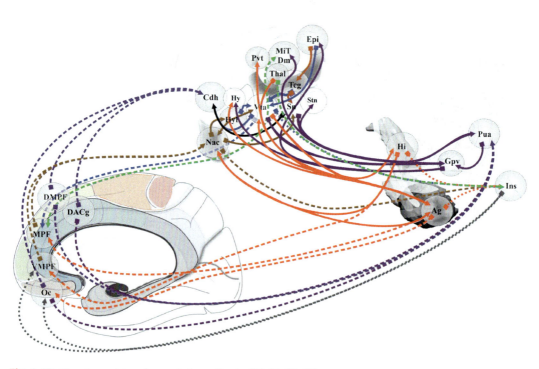

Fig. 1.13 Neural correlates of reward. According to [36, 91, 95, 97]

Fig. 1.14 Memory circuit

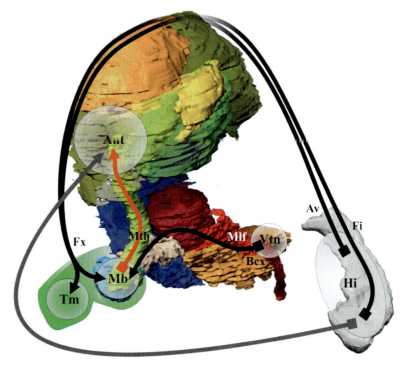

List of Abbreviations Used in Figures

AC	Anterior commissure
ACc	Anterior cingulate cortex
Ach	Acetylcholine
Ag	Amygdala
Al	Ansa lenticularis
Alat	Anterolateral nucleus (Thalamus)
Am	Anteromedial nucleus (Thalamus)
Ant	Anterior thalamus
Ap	Anterior perforate region
Ar	Arcuate nucleus (hypothalamus)
Av	Alveus
Bfb	Basal forebrain bundle
Bst	Bed of stria terminalis
CAg	Centromedial amygdala
Cc	Corpus callosum
Clau	Claustrum
Cd, h, t	Caudate nucleus, head, tale
Cg	Cingulate (gyrus)
Ci	Cingulum (longitudinal fascicle of the gyrus limbici)
Cao	Carrefour olfactif of Broca (para-olfactory area)
Cs	Cingulate sulcus
D1, 2	Dopamine receptor: types 1 and 2
DA	Dopamine neuron
DACg	Dorsal anterior cingulate
Db	Diagonal band of Broca
Dl	Dorsolateral nucleus (thalamus)
DLPF	Dorsolateral prefronal cortex
DMPF	Dorsomedial prefronal cortex
Dm	Dorsomedial nucleus (thalamus)
Dom	Dorsomedial nucleus (hypothalamus)
DPM	Dorsal premotor cortex
Ea	Extended amygdala
ECg	External cingulate gyrus
Ep	Epithalamus
Epl	Lateral habenula
Ent	Entorhinal cortex
Fa	Fascicle angularis
Fbc	Fronto-basal cortex
FEF	Frontal eye field
Fi	Fimbria
Fo	Fascicle olfactorius, diagonal band of Broca
FPc	Frontopolar cortex
Fr	Fascicle retroflexus
Fx	Fornix
Gaba	Gamma-aminobutyric acid neuron
Glu	Glutamate
gR	Gyrus rectus
Gp, e, i, v	Globus pallidum extern, intern, ventral
Hi	Hippocampus
Hy, l	Hypothalamus, lateral
Ical	Internal capsule anterior limb
Ida	Insular dysgranular area
Ifs	Inferior frontal gyrus
Ins	Insula
Ipn	Interpeduncular nucleus
Isth	Isthmus
Lat	Lateral nucleus (hypothalamus)
Lgb	Lateral geniculate body
LBco	Laterobasal complex of amygdala
M-I	Primary motor area
M-II, SMA	Supplementary motor area
Mb	Mammilary body
MCc	Midcingulate cortex
MFc	Motor frontal cortex

MiT	Midline thalamus	Rn	Red nucleus
MPF	Medial prefrontal cortex	Rrn	Retrorubral nucleus or field
Msn	Medium spiny neuron	Sc	Suprachiasmatic nucleus (hypothalamus)
Mtb	Mamillo-thalamic bundle		
Nac (c, s)	Nucleus accumbens (core, shell)	SCg	Subcallosal gyrus
Nal	Nucleus ansa lenticularis	Se	Septum (nuclei)
NM	Nucleus of Meynert	Ser	Serotonine or 5-hydroxytryptamine
Mt	Mammillo-tegmental fascicle	Si	Substantia innominata
Oc	Orbitofrontal cortex	Sm	Stria medullaris
OFg	Orbitofrontal gyri	So	Supraoptic nucleus (hypothalamus)
Ol	Ofactive system		
Ot	Optical tract	Sos	Supraorbitaris sulci
Ox	Optic chiasma	Spl	Splenium of the corpus callosum
ParaHg	Parahypoccampal gyrus	Sq	Substance Q
PCc	Posterior cingulate cortex	St	Stria terminalis
PCs	Paracingulate sulcus	Stn	Subthalamic nucleus
Pf	Parafascicular nucleus (thalamus)	Std	Dorsal striatum
Pfo	Perifornical nucleus (hypothalamus)	Stv	Ventral striatum
		Sn, c, r	Substantia nigra, compacta, reticulata
PFc	Prefrontal cortex		
Pol	Temporo-polar region	Teg	Tegmentum
Pos	Paraolfactive or subcallosal sulcus	Thal	Thalamus
Post	Posterior nucleus (hypothalamus)	Tm	Nucleus tuberomammillaris (hypothalamus)
Pr	Preoptic nucleus (hypothalamus)		
PreCuneus	Pre cuneus of the medial parieto-cingulate region	Trg	Transverse gyri
		VLPF	Ventrolateral prefrontal cortex
Pu, a	Putamen, anterior	VMPF	Ventromedial prefrontal cortex
Pul	Pulvinar	Vc	Thalamus ventro-caudal
Pv	Periventricular nucleus (hypothalamus)	Vm	Ventromedial nucleus (hypothalamus)
Pvg	Paraventricular grey matter	Vo	Thalamus ventro-oral
Pvt	Paraventricular thalamus	VPM	Ventral premotor cortex
RCc	Radiation of the corpus callosum	Vta, L, CM	Ventral tegmental area, lateral and caudo-medial parts
RSC	Retrosplenial cingulate cortex		
Ro	Olfactive radiation	Zi	Zona incerta

References

1. Aggleton JP. Multiple anatomical systems embedded within the primate medial temporal lobe: Implications for hippocampal function. Neurosci Biobehav Rev. 2012;36:1579–96.
2. Agnati LF, Guidolin D, Guescini M, Genedani S, Fuxe K. Understanding wiring and volume transmission. Brain Res Rev. 2010;64:137–59.
3. Alexander GE, DeLong MR, Strick PL. Parallel organization of functionally segregated circuits linking basal ganglia and cortex. Annu Rev Neurosci. 1986;9:357–81.
4. Andrés P. Frontal cortex as the central executive of working memory: time to revise our view. Cortex J Devoted Stud Nerv Syst Behav. 2003;39:871–95.
5. Avery JA, Drevets WC, Moseman SE, Bodurka J, Barcalow JC, Simmons WK. Major depressive disorder is associated with abnormal interoceptive activity and functional connectivity in the insula. Biol Psychiatry. 2013.
6. Barbizet J. Defect of memorizing of hippocampal-mammillary origin: A review. J Neurol Neurosurg Psychiatry. 1963;26:127–35.
7. Bewernick BH, Hurlemann R, Matusch A, Kayser S, Grubert C, Hadrysiewicz B, Axmacher N, Lemke M, Cooper-Mahkorn D, Cohen MX, Brockmann H, Lenartz D, Sturm V, Schlaepfer TE. Nucleus accumbens deep brain stimulation decreases ratings of depression and anxiety in treatment-resistant depression. Biol Psychiatry. 2010;67:110–6.
8. Bonini F, Burle B, Liégeois-Chauvel C, Régis J, Chauvel P, Vidal F. Action monitoring and medial frontal cortex: Leading role of supplementary motor area. Science. 2014;343:888–91.
9. Borisovska M, Bensen AL, Chong G, Westbrook GL. Distinct modes of dopamine and GABA release in a dual transmitter neuron. J Neurosci Off J Soc Neurosci. 2013;33:1790–6.
10. Britt JP, Bonci A. Optogenetic interrogations of the neural circuits underlying addiction. Curr Opin Neurobiol. 2013;23:539–45.
11. Broca P. Sur la circonvolution limbique et la scissure limbique. Bull Société Anthr Paris. 1877;12:646–57.
12. Brüstle O. Developmental neuroscience: miniature human brains. Nature. 2013;501:319–20.
13. Creed MC, Ntamati NR, Tan KR. VTA GABA neurons modulate specific learning behaviors through the control of dopamine and cholinergic systems. Front Behav Neurosci. 2014;8:8.
14. Dani A, Huang B, Bergan J, Dulac C, Zhuang X. Superresolution imaging of chemical synapses in the brain. Neuron. 2010;68:843–56.
15. De Smet HJ, Paquier P, Verhoeven J, Mariën P. The cerebellum: its role in language and related cognitive and affective functions. Brain Lang. 2013;127:334–42.
16. Dejerine J. Anatomie des centres nerveux (Tomes 1 and 2), Rueff et Cie. ed. Paris; 1901.
17. Drevets WC, Price JL, Simpson JR Jr, Todd RD, Reich T, Vannier M, Raichle ME. Subgenual prefrontal cortex abnormalities in mood disorders. Nature. 1997;386:824–7.
18. Drevets WC, Savitz J, Trimble M. The subgenual anterior cingulate cortex in mood disorders. CNS Spectr. 2008;13:663–81.
19. Duvernoy H, Cabanis E-A, Iba-Zizen M-T, Tamraz J, Guyot J. Le cerveau humain: surfaces, coupes sériées tridimentionelles et IRM. Paris: Springer; 1992.
20. Euston DR, Gruber AJ, McNaughton BL. The role of medial prefrontal cortex in memory and decision making. Neuron. 2012;76:1057–70.
21. Ferrarelli F, Tononi G. The thalamic reticular nucleus and schizophrenia. Schizophr Bull. 2011;37:306–15.
22. Ferreira JGP, Del-Fava F, Hasue RH, Shammah-Lagnado SJ. Organization of ventral tegmental area projections to the ventral tegmental area-nigral complex in the rat. Neuroscience. 2008;153:196–213.
23. Fontaine D, Lanteri-Minet M, Ouchchane L, Lazorthes Y, Mertens P, Blond S, Geraud G, Fabre N, Navez M, Lucas C, Dubois F, Sol JC, Paquis P, Lemaire JJ. Anatomical location of effective deep brain stimulation electrodes in chronic cluster headache. Brain J Neurol. 2010;133:1214–23.
24. Fossati P. Neural correlates of emotion processing: from emotional to social brain. Eur Neuropsycho pharmacol. 2012;22:S487–91.
25. Fudge JL, Emiliano AB. The extended amygdala and the dopamine system: another piece of the dopamine puzzle. J Neuropsychiatry Clin Neurosci. 2003;15:306–16.
26. Fudge JL, Haber SN. Bed nucleus of the stria terminalis and extended amygdala inputs to dopamine subpopulations in primates. Neuroscience. 2001;104:807–27.
27. Fudge JL, deCampo DM, Becoats KT. Revisiting the hippocampal–amygdala pathway in primates: association with immature-appearing neurons. Neuroscience. 2012;212:104–19.
28. Garavan H. Insula and drug cravings. Brain Struct Funct. 2010;214:593–601.
29. Ge J-F, Qi C-C, Zhou J-N. Imbalance of leptin pathway and hypothalamus synaptic plasticity markers are associated with stress-induced depression in rats. Behav Brain Res. 2013;249:38–43.
30. Geyer S, Luppino G, Rozzi S. Motor cortex. In: Mai JK, Paxinos G, editors. The human nervous system; 3rd ed. Elsevier: London; 2012. p. 1012–1035.
31. Goldman-Rakic PS, Selemon LD, Schwartz ML. Dual pathways connecting the dorsolateral prefrontal cortex with the hippocampal formation and parahippocampal cortex in the rhesus monkey. Neuroscience. 1984;12:719–43.
32. Govindaiah G, Wang Y, Cox CL. Substance P selectively modulates GABA(A) receptor-mediated synaptic transmission in striatal cholinergic interneurons. Neuropharmacology. 2010;58:413–22.

33. Greenberg BD, Malone DA, Friehs GM, Rezai AR, Kubu CS, Malloy PF, Salloway SP, Okun MS, Goodman WK, Rasmussen SA. Three-year outcomes in deep brain stimulation for highly resistant obsessive-compulsive disorder. Neuropsychopharmacol Off Publ Am Coll Neuropsychopharmacol. 2006;31:2384–93.
34. Haber SN. The primate basal ganglia: parallel and integrative networks. J Chem Neuroanat. 2003;26:317–30.
35. Haber SN, Calzavara R. The cortico-basal ganglia integrative network: the role of the thalamus. Brain Res Bull. 2009;78:69–74.
36. Haber SN, Knutson B. The reward circuit: Linking primate anatomy and human imaging. Neuropsychopharmacology. 2009;35:4–26.
37. Haber SN, Adler A, Bergman H. The basal ganglia. In: Mai JK, Paxinos G, editors. The human nervous system. 3rd ed. Amsterdam: Academic Press; 2011. p. 678–738.
38. Haynes WIA, Haber SN. The organization of prefrontal-subthalamic inputs in primates provides an anatomical substrate for both functional specificity and integration: implications for Basal Ganglia models and deep brain stimulation. J Neurosci Off J Soc Neurosci. 2013;33:4804–14.
39. Heimer L. Basal forebrain in the context of schizophrenia. Brain Res Brain Res Rev. 2000;31:205–35.
40. Heimer L, Harlan RE, Alheid GF, Garcia MM, de Olmos J. Substantia innominata: a notion which impedes clinical-anatomical correlations in neuropsychiatric disorders. Neuroscience. 1997;76:957–1006.
41. Heng S, Song AW, Sim K. White matter abnormalities in bipolar disorder: insights from diffusion tensor imaging studies. J Neural Transm. 2010;1996(117):639–54.
42. Hryhorczuk C, Sharma S, Fulton SE. Metabolic disturbances connecting obesity and depression. Front Neurosci. 2013;7:177.
43. Ikemoto S. Dopamine reward circuitry: two projection systems from the ventral midbrain to the nucleus accumbens-olfactory tubercle complex. Brain Res Rev. 2007;56:27–78.
44. Ikemoto S, Wise RA. Mapping of chemical trigger zones for reward. Neuropharmacology. 2004;47(1):190–201.
45. Ikemoto S, Bonci A. Neurocircuitry of drug reward. Neuropharmacology. 2014;76:329–341.
46. Jones DK, Christiansen KF, Chapman RJ, Aggleton JP. Distinct subdivisions of the cingulum bundle revealed by diffusion MRI fibre tracking: implications for neuropsychological investigations. Neuropsychologia. 2013;51:67–78.
47. Karachi C, François C, Parain K, Bardinet E, Tandé D, Hirsch E, Yelnik J. Three-dimensional cartography of functional territories in the human striatopallidal complex by using calbindin immunoreactivity. J Comp Neurol. 2002;450:122–34.
48. Kash TL. The role of biogenic amine signaling in the bed nucleus of the stria terminals in alcohol abuse. Alcohol. 2012;46:303–8.
49. Kha HT, Finkelstein DI, Pow DV, Lawrence AJ, Horne MK. Study of projections from the entopeduncular nucleus to the thalamus of the rat. J Comp Neurol. 2000;426:366–77.
50. Klingler J. Erleichterung des makroskopischen praeparation des gehirns durch den gefrierprozess. Schweiz Arch Neurol Psychiatr. 1935;36:247–56.
51. Laxton AW, Tang-Wai DF, McAndrews MP, Zumsteg D, Wennberg R, Keren R, Wherrett J, Naglie G, Hamani C, Smith GS, Lozano AM. A phase I trial of deep brain stimulation of memory circuits in Alzheimer's disease. Ann Neurol. 2010;68:521–34.
52. LeDoux J. The emotional brain, fear, and the amygdala. Cell Mol Neurobiol. 2003;23:727–38.
53. LeDoux J. The amygdala. Curr Biol. 2007;17:R868–74.
54. Lemaire J, Sakka L, Ouchchane L, Caire F, Gabrillargues J, Bonny J. Anatomy of the human thalamus based on spontaneous contrast and microscopic voxels in high-field magnetic resonance imaging. Neurosurgery. 2010;66:161–72.
55. Lemaire J-J, Frew AJ, McArthur D, Gorgulho AA, Alger JR, Salomon N, Chen C, Behnke EJ, De Salles AAF. White matter connectivity of human hypothalamus. Brain Res. 2011;1371:43–64.
56. Lipsman N, Woodside DB, Giacobbe P, Hamani C, Carter JC, Norwood SJ, Sutandar K, Staab R, Elias G, Lyman CH, Smith GS, Lozano AM. Subcallosal cingulate deep brain stimulation for treatment-refractory anorexia nervosa: a phase 1 pilot trial. Lancet. 2013;381:1361–70.
57. Lucassen PJ, Pruessner J, Sousa N, Almeida OFX, Van Dam AM, Rajkowska G, Swaab DF, Czéh B. Neuropathology of stress. Acta Neuropathol (Berl). 2014;127:109–35.
58. MacLean PD. Psychosomatic disease and the visceral brain; recent developments bearing on the Papez theory of emotion. Psychosom Med. 1949;11:338–53.
59. Mallet L, Schüpbach M, N'Diaye K, Remy P, Bardinet E, Czernecki V, Welter M-L, Pelissolo A, Ruberg M, Agid Y, Yelnik J. Stimulation of subterritories of the subthalamic nucleus reveals its role in the integration of the emotional and motor aspects of behavior. Proc Natl Acad Sci USA. 2007;104:10661–6.
60. Mallet L, Polosan M, Jaafari N, Baup N, Welter M-L, Fontaine D, du Montcel ST, Yelnik J, Chéreau I, Arbus C, Raoul S, Aouizerate B, Damier P, Chabardès S, Czernecki V, Ardouin C, Krebs M-O, Bardinet E, Chaynes P, Burbaud P, Cornu P, Derost P, Bougerol T, Bataille B, Mattei V, Dormont D, Devaux B, Vérin M, Houeto J-L, Pollak P, Benabid A-L, Agid Y, Krack P, Millet B, Pelissolo A. STOC Study Group. Subthalamic nucleus stimulation in severe obsessive-compulsive disorder. N Engl J Med. 2008;359:2121–34.

61. Malone DA Jr, Dougherty DD, Rezai AR, Carpenter LL, Friehs GM, Eskandar EN, Rauch SL, Rasmussen SA, Machado AG, Kubu CS, Tyrka AR, Price LH, Stypulkowski PH, Giftakis JE, Rise MT, Malloy PF, Salloway SP, Greenberg BD. Deep brain stimulation of the ventral capsule/ventral striatum for treatment-resistant depression. Biol Psychiatry. 2009;65:267–75.
62. Marchand WR. Cortico-basal ganglia circuitry: a review of key research and implications for functional connectivity studies of mood and anxiety disorders. Brain Struct Funct. 2010;215:73–96.
63. Markram H. The blue brain project. Nat Rev Neurosci. 2006;7:153–60.
64. Mayberg HS, Lozano AM, Voon V, McNeely HE, Seminowicz D, Hamani C, Schwalb JM, Kennedy SH. Deep brain stimulation for treatment-resistant depression. Neuron. 2005;45:651–60.
65. McCollum LA, Roche JK, Roberts RC. Immunohistochemical localization of enkephalin in the human striatum: a postmortem ultrastructural study. Synapse. 2012;66:204–19.
66. McGaugh JL. The amygdala modulates the consolidation of memories of emotionally arousing experiences. Annu Rev Neurosci. 2004;27:1–28.
67. Melega WP, Lacan G, Gorgulho AA, Behnke EJ, De Salles AAF. Hypothalamic deep brain stimulation reduces weight gain in an obesity-animal model. PLoS One. 2012;7:e30672.
68. Menon V, Uddin LQ. Saliency, switching, attention and control: a network model of insula function. Brain Struct Funct. 2010;214:655–67.
69. Mignarri A, Tessa A, Carluccio MA, Rufa A, Storti E, Bonelli G, Marcotulli C, Santorelli FM, Leonardi L, Casali C, Federico A, Dotti MT. Cerebellum and neuropsychiatric disorders: insights from ARSACS. Neurol Sci. 2013.
70. Miyawaki E, Perlmutter JS, Tröster AI, Videen TO, Koller WC. The behavioral complications of pallidal stimulation: a case report. Brain Cogn. 2000;42:417–34.
71. Mohr P, Rodriguez M, Slavíčková A, Hanka J. The application of vagus nerve stimulation and deep brain stimulation in depression. Neuropsychobiology. 2011;64:170–81.
72. Naidich TP, Duvernoy HM, Delman BN, Sorensen AG, Kollias SS, Haache EM. Duvernoy's atlas of the human brain stem and cerebellum. Austria: Springer; 2009.
73. Nambu A, Tokuno H, Takada M. Functional significance of the cortico-subthalamo-pallidal "hyperdirect" pathway. Neurosci Res. 2002;43: 111–7.
74. Niciu MJ, Kelmendi B, Sanacora G. Overview of glutamatergic neurotransmission in the nervous system. Pharmacol Biochem Behav. 2012; 100:656–64.
75. Nieh EH, Kim S-Y, Namburi P, Tye KM. Optogenetic dissection of neural circuits underlying emotional valence and motivated behaviors. Brain Res. 2013;1511:73–92.
76. Oades RD, Halliday GM. Ventral tegmental (A10) system: neurobiology. 1. Anatomy and connectivity. Brain Res Rev. 1987;12:117–65.
77. Okun MS, Mann G, Foote KD, Shapira NA, Bowers D, Springer U, Knight W, Martin P, Goodman WK. Deep brain stimulation in the internal capsule and nucleus accumbens region: responses observed during active and sham programming. J Neurol Neurosurg Psychiatry. 2007;78:310–4.
78. Oldenburg IA, Ding JB. Cholinergic modulation of synaptic integration and dendritic excitability in the striatum. Curr Opin Neurobiol. 2011;21(3):425−432.
79. Papez JW. A proposed mechanism of emotion. Arch Neurol Psychiatry. 1937;38:725–43.
80. Parent A, Hazrati LN. Functional anatomy of the basal ganglia. I. The cortico-basal ganglia-thalamo-cortical loop. Brain Res Rev. 1995;20:91–127.
81. Perry RH, Candy JM, Perry EK, Thompson J, Oakley AE. The substantia innominata and adjacent regions in the human brain: histochemical and biochemical observations. J Anat. 1984;138(Pt 4):713–32.
82. Petrides M, Pandya DN. The frontal cortex. In: Mai JK, Paxinos G, editors. The human nervous system, 3rd ed. London; 2012. p. 988–1011.
83. Phillips ML, Drevets WC, Rauch SL, Lane R. Neurobiology of emotion perception I: the neural basis of normal emotion perception. Biol Psychiatry. 2003;54:504–14.
84. Phillips ML, Ladouceur CD, Drevets WC. A neural model of voluntary and automatic emotion regulation: implications for understanding the pathophysiology and neurodevelopment of bipolar disorder. Mol Psychiatry. 2008;13(829):833–57.
85. Pirone A, Cozzi B, Edelstein L, Peruffo A, Lenzi C, Quilici F, Antonini R, Castagna M. Topography of Gng2- and NetrinG2-expression suggests an insular origin of the human claustrum. PLoS One. 2012;7: e44745.
86. Price JL, Drevets WC. Neurocircuitry of mood disorders. Neuropsychopharmacol: Neuropsychopharmacol Off Publ Am Coll; 2009.
87. Price JL, Drevets WC. Neural circuits underlying the pathophysiology of mood disorders. Trends Cogn Sci. 2012;16:61–71.
88. Rieu I, Derost P, Ulla M, Marques A, Debilly B, De Chazeron I, Chéreau I, Lemaire JJ, Boirie Y, Llorca PM, Durif F. Body weight gain and deep brain stimulation. Sci: J Neurol; 2011.
89. Riley H. An atlas of the basal ganglia, brain stem and spinal cord. Williams & Wilkins: Baltimore; 1953.
90. Rive MM, van Rooijen G, Veltman DJ, Phillips ML, Schene AH, Ruhé HG. Neural correlates of dysfunctional emotion regulation in major depressive disorder. A systematic review of neuroimaging studies. Neurosci Biobehav Rev. 2013.

91. Russo SJ, Nestler EJ. The brain reward circuitry in mood disorders. Nat Rev Neurosci. 2013;14:609–25.
92. Rück C, Karlsson A, Steele JD, Edman G, Meyerson BA, Ericson K, Nyman H, Asberg M, Svanborg P. Capsulotomy for obsessive-compulsive disorder: long-term follow-up of 25 patients. Arch Gen Psychiatry. 2008;65:914–21.
93. Sadikot AF, Rymar VV. The primate centromedian-parafascicular complex: anatomical organization with a note on neuromodulation. Brain Res Bull. 2009;78:122–30.
94. Schaltenbrand G, Bailey P, editors. Introduction to stereotaxis with an atlas of the human brain, Georg Thieme: Stuttgart; 1959.
95. Sinha R. Disgust, insula, immune signaling, and addiction. Biol Psychiatry. 2014;75:90–1.
96. Solomon MB, Furay AR, Jones K, Packard AEB, Packard BA, Wulsin AC, Herman JP. Deletion of forebrain glucocorticoid receptors impairs neuroendocrine stress responses and induces depression-like behavior in males but not females. Neuroscience. 2012;203:135–43.
97. Stamatakis AM, Sparta DR, Jennings JH, McElligott ZA, Decot H, Stuber GD. Amygdala and bed nucleus of the stria terminalis circuitry: implications for addiction-related behaviors. Neuropharmacology. 2014; 76:320–328.
98. Strakowski SM, Adler CM, Almeida J, Altshuler LL, Blumberg HP, Chang KD, DelBello MP, Frangou S, McIntosh A, Phillips ML, Sussman JE, Townsend JD. The functional neuroanatomy of bipolar disorder: a consensus model. Bipolar Disord. 2012;14:313–25.
99. Strutt AM, Simpson R, Jankovic J, York MK. Changes in cognitive-emotional and physiological symptoms of depression following STN-DBS for the treatment of Parkinson's disease. Eur J Neurol Off J Eur Fed Neurol Soc. 2012;19:121–7.
100. Suthana N, Haneef Z, Stern J, Mukamel R, Behnke E, Knowlton B, Fried I. Memory enhancement and deep-brain stimulation of the entorhinal area. N Engl J Med. 2012;366:502–10.
101. Ting JT, Feng G. Neurobiology of obsessive-compulsive disorder: insights into neural circuitry dysfunction through mouse genetics. Curr Opin Neurobiol. 2011;21:842–8.
102. Tsuchida A, Fellows LK. Are core component processes of executive function dissociable within the frontal lobes? Evidence from humans with focal prefrontal damage. Cortex. J Devoted Stud Nerv Syst Behav. 2013;49:1790–800.
103. Ulla M, Thobois S, Llorca P-M, Derost P, Lemaire J-J, Chereau-Boudet I, de Chazeron I, Schmitt A, Ballanger B, Broussolle E, Durif F. Contact dependent reproducible hypomania induced by deep brain stimulation in Parkinson's disease: clinical, anatomical and functional imaging study. J Neurol Neurosurg Psychiatry. 2010.
104. Van Domburg PH, ten Donkelaar HJ. The human substantia nigra and ventral tegmental area. A neuroanatomical study with notes on aging and aging diseases. Adv Anat Embryol Cell Biol. 1991;121:1–132.
105. Van Wieringen J-P, Booij J, Shalgunov V, Elsinga P, Michel MC. Agonist high- and low-affinity states of dopamine D_2 receptors: methods of detection and clinical implications. Naunyn Schmiedebergs Arch Pharmacol. 2013;386:135–54.
106. Vann SD. Gudden's ventral tegmental nucleus is vital for memory: re-evaluating diencephalic inputs for amnesia. Brain J Neurol. 2009;132:2372–84.
107. Vogt BA, Palomero-Gallagher N. Cingulate cortex, In: Mai JK, Paxinos G, editors. The human nervous system. 3rd ed. Elsevier: London; 2012. p. 943–987.
108. Voorn P, Brady LS, Berendse HW, Richfield EK. Densitometrical analysis of opioid receptor ligand binding in the human striatum—I. Distribution of μ opioid receptor defines shell and core of the ventral striatum. Neuroscience. 1996;75:777–92.
109. Weltens N, Zhao D, Van Oudenhove L. Where is the comfort in comfort foods? Mechanisms linking fat signaling, reward, and emotion. Neurogastroenterol Motil Off J Eur Gastrointest Motil Soc. 2014; 26:303–15.
110. Whiting DM, Tomycz ND, Bailes J, de Jonge L, Lecoultre V, Wilent B, Alcindor D, Prostko ER, Cheng BC, Angle C, Cantella D, Whiting BB, Mizes JS, Finnis KW, Ravussin E, Oh MY. Lateral hypothalamic area deep brain stimulation for refractory obesity: a pilot study with preliminary data on safety, body weight, and energy metabolism. J Neurosurg. 2013;119:56–63.
111. Zhou Y, Chen C-C, Weber AE, Zhou L, Baker LA, Hou J. Potentiometric-scanning ion conductance microscopy for measurement at tight junctions. Tissue Barriers. 2013;1:e25585.

High-angular diffusion MRI in reward-based psychiatric disorders

2

Wenwen Yu, Qiming Lv, Chencheng Zhang, Zhuangming Shen, Bomin Sun and Zheng Wang

Abstract

The structural mapping of the complex brain networks under healthy and diseased states is of great importance to understand the working mechanism of the brain function. Diffusion weighted magnetic resonance imaging and its derivative methods are currently the only way to measure macroscopic axonal organization in nervous system tissues, in vivo and non-invasively. Nevertheless, it has revealed tremendous unprecedented details about the brain architecture and inspired unlimited expectation on its future development. In this chapter, we first explain the basic principles of diffusion tensor imaging (DTI), and then discuss the strategies for resolving multiple fibers within one voxel, in particular on the diffusion spectrum imaging (DSI) method. We further introduce the pipeline of data analysis including quantification of whole brain white matter and visualization of specific microstructural tracts, and conclude with their recent applications in psychiatric disorders.

Keywords

Magnetic resonance imaging · Diffusion tensor imaging · Diffusion spectrum imaging · Tractography · Fiber crossing · Neuroanatomy

2.1 Introduction

Diffusion-weighted magnetic resonance imaging (DW-MRI) is an emerging magnetic resonance imaging (MRI) method ever since the mid-1980s [7, 37, 62], which allows the detecting of the diffusion process of water molecules in biological tissues, in vivo and non-invasively. By calculating the biophysical trajectory of water diffusion to infer the architecture of the white matter, diffusion tensor imaging (DTI) has become one of the most valuable MRI techniques

W. Yu · Q. Lv · Z. Shen · Z. Wang (✉)
Institute of Neuroscience, Shanghai Institutes for Biological Sciences, Chinese Academy of Sciences, 320 Yueyang Road, Shanghai 200031, China
e-mail: zheng.wang@ion.ac.cn

C. Zhang · B. Sun
Department of Functional Neurosurgery, Ruijin Hospital, School of Medicine, Shanghai Jiaotong University, Shanghai 200025, China

B. Sun and A. De Salles (eds.), *Neurosurgical Treatments for Psychiatric Disorders*, DOI 10.1007/978-94-017-9576-0_2
© Shanghai Jiao Tong University Press, Shanghai and Springer Science+Business Media Dordrecht 2015

of pursuing the working mechanism of brain architecture [26, 33, 43, 56]. Furthermore, assessment of the microstructural integrity of the axonal fibers using a variety of diffusion indices has absorbed an increasing attention in the study of neurological diseases or psychiatric disorders [4, 5, 13, 25, 32, 45].

This chapter starts from some theoretical background of diffusion derived MRI methods including the widely-accepted DTI and newly-developed diffusion spectrum imaging (DSI), and introduces some popular algorithms available for in vivo constructing tractography, as illustrated with some classic white matter (WM) fiber tracts. Finally it concludes with short summary of their current clinical applications in a wide range of psychiatric disorders. It is reasonably expected that such kind of discussion could catalyze the technological development in the light of meeting the clinical needs, and vice versa foster more potential applications for various categories of diagnostic purposes.

2.2 How DTI Works

The human body is made up of over 70 % water, in which the incessant random motion of water molecules is influenced by distinct kinds of restricted factors such as cell membranes, cytoskeleton, and macromolecules [26]. Because diffusional processes are influenced by the geometrical structure of the biological environment, diffusion MRI, has been successfully demonstrated to characterize diffusion displacement of water molecules and reveal the underlying microstructure in vivo [14, 16, 53, 66]. In spite of its recent introduction to brain imaging, tensor-based diffusion MRI has inspired a rising wave of biomedical applications of quantifying the diffusional characteristics of a wide range of specimens. In particular, for brain diseases diagnostics, DTI has been successfully used to demonstrate subtle abnormalities in a variety of neurological diseases (including stroke, multiple sclerosis, dyslexia, schizophrenia, and Alzheimer's disease) and is currently becoming an

indispensable part of many routine clinical protocols [4, 13, 25, 32, 34, 40, 48, 50, 63]. The diffusion pattern of water molecules can be simplified by the diffusion tensor model, which makes it feasible to show the gross fiber orientation and provide quantitative descriptions such as fractional anisotropy (FA) and diffusivity [54]. As such, more unique insights into tissue microstructure can be gained through the use of these indices: diffusion anisotropy as a useful index of white matter integrity and estimated orientation of the principal direction of axon fibers to enable tractography [21, 23]. These unprecedented information obtained from DTI studies are hence increasingly invaluable to both clinical physicians and scientific researchers.

Here we present a brief overview of the basic principles of DTI method and the readers can consult to the literature for more in-depth technical details [10, 26]. In essence, diffusion MRI measures the dephasing of spins of protons in the presence of a spatially-varying magnetic field ('gradient'), which changes their Larmor frequency [37, 59, 62]. The intuitive mechanism here is the phase change resulting from components of incoherent displacement of spins along the axis of the applied field gradient. For stationary (non-diffusing) molecules, the phases induced by both gradient pulses will completely cancel so as to lead the maximally coherent magnetization and there will be no signal loss from diffusion [27]. In the case of coherent flow in the direction of the applied gradient, the bulk motion will cause the signal phase to change by different amounts regarding to each pulse so that there will be a net phase difference. Therefore, in the presence of diffusion gradients, water molecules will accumulate different phases, and the phase dispersion from diffusion will cause signal attenuation, S.

$$S = S_0 e^{-bD} \qquad (2.1)$$

where S is the DW signal, S_0 is the signal without any DW gradients (but otherwise identical imaging parameters), D is the apparent diffusion coefficient, and b is so-called "b-factor". MRI signals are proportional to the sum of magnetization components from all water molecules in a voxel, which is closely associated with the area of the diffusion gradient pulses defined by the amplitude of the magnetic field gradient pulses, G, and the temporal duration, δ, and the temporal spacing between the pulses, Δ. The effects of all these parameters are indeed ascribed to a coarse term "b-factor" as below:

$$b = \gamma^2 G^2 \delta^2 (\Delta - \delta/3) \qquad (2.2)$$

where γ is the gyromagnetic ratio.

By applying the appropriate magnetic field gradients, MR imaging may be sensitized to the random, thermally driven motion (diffusion) of water molecules in the direction of the field gradient. Diffusion is anisotropic (directionally dependent) in WM fiber tracts, as axonal membranes and myelin sheaths present barriers to the motion of water molecules in directions not parallel to their own orientation. The direction of maximum diffusivity has been shown to coincide with the orientation of WM fiber tracts [44].

In short, the fundamental concept behind DTI is that water molecules diffuse differently in the tissues heavily depending on its type, integrity, architecture, and presence of barriers, generating information about its orientation and quantitative anisotropy embodied by the diffusion tensors [9, 14, 44]. DTI may be used to map and characterize the three-dimensional diffusion pattern as a function of spatial location, which can further be taken advantage of estimating the connectivity properties of the whole brain WM networks, using the diffusion anisotropy and the principal diffusion directions [23].

Undoubtedly, DTI holds a unique and unparalleled sensitivity to water movements of painting the blueprint of brain architecture [26, 33, 43, 56], as uses existing MRI technology without the necessity of investing new equipment, contrast agents, or even radiochemical tracers. However, there remain many technical issues with regard to the performance of the tool, practical considerations of working on biological specimens, and the interpretation of DTI tractography images. For instance, within each voxel of diffusion-encoded images, it can only resolve the single (the most dominant) fiber direction and cannot differentiate the kissing/crossing/branching fibers in the complex cerebral regions [1, 71]. Consequently it estimates the fiber orientation to be the mean of the underlying fiber directions, even though the mean direction will not be representative of the true fiber directions [3]. Nevertheless, it is not capable of determining with accuracy the origin and destination of fibers, which requires further comprehensive evidence to corroborate, even in combination with employing other advanced technologies [5, 58].

2.3 Diffusion Spectrum MRI (DSI)

Recent technological development of MRI methods has been devoted to solving the aforementioned issues, so as to better characterize the complicated fiber patterns and discern fiber orientations. As matter of a fact, either model-based or model-free methods have been acknowledged that have the capacity to resolve heterogeneity of fiber orientations in each resolved volume of tissue (voxel) [65, 68], and provide detailed views into the precise organization of cerebral white matter tracts [69]. Here we will focus on the model-free derivations of diffusion MRI technique.

Model-free methods, also called q-space imaging methods [11, 16, 59], measure the microscopic diffusion function directly without any assumptions on the form of the underlying diffusion function, even though they still have to count on the Fourier transform relation between the diffusion MR signals and the underlying diffusion displacement [31]. Firstly the probability density function (PDF) or orientation distribution function (ODF) of the diffusion displacement in the three biophysical dimension are obtained. One can then calculate a common quantitative scalar measure, generalized fractional anisotropy (GFA) in DSI, physiologically equivalent to FA [19], so as to implicate the microstructure property. Worthy to mention, FA, an index derived from the diffusion tensor that reflects the degree of directional coherence, myelination, and diameter of axonal fibers has been widely used to examine the integrity of white matter tracts in DTI [4, 26]. Simply put, higher FA or GFA values imply higher coherence of fiber directions, more myelination or larger axonal diameters in the white matter at the microstructural level.

More frequently the connections of each ODF will be explored to infer the underlying linking patterns of the fibers [22]. Here in after, we briefly discuss two commonly used q-space (diffusion-encoding space) reconstruction methods to estimate the ODF from the acquired diffusion MR signals, with particular emphasis on the DSI method.

Q-ball imaging (QBI): Tuch and his co-workers introduced q-ball imaging (QBI) [64], which usually used the Funk–Radon transform (also known as the spherical Radon transform) to reconstruct ODF at the cost of large pulsed field gradient and time-intensive sampling. It is also feasible to resolve intravoxel fiber crossing through using a high angular resolution diffusion imaging (HARDI) scheme, which samples data on a shell in the diffusion encoding space. The Funk–Radon transform relation forms the core basis of the QBI reconstruction method to avoid any assumptions on the diffusion process like Gaussianity or multi-Gaussianity and to achieve better accuracy and efficiency [17].

Diffusion spectrum imaging (DSI): Wedeen and his colleagues proposed to acquire the diffusion MR signals by using the grid sampling scheme, and then applied the Fourier transform on the q-space data to estimate the underlying diffusion displacement pattern for further calculation of the ODF [15, 21, 31, 61, 65, 68–70, 72]. The sampling scheme of DSI produces a cluster of grid points distributed on a sphere in the q-space. Each grid point corresponds to a specific value of diffusion sensitivity (b-value) and direction, and the b-value increases incrementally from 0 to a maximal b-value (b-max). When all the diffusion-encoding samples in the q-space have been collected, the Fourier transform (FT) is performed to obtain the PDF as the diffusion-encoding samples $S(q)$ and their corresponding PDFs constitute a Fourier pair [10]. In sum, DSI measures the ODF by acquiring hundreds of diffusion-weighted images (DWI) with different diffusion-encoding gradients, each with different strength and direction [5, 21]. In this manner, it is possible to infer the number of fiber-compartments and their relative amplitude as well as spatial orientations by reconstructing the ODF local maxima. It enables DSI to resolve kissing or crossing or bending fiber orientations at single voxel-based level, as shown in Fig. 2.1.

Bear in mind, though, some precautions should be carefully exercised when implementing these two q-space imaging methods to derive diffusion ODF. One caveat of the QBI method is that the acquired diffusion MR signal is in fact contributed by the diffusion displacements in all directions, not just the displacements perpendicular to the diffusion gradient vector. Consequently the q-ball ODF can only be deemed as good approximation since it doesn't consider all diffusion displacements in the three-dimensional space [62]. On the other hand, DSI is able to characterize the diffusion probability density function by applying the Fourier transform to the MR signals in the q-space; however, it still relies on numerical estimation to calculate the ODF. The mathematical estimation often encounters the truncation artifacts in the Fourier transform, as entails additional treatment like a Hanning filter smoothing on the PDF [22, 31].

Generalized-sampling imaging (GQI): Recently the spin distribution function (SDF) has been defined to quantitatively describe a distribution of the spins undergoing diffusion on the voxel basis, which is unlike the diffusion ODF representing a probability distribution of the diffusion displacement [72]. This relation leads to an imaging method named generalized q-sampling imaging (GQI) which is readily applicable to a wide range of q-space datasets including those acquired by the shell or grid sampling schemes. Taking a closer look at the reconstruction equations of GQI and DSI, they share the same theoretical basis. Hence GQI and DSI reconstruction could result in similar diffusion patterns. Note that the reconstruction process of GQI does not require deconvolution procedures and the SDF values can be compared across voxels [72].

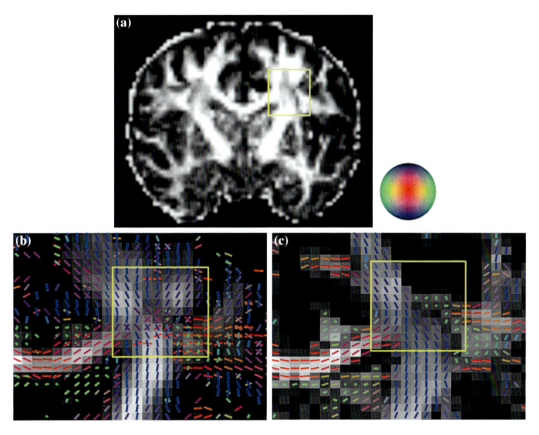

Fig. 2.1 Comparison on the fiber orientations of the centrum semiovale resolved by DTI and DSI on the same subject. **b** Using DSI, fibers coursing towards the corpus callosum (*red*) intersect with vertically oriented corona radiata fibers (*blue*) and rostro-caudally oriented long association fibers (*green*). In contrast to using DTI (**c**), only one fiber orientation is seen within one voxel. **a** DTI-derived FA map. The area within *yellow boxes* of each image **a**, **b**, **c** is the centrum semiovale. The directions of the ODF or SDF are pseudo-colored: *red* in the left–right direction, *green* in the anterior-posterior direction, and *blue* in the axial superior-inferior direction, illustrated by the color ball. The *gray* background represents the calculated values of GFA (**b**) and FA (**c**), respectively

2.4 Diffusion MR Tractography

Tractography hasbeen developed to improve the depiction of data from diffusion imaging of the brain and aid the image interpretation [8, 67]. The primary purpose of tractography is to clarify the orientational architecture of nerve fibers by integrating pathways of maximum diffusion coherence. The computational algorithms normally track the diffusion maximum from voxel to voxel in such a way of simulating the fibers growing across the brain. The fibers offered by tractography are often accepted to represent individual axons or nerve fibers, but they are more accurately viewed as lines of dominant diffusion that follow or parallel the local diffusion maxima [43]. This distinction is vital because, given with certain imaging resolution and signal-to-noise level, lines of maximum diffusion coherence may differ from the axonal architecture in some brains [42]. For example, DTI provides a Gaussian approximation of the actual displacement distribution, and since the representation of that distribution is restricted to variations of an ellipsoid, this method creates various biases in the resulting tractography [27]. Also the tractography results depend on the tracking algorithm used. Deterministic fiber tracking from DTI uses the principal direction of diffusion to integrate trajectories

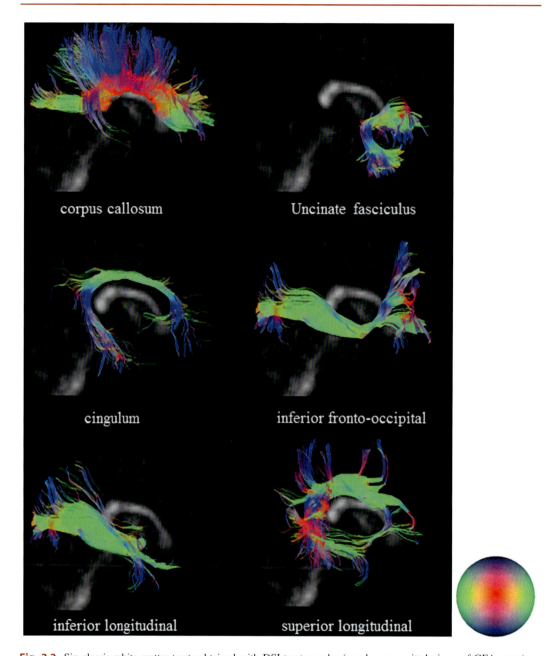

Fig. 2.2 Six classic white matter tracts obtained with DSI tractography (overlay on sagittal views of GFA maps)

over the image but ignores the fact that fiber orientation is often undetermined in the diffusion tensor imaging data [42].

The fact is that the connectivity maps obtained with tractography vary according to the diffusion imaging modality used to obtain the diffusion datasets. Hagmann and colleagues investigated statistical fiber tracking methods based on consideration of the tensor as a probability distribution of fiber orientation [23]. The application of fiber tractography to data such as those obtained with DSI or QBI results in the depiction of a large set of fiber tracts with a more complex geometry. Such greater complexity obtained with this method is due to the consideration of numerous intersections between fibers that can be resolved or differentiated. In such sense, DSI tractography overcomes some above biases and allows more realistic mapping of connectivity [21, 31, 69, 70]. Figure 2.2 presents typical examples of six major white matter tracts reconstructed by DSI.

Nonetheless, tractography provides more interesting and valuable information for depicting the human neuroanatomy in vivo.

2.5 Procedure of Data Analysis

Here we used the DSI image dataset collected by Functional Brain Imaging Platform (FBIP) at Institute of Neuroscience, Chinese Academy of Sciences, Shanghai, to demonstrate the procedure widely-used in the analysis of the diffusion MRI data. It will lend the support to those who are interested in applying these neuroimaging techniques to solve those clinically-driven problems during diagnostics and therapy of psychiatric disorders. A schematic workflow diagram of diffusion MRI processing is illustrated in Fig. 2.3.

The detailed imaging protocol will be described in other places and summarized shortly here. T1-weighted structural MRI images were acquired on a 3T MR imaging system (Magnetom Trio; Siemens, Erlangen, Germany) using a 12-channel phased array head coil (TR = 2,300 ms, TE = 3 ms, TI = 1,000 ms, flip angle = 9°, FOV = 256 × 256 mm^2, voxel size = 1.0 × 1.0 × 1.0 mm^3, 176 slices, no slice gap). Earplugs were used, and movement was minimized by stabilizing the head with cushions. Diffusion spectrum imaging was acquired using a twice-refocused spin-echo EPI pulse sequence [55]. The diffusion-encoding scheme used in this study followed the framework of DSI in which diffusion-weighted images were acquired with diffusion gradients of different b values corresponding to the grid points filled within a sphere in the 3D diffusion-encoding space (q-space) [68]. TR = 9,500 ms,

TE = 152 ms, flip angle = 90°, FOV = 80 × 80 mm^2, voxel size = 2.4 × 2.4 × 2.4 mm^3, b-max = 7,000 s/mm^{-2}. To reduce the scan time, we only recorded half-sphere DSI data [20, 21]. Specifically, the DSI data were acquired with 128 diffusion-encoding directions corresponding to grid points filled in the half sphere of the q-space. Acquisition time for the half-scheme acquisition was 21 min. To correct for image distortion resulting from magnetic susceptibility, field maps were acquired using a GRE sequence with two TEs (acquisition time, 91 s, TR/TE = 500/3.38 and 5.84 ms). The matrix size and FOV of the field maps were the same as those used in the DSI dataset.

The half-sphere data were extrapolated to the other half of the sphere based on the symmetry property of the data in the q-space, and the eight corners of the cube that were unsampled were zero-filled. The susceptibility-induced distortion on each DSI image was first corrected using the acquired field maps [24], and then subjected to the motion correction and eddy current compensation using the software based on FSL (http://www.fmrib.ox.ac.uk/fsl). The following DSI data reconstruction was conducted through using the generalized q-sampling imaging approach available in the software of DSI Studio (http://dsi-studio.labsolver.org) [15]. The ODFs were reconstructed to 162 discrete sampling directions (corresponding to the vertices of a 4-fold regularly tessellated icosahedron projected onto the sphere). The diffusion deconvolution was then applied to the diffusion ODFs generated from GQI to increase the angular resolution of the resolved fiber. Having obtained the ODF, the GFA (similar to FA) was derived to quantify the directionality of the diffusion on a scale from zero (when the diffusion was totally random) to one (when the diffusion was along one direction only). The formula of deriving the value of GFA is defined as the ratio of the standard deviation of ODF and its root mean square [64]. Like FA, GFA has been used to infer microstructure integrity of the white matter fiber tracts.

Fig. 2.3 A schematic diagram of typical DSI data-processing workflow. Step 1: Data acquisition (*A*). Step 2: Preprocessing includes the conversion of original dataformat (*B*), eddy and motion correction (*C*), and skull stripping (*D*). Step 3: Image reconstruction. Some commonly-used reconstruction approaches are listed here like DSI, GQI or QSDR (*E*). The ODFs or GFA are calculated for further analysis (*F*). Step 4: Fiber tracking. Either the whole-brain (*G*) or ROI-based fiber tracking (*H*) can be chosen for distinct research objectives. Step 5: Data analysis. Statistical comparison of fiber tracts can be conducted at group-level (*I* and *J*) and the network-level analysis can be used to extract more features from the structural connectivity matrix

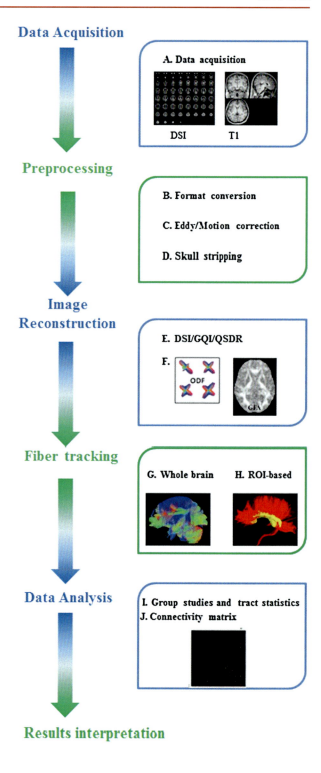

In addition to subject-specific reconstruction approach, we also reconstructed the DSI data in MNI-152 space (a standard space introduced by the International Consortium for Brain Mapping, http://www.bic.mni.mcgill.ca/ServicesAtlases/ICBM152NLin2009) using q-space diffeomorphic reconstruction (QSDR) [15], which provides a direct approach to analyze the group difference and also facilitates the comparison using fiber tracking. QSDR is the generalization of GQI that allows users to construct ODFs in any given template space (e.g. MNI space). DSI Studio first calculates the quantitative anisotropy (QA) mapping and then normalizes it to the NTU-90 QAmap. The NTU-90 atlas is the average of the normalized subject data in the MNI-152 space.

For the fiber-tracking datasets, all fiber tracking was performed using the DSI Studio. In most of clinical studies, an ODF-streamlined region of interest (ROI)-based approach are frequently chosen to discern the difference between the patient and control groups [15]. Depending on various kinds of research objectives, there are several ways available to define the ROIs of the subjects. In QSDR reconstruction approach, we used the normalized ROIs from the JHU White Matter tractography atlas provided by DSI studio [67]; In GQI reconstruction approach, we used the selected ROIs from the JHU atlas and warped it to the subject T1-weighted image space by linear registration. Tracts were generated using an ODF-streamline version of the FACT deterministic tractography algorithm [8, 15], and left and right hemispheres were investigated separately. If an ODF had more than one peak orientation, the initial direction was the primary fiber from the resolved orientations. The advantage of "primary" is the stableness and consistency of the results. Trilinear interpolation was used to estimate the propagation direction. Fiber progression continued with a certain step size like 1 mm (half the spacing for QSDR reconstruction approach), minimum fiber length like 40 mm, and turning angle threshold (usually set at $40°–70°$). To smooth each track, the next moving directional estimate of each voxel was weighted by a combination of the previous incoming direction and the nearest fiber orientation. Once tracked, all streamlines were saved in the TrackVis file format. Segmentation of the fiber tracts was performed with TrackVis software (http://trackvis.org).

2.6 Diffusion MRI Applications in Psychiatric Disorders

Diffusion MRI has been becoming an indispensable tool to investigate a variety of psychiatric disorders such as schizophrenia, major depressive disorder, eating disorders, attention deficit disorder and addictions and so on. It has shed insightful light on our understanding of neural connectivity and how abnormalities in connectivity may contribute to the pathogenesis of psychiatric illnesses. This section will concisely summarize recent applications on those psychiatric diseases with DTI/DSI techniques, specifically restricting our attention to the reward-circuitry based brain disorders.

Obsessive-Compulsive Disorder (OCD): Alterations in the WM tracts within the classic cortico-striato-thalamo-cortical (CSTC) circuitry, which has long been implicated in the pathogenesis of OCD [39], were always observed in the literature with DTI method. There have been reported that alterations of FA were observed in many brain regions of OCD patients, such as the anterior cingulate [12, 60], internal capsule [12, 73], white matter in the area superolateral to the right caudate [73], corpus callosum [57, 73], and the right inferior parietal and medial frontal regions [36], the bilateral semiovalcenter extending to the subinsular white matter [45]. However, the conclusions drawn from these current studies have been inconsistent. For example, findings in the FA of the anterior cingulate were particularly mysterious, showing higher values [12], lower values [60], or no changes [36, 45, 73] in OCD patients in comparison to normal subjects.

Findings concerning the anterior thalamic radiations (ATR) seem to be inconsistent as well. Cannistraro et al. [12] reported an increased FA value in the left anterior limb of the internal-capsule, whereas Yoo et al. [73] found increases in FA in the superolateral area of the right caudate that were penetrated by the ATR. These divergent observations by the DTI could be caused by the notoriously complicated structure of the brain network, in which the presence of crossing fibers has been robustly demonstrated by the DSI-based tractography in both nonhuman primate and human [21, 58, 69]. Therefore, Chiu and his co-workers applied the GFA value to describe the microstructural integrity of the white matter tracts [15]. They found significantly lower mean GFA in the right ATR and the left the anterior segment of cingulum bundles in OCD subjects compared to the ATRs and cingulum bundles of normal controls. In addition to the GFA measure, asymmetry of the mean GFA between the left and right tracts was also calculated [15], which might provide a parsimonious explanation to the above discrepancy observed in different reports. Notwithstanding the new evidence, it requires further research to fully elucidate those apparent contradictory results. Besides that, more widespread WM abnormalities like the microstructural alterations in the fronto-basal pathways targeting the orbitofrontal cortex and the anterior cingulate cortex have been proposed to be involved in OCD [39]. Menzies and colleagues reported that the anatomical connectivity between lateral frontal and parietal regions was altered as well as microstructural abnormalities in intra-hemispheric bundles linking distinctive areas of the prefrontal cortex to posterior parietal and occipital association cortices [36].

Major depressive disorder (***MDD***): Decrease in FA was found in the right middle frontal gyrus, left occipitotemporal gyrus, and the subgyral and angular gyri of the right parietal lobe in medication-free young adults with MDD [2]. Lower FA in regions lateral to the anterior cingulate was associated with lower occurring rates of remission in geriatric depression [4]. Older patients with MDD have been shown to demonstrate lower FA in the dorsolateral prefrontal cortex and anterior cingulate cortex [6], and diffuse frontal [2, 47, 63] and temporal lobe [47]. Interestingly, after electroconvulsive therapy (ECT), depressed geriatric patients had an increase in frontal FA associated with the improvement of their clinical symptoms [46], but not in the temporal WM regions. Diminished FA in white matter regions including anterior cingulate and dorsolateral frontal pathways in patients with late life depression was found to be a strong predictor of poor response to the antidepressant Citalopram [4]. In the future growing psychiatric research with diffusion MRI that points to predicting the disease risks and response factors (ultimately for early intervention or prevention) can be much of translational utility [2].

Eating Disorder (***ED***): Eating disorder is a severe psychiatric disorder associated with self-driven food refusal and emaciation, altered body perception and preoccupations with weight, which generally includes three major categories: Anorexia Nervosa (AN), Bulimia Nervosa (BN) and Eating Disorder Not Otherwise Specified (EDNOS) [29]. In AN patients, Kim and Whalen found that left ventral amygdala responses to fearful versus neutral faces were positively correlated with local FA values along the white matter fibers located within the amygdala-ventromedial prefrontal cortex pathway. Intriguingly, these significantly correlated voxel clusters extended into the left ventral striatum and terminated at the left medial orbitofrontal cortex [30]. The abnormal WM integrity of the limbic and association pathways in AN patients has been found to account for disturbed feeding, emotion processing and body perception. Moreover, changes of FA in the left and right fimbria-fornix were allowed to predict the harm avoidance behavior of AN patients, which suggested that the fimbria-fornix WM pathway is possibly involved in high anxiety level of AN [28]. Frieling and his coworkers identified disturbances of associational and commissural fibers in the bilateral occipitotemporal white matter, suggesting that the distortion of self-body image could be related to microstructural alterations of white matter tracts connecting the extrastriate visual cortex with other brain regions involved in body perception [18]. Moreover, they identified in AN patients bilateral reductions of FA maps in the posterior thalamic radiation including the optic radiation and the left mediodorsal thalamus [18]. On the other hand, widespread decrease in FA values of BN patients were observed in the bilateral corona radiata extending into the posterior limb of the internal capsule, the corpus callosum, the right subinsular WM, and right fornix. The result suggested that the integrity of WM fiber tracts was largely altered in BN, especially in the corona radiata which was deemed to account for taste and brain reward processing [38].

Substance Dependence (SD): Compared with normal controls, both men and women with chronic alcoholism show a decrease in FA in the genu of the CC and the centrum semiovale [48–52]. FA decreases in the splenium of the CC was also found in male subjects [48, 51]. The decrease in FA in the genu was associated with decreased volume of both the genu and the body of the CC, and decreases in FA have been shown to correlate with the amount of alcohol consumption and with comorbid human immunodeficiency syndrome infection [50]. Men with alcohol dependence showed lower generalized FA values on all segments of the corpus callosum. The segment interconnecting the bilateral orbitofrontal cortices was the most affected [15].

Another major SD in our daily life is cocaine use, which can result in a number of neurological complications including headaches, seizures, and strokes. There is evidence that cocaine adversely disrupted the myelin sheaths [41]. DTI studies of cocaine abuse patients reveal a decrease in frontal FA and the genu and rostral body of the CC, and the FA measures in the CC were inversely correlated with impulsivity [35, 36, 40, 70].

2.7 Conclusion

The high sensitivity of diffusion MRI technique enables its rising popularity in the diagnosis of psychiatric illnesses and the monitoring of the brain response to therapeutic interventions. One attractive perspective is to follow subjects longitudinally to determine how the microstructural properties of the tissue change over time if each subject serves as their own baseline reference. In

this way, the abnormality at different stage can be well characterized and the therapeutic effects are readily predicted. Diffusion image-based prognostic indicators of disease course and response to therapy would be extremely valuable to assess the responsiveness of patients to specific therapies, since predictive imaging measures would enable earlier interventions. Up to date, there are only a handful of DSI studies to examine the brain architecture and connectivity in psychiatric disorders. Due to differences in methodologies, scanner sequences, and image processing algorithms, it requires more cautions to interpret the physiological meaning of results obtained by the diffusion MRI methods in clinical psychiatric research.

Acknowledgments This work was partially supported by The Hundred Talent Program (Technology), Chinese Academy of Sciences (ZW). We thank Franz Schmitt, Renate Jerecic, Thomas Benner, Kecheng Liu, Ignacio Vallines, and Hui Liu for their help and contribution to the construction of our custom-tuned gradient-insert MRI facility.

References

1. Alexander AL. Analysis of partial volume effects in diffusion-tensor MRI. Magn Reson Med. 2001;45: 770–80.
2. Alexander AL, Lee JE, Lazar M, Field AS. Diffusion tensor imaging of the brain. Neurotherapeutics. 2007;4:316–29.
3. Alexander DC, Barker GJ. Optimal imaging parameters for fiber-orientation estimation in diffusion MRI. Neuroimage. 2005;27:357–67.
4. Alexopoulos GS, Kiosses DN, Choi SJ, Murphy CF, Lim KO. Frontal white matter microstructure and treatment response of late-life depression: a preliminary study. Am J Psychiatry. 2002;159: 1929–32.
5. Ardekani BA, Nierenberg J, Hoptman MJ, Javitt DC, Lim KO. MRI study of white matter diffusion anisotropy in schizophrenia. Neuroreport. 2003; 14:2025–9.
6. Bae JN, MacFall JR, Krishnan KR, Payne ME, Steffens DC, Taylor WD. Dorsolateral prefrontal cortex and anterior cingulate cortex white matter alterations in late-life depression. Biol Psychiatry. 2006;60:1356–63.
7. Basser PJ, Mattiello J, LeBihan D. MR diffusion tensor sepctroscopy and imaging. Biophys J. 1994;66:259–67.

8. Basser PJ, Pajevic S, Pierpaoli C, Duda J, Aldroubi A. In vivo fiber tractography using DT-MRI data. Magn Reson Med. 2000;44:625–32.
9. Beaulieu C. The basis of anisotropic water diffusion in the nervous system—a technical review. NMR Biomed. 2002;15:435–55.
10. Callaghan PT. Principles of Nuclear Magnetic Resonance Microscopy. Oxford: Oxford University Press; 1993.
11. Callaghan PT, Eccles CD, Xia Y. NMR microscopy of dynamic displacements—K-Space and Q-Space Imaging. J Phys E: Sci Instrum. 1988;21:820–2.
12. Cannistraro PA, Makris N, Howard JD, Wedig MM, Hodge SM, et al. A diffusion tensor imaging study of white matter in obsessive-compulsive disorder. Depress Anxiety. 2007;24:440–6.
13. Catani M. Diffusion tensor magnetic resonance imaging tractography in cognitive disorders. Curr Opin Neurol. 2006;19:599–606.
14. Chenevert TL, Brunberg JA, Pipe JG. Anisotropic diffusion in human white matter: demonstration with MR techniques in vivo. Radiology. 1990;171:401–5.
15. Chiu CH, Lo YC, Tang HS, Liu IC, Chiang WY, et al. White matter abnormalities of fronto-striato-thalamic circuitry in obsessive-compulsive disorder: a study using diffusion spectrum imaging tractography. Psychiatry Res. 2011;192:176–82.
16. Cory DG, Garroway AN. Measurement of translational displacement probabilities by NMR—an indicator of compartmentation. Magn Reson Med. 1990;14:435–44.
17. Descoteaux M, Angelino E, Fitzgibbons S, Deriche R. Regularized, fast, and robust analytical Q-ball imaging. Magn Reson Med. 2007;58:497–510.
18. Frieling H, Fischer J, Wilhelm J, Engelhorn T, Bleich S, et al. Microstructural abnormalities of the posterior thalamic radiation and the mediodorsal thalamic nuclei in females with anorexia nervosa—a voxel based diffusion tensor imaging (DTI) study. J Psychiatr Res. 2012;46:1237–42.
19. Gorczewski K, Mang S, Klose U. Reproducibility and consistency of evaluation techniques for HARDI data. MAGMA. 2009;22:63–70.
20. Granziera C, Schmahmann JD, Hadjikhani N, Meyer H, Meuli R, et al. Diffusion spectrum imaging shows the structural basis of functional cerebellar circuits in the human cerebellum in vivo. PLoS One. 2009;4: e5101.
21. Hagmann P, Cammoun L, Gigandet X, Meuli R, Honey CJ, Wedeen VJ. Mapping the structural core of human cerebral cortex. PLoS Biol. 2008.
22. Hagmann P, Jonasson L, Deffieux T, Meuli R, Thiran JP, Wedeen VJ. Fibertract segmentation in position orientation space from high angular resolution diffusion MRI. Neuroimage. 2006;32:665–75.
23. Hagmann P, Thiran JP, Jonasson L, Vandergheynst P, Clarke S, et al. DTI mapping of human brain connectivity: statistical fibre tracking and virtual dissection. Neuroimage. 2003;19:545–54.
24. Hsu YC, Hsu CH, Tseng WYI. Correction for susceptibility-induced distortion in echo-planar imaging using field maps and model-based point spread function. IEEE Trans Med Imaging. 2009;28:1850–7.
25. Johansen-Berg H. Behavioural relevance of variation in white matter microstructure. Curr Opin Neurol. 2010;23:351–8.
26. Johansen-Berg H, Behrens TEJ. Diffusion MRI: from quantitative measurement to in-vivo neuroanatomy. In: Johansen-Berg H, Behrens TEJ, editors. Diffusion MRI. San Diego: Academic Press; 2009.
27. Jones DK, Knosche TR, Turner R. White matter integrity, fiber count, and other fallacies: the do's and don'ts of diffusion MRI. Neuroimage. 2013;73:239–54.
28. Kazlouski D, Rollin MD, Tregellas J, Shott ME, Jappe LM, et al. Altered fimbria-fornix white matter integrity in anorexia nervosa predicts harm avoidance. Psychiatry Res. 2011;192:109–16.
29. Keel PK, Brown TA, Holland LA, Bodell LP. Empirical classification of eating disorders. Annu Rev Clin Psychol. 2012;8:381–404.
30. Kim MJ, Whalen PJ. The structural integrity of an amygdala-prefrontal pathway predicts trait anxiety. J Neurosci. 2009;29:11614–8.
31. Kuo LW, Chen JH, Wedeen VJ, Tseng WY. Optimization of diffusion spectrum imaging and q-ball imaging on clinical MRI system. Neuroimage. 2008;41:7–18.
32. Kyriakopoulos M, Frangou S. Recent diffusion tensor imaging findings in early stages of schizophrenia. Curr Opin Psychiatry. 2009;22:168–76.
33. Le Bihan D. Looking into the functional architecture of the brain with diffusion MRI. Nat Rev Neurosci. 2003;4:469–80.
34. Le Bihan D, Breton E, Lallemand D, Grenier P, Cabanis E, Laval-Jeantet M. MR imaging of intravoxel incoherent motions: application to diffusion and perfusion in neurologic disorders. Radiology. 1986;161:401–7.
35. Lim KO, Wozniak JR, Mueller BA, Franc DT, Specker SM, et al. Brain macrostructural and microstructural abnormalities in cocaine dependence. Drug Alcohol Depend. 2008;92:164–72.
36. Menzies L, Chamberlain SR, Laird AR, Thelen SM, Sahakian BJ, Bullmore ET. Integrating evidence from neuroimaging and neuropsychological studies of obsessive-compulsive disorder: the orbitofronto-striatal model revisited. Neurosci Biobehav Rev. 2008;32:525–49.
37. Merboldt K-D, Hanicke W, Frahm J. Self-diffusion NMR imaging using stimulated echoes. J Magn Reson. 1985;64:479–86.
38. Mettler LN, Shott ME, Pryor T, Yang TT, Frank GK. White matter integrity is reduced in bulimia nervosa. Int J Eat Disord. 2013;46:264–73.
39. Milad MR, Rauch SL. Obsessive-compulsive disorder: beyond segregated cortico-striatal pathways. Trends Cogn Sci. 2012;16:43–51.

40. Moeller FG, Hasan KM, Steinberg JL, Kramer LA, Dougherty DM, et al. Reduced anterior corpus callosum white matter integrity is related to increased impulsivity and reduced discriminability in cocaine-dependent subjects: diffusion tensor imaging. Neuropsychopharmacology. 2005;30:610–7.

41. Moeller FG, Hasan KM, Steinberg JL, Kramer LA, Valdes I, et al. Diffusion tensor imaging eigenvalues: preliminary evidence for altered myelin in cocaine dependence. Psychiatry Res. 2007;154:253–8.

42. Mori S, van Zijl PCM. Fiber tracking: principles and strategies—a technical review. NMR Biomed. 2002;15:468–80.

43. Mori S, Zhang J. Principles of diffusion tensor imaging and its applications to basic neuroscience research. Neuron. 2006;51:527–39.

44. Moseley ME, Cohen Y. Diffusion-weighted MR imaging of anisotropic water diffusion in cat central nervous system. Radiology. 1990;176:439–45.

45. Nakamae T, Narumoto J, Shibata K, Matsumoto R, Kitabayashi Y, et al. Alteration of fractional anisotropy and apparent diffusion coefficient in obsessive-compulsive disorder: a diffusion tensor imaging study. Prog Neuropsychopharmacol Biol Psychiatry. 2008;32:1221–6.

46. Nobuhara K, Okugawa G, Minami T, Takase K, Yoshida T, et al. Effects of electroconvulsive therapy on frontal white matter in late-life depression: a diffusion tensor imaging study. Neuropsychobiology. 2004;50:48–53.

47. Nobuhara K, Okugawa G, Sugimoto T, Minami T, Tamagaki C, et al. Frontal white matter anisotropy and symptom severity of late-life depression: a magnetic resonance diffusion tensor imaging study. J Neurol Neurosurg Psychiatry. 2006;77:120–2.

48. Pfefferbaum A, Adalsteinsson E, Sullivan EV. Dysmorphology and microstructural degradation of the corpus callosum: interaction of age and alcoholism. Neurobiol Aging. 2006;27:994–1009.

49. Pfefferbaum A, Adalsteinsson E, Sullivan EV. Supratentorial profile of white matter microstructural integrity in recovering alcoholic men and women. Biol Psychiatry. 2006;59:364–72.

50. Pfefferbaum A, Rosenbloom MJ, Adalsteinsson E, Sullivan EV. Diffusion tensor imaging with quantitative fibre tracking in HIV infection and alcoholism comorbidity: synergistic white matter damage. Brain. 2007;130:48–64.

51. Pfefferbaum A, Sullivan EV. Microstructural but not macrostructural disruption of white matter in women with chronic alcoholism. Neuroimage. 2002; 15:708–18.

52. Pfefferbaum A, Sullivan EV. Disruption of brain white matter microstructure by excessive intracellular and extracellular fluid in alcoholism: evidence from diffusion tensor imaging. Neuropsychopharmacology. 2005;30:423–32.

53. Pierpaoli C. Diffusion tensor MR imaging of the human brain. Radiology. 1996;201:637–48.

54. Pierpaoli C, Basser PJ. Toward a quantitative assessment of diffusion anisotropy. Magn Reson Med. 1996;36:893–906.

55. Reese TG, Heid O, Weisskoff RM, Wedeen VJ. Reduction of eddy-current-induced distortion in diffusion MRI using a twice-refocused spin echo. Magn Reson Med. 2003;49:177–82.

56. Roberts RE, Anderson EJ, Husain M. White matter microstructure and cognitive function. Neuroscientist. 2013;19:8–15.

57. Saito Y, Nobuhara K, Okugawa G, Takase K, Sugimoto T, et al. Corpus callosum in patients with obsessive-compulsive disorder: diffusion-tensor imaging study. Radiology. 2008;246:536–42.

58. Schmahmann JD, Pandya DN, Wang R, Dai G, D'Arceuil HE, et al. Association fibre pathways of the brain: parallel observations from diffusion spectrum imaging and autoradiography. Brain. 2007;130: 630–53.

59. Stejskal EO, Tanner JE. Spin diffusion measurements: spin echoes in the presence of a time-dependent field gradient. J Chem Phys. 1965;42:288–292.

60. Szeszko PR, MacMillan S, McMeniman M, Lorch E, Madden R, et al. Amygdala volume reductions in pediatric patients with obsessive-compulsive disorder treated with paroxetine: preliminary findings. Neuropsychopharmacology. 2004;29:826–32.

61. Tang PF, Ko YH, Luo ZA, Yeh FC, Chen SH, Tseng WY. Tract-specific and region of interest analysis of corticospinal tract integrity in subcortical ischemic stroke: reliability and correlation with motor function of affected lower extremity. Am J Neuroradiol. 2010;31:1023–30.

62. Taylor DG, Bushell MC. The spatial-mapping of translational diffusion-coefficients by the NMR imaging technique. Phys Med Biol. 1985;30:345–9.

63. Taylor WD, MacFall JR, Payne ME, McQuoid DR, Provenzale JM, et al. Late-life depression and microstructural abnormalities in dorsolateral prefrontal cortex white matter. Am J Psychiatry. 2004;161:1293–6.

64. Tuch DS. Q-ball imaging. Magn Reson Med. 2004;52:1358–72.

65. Tuch DS, Reese TG, Wiegell MR, Makris N, Belliveau JW, Wedeen VJ. High angular resolution diffusion imaging reveals intravoxel white matter fiber heterogeneity. Magn Reson Med. 2002; 48:577–82.

66. Tuch DS, Reese TG, Wiegell MR, Wedeen VJ. Diffusion MRI of complex neural architecture. Neuron. 2003;40:885–95.

67. Wakana S, Caprihan A, Panzenboeck MM, Fallon JH, Perry M, et al. Reproducibility of quantitative tractography methods applied to cerebral white matter. Neuroimage. 2007;36:630–44.

68. Wedeen VJ, Hagmann P, Tseng WY, Reese TG, Weisskoff RM. Mapping complex tissue architecture with diffusion spectrum magnetic resonance imaging. Magn Reson Med. 2005;54:1377–86.

69. Wedeen VJ, Rosene DL, Wang R, Dai G, Mortazavi F, et al. The geometric structure of the brain fiber pathways. Science. 2012;335:1628–34.
70. Wedeen VJ, Wang RP, Schmahmann JD, Benner T, Tseng WY, et al. Diffusion spectrum magnetic resonance imaging (DSI) tractography of crossing fibers. Neuroimage. 2008;41:1267–77.
71. Wiegell MR. Fiber crossing in human brain depicted with diffusion tensor MR imaging. Radiology. 2000;217.
72. Yeh FC, Wedeen VJ, Tseng WY. Generalized q-sampling imaging. IEEE Trans Med Imaging. 2010;29:1626–35.
73. Yoo SY, Jang JH, Shin YW, Kim DJ, Park HJ, et al. White matter abnormalities in drug-naive patients with obsessive-compulsive disorder: a diffusion tensor study before and after citalopram treatment. Acta Psychiatr Scand. 2007;116:211–9.

Neuroimaging in Psychiatry

3

Chuantao Zuo and Huiwei Zhang

3.1 Introduction

Psychiatric disorders are generally defined by a combination of how a person feels, behaves, thinks, or perceives. The disorders may be associated with particular brain regions or functional units or with the nervous system as a whole, and are often diagnosed within a particular social context. In the past few decades, neuroimaging modalities have been developed to investigate specific brain regions thought to be involved in particular disorders. Neuroimaging has been applied in the differential diagnosis of neuropsychiatric syndromes and disorders, especially in otherwise difficult clinical contexts. Neuroimaging methodologies can also provide information about neural mechanisms and abnormal neural circuitry involved in various psychiatric disorders. Additionally, neuroimaging is an important tool for drug discovery and development.

With the advancement of neuroimaging techniques and softwares, it is now possible to reliably segment the brain into gray matter (GM), white matter (WM), and cerebrospinal fluid (CSF) with little effort. Imaging studies can be divided into structural gray matter studies, studies examining the white matter connectivity, functional magnetic resonance imaging (fMRI) studies, and studies measuring neurotransmitter and neurotransmitter receptor changes. Structural brain imaging studies can be broadly divided into region of interest (ROI) studies and voxel-based morphometric (VBM) analyses. In the former, a brain region is chosen and using specific tracing guidelines, the region is then demarcated with subsequent volume calculation and comparison, for example, between patients with schizophrenia and healthy subjects. The latter (i.e., VBM) is more automated with easier methods for segmentation and volume comparisons. The basic principle underlying diffusion tensor imaging (DTI), which is used to assess white matter integrity, is that the diffusion of water molecules is restricted equally in all directions in the CSF (isotropic diffusion) but not in the white and grey matter; water exhibits strong anisotropic diffusion in the white matter, whereas in gray matter, it exhibits weak anisotropic diffusion. There has been a rapid increase in the number of fMRI studies on psychiatric disorders. fMRI helps in understanding the relationship between brain and behavior. An essential aim of a study using fMRI is to show how a failure to stimulate a neural system (as evidenced by reduced blood flow in test subjects during attempts to stimulate the system relative to control patients) leads to behavioral deficits in patients. Magnetic resonance spectroscopy (MRS) is a non-invasive analytical technique that has been used to study metabolic changes in the brain. This technique is used to study metabolites that reflect specific

---

C. Zuo (✉) · H. Zhang
PET Center, Huashan Hospital, Fudan University,
Shanghai, China
e-mail: zuoct_cn2000@126.com

B. Sun and A. De Salles (eds.), *Neurosurgical Treatments for Psychiatric Disorders*,
DOI 10.1007/978-94-017-9576-0_3
© Shanghai Jiao Tong University Press, Shanghai and Springer Science+Business Media Dordrecht 2015

brain functions. In addition, the introduction of techniques such as positron emission tomography (PET) and single photon emission tomography (SPECT) has allowed direct in vivo examination of neurotransmitter functioning in the brain. PET/SPECT have been employed in many studies to quantify metabolism or blood flow in different brain regions, measure neurotransmitter receptor binding potential, quantify regional density of receptors of a given type, determine receptor binding displacement during pharmacological or physiological challenge, as well as to quantify neurotransmitter release.

3.2 Schizophrenia

Magnetic resonance imaging (MRI) studies have examined various aspects of schizophrenia ranging from establishing structural brain deficits to brain connectivity impairments down to the level of functional impairment apart from neurotransmitter and receptor changes. Structural MRI represents a useful tool in understanding the biological underpinnings of schizophrenia and in planning focused interventions, thus assisting clinicians especially in the early phases of the illness [1]. The current concept of pathophysiology of schizophrenia has shifted towards abnormalities in pathways rather than a region-specific lesion, even though it is difficult to definitively state that a specific pathway is affected. The neuropsychological deficits consistently reported in schizophrenia are executive function impairments in tests such as rule set shifting, response inhibition, and selective attention. Deficits in processing speed, language abilities, working memory, and verbal and visual memory are also reported. The diversity of symptoms could also reflect multiple brain region involvement [2].

Studies using VBM or other quantitative structural MRI techniques have shown that patients with first-episode schizophrenia (FES) have significant regional gray matter reduction in the prefrontal cortex, temporal cortex, and hippocampus, as well as in the anteromedial thalamus [3–5]. Similar structural changes can be effected by the use of antipsychotic medication [6]. A VBM study on patients with schizophrenia and their unaffected siblings revealed that they might share decreases in the gray matter volume of the left middle temporal gyrus. This regional reduction might be a potential endophenotype of schizophrenia [5]. However, a meta-analyses study argued that the GM changes in patients with schizophrenia and their unaffected relatives are largely different, although there is subtle overlap in some regions [7].

fMRI has been utilized to evaluate many aspects such as cognition [8], emotional processing [9], and social cognition [10] in schizophrenia, in addition to identifying substrates of psychopathology [11]. fMRI studies have examined and demonstrated functional brain abnormalities at rest and during various postulated cognitive aberrations due to schizophrenia. They have also been able to provide insights regarding the neural basis of some important and classical schizophrenia-related symptoms such as auditory hallucinations [12]. In addition, by examining the relationship between specific eye movement and neuropsychological measures, antisaccade errors were suggested to be a sign of a generalized neuropsychological deficit in patients with schizophrenia [13]. fMRI and $H_2^{15}O$ PET scans have revealed abnormal activation in the prefrontal and cingulate cortex and the medial temporal lobe in these patients as well as abnormal interaction between these structures [14, 15]. Decreased suppression of the resting state brain network during stimulation paradigms has also been reported in schizophrenia [16].

Structural volumetric MRI studies have focused on a priori relevant brain regions in schizophrenia. VBM studies have also identified the areas implicated in the cortico-cerebello-thalamo-cortical circuit. This circuit and its components have been implicated in monitoring and coordinating the smooth execution of mental activity. Disruption in this circuit has been proposed as to cause "cognitive dysmetria" leading to disordered cognition and symptoms of schizophrenia. DTI studies have provided evidence for cortico-cortical and cortico-subcortical disconnectivity in schizophrenia. These changes appear to be widespread, and structural data supplement the evidence of extensive abnormalities in cortical areas demonstrated by VBM studies.

Neurotransmitters, including dopamine (DA), serotonin, gamma-aminobutyric acid (GABA) and glutamate, have been evaluated in the context of schizophrenia. DA function has been studied at several levels: (1) at a presynaptic level, neuroimaging studies investigating DOPA uptake capacity clearly show increased DA synthesis in patients with schizophrenia (meta-analysis showed consistently increased striatal dopamine synthesis capacity in schizophrenia, with a 14 % elevation in patients compared with healthy controls [17, 18]; (2) at a synaptic level, neuroimaging studies investigating dopamine transporter availability (DAT) do not show any evidence of dysfunction; (3) at a DA receptor level, neuroimaging studies investigating DA receptor density show a mild increase of dopamine D2 receptor density in basic condition and a hyper-reactivity of the DA system in dynamic conditions. Striatal DA abnormalities are now clearly demonstrated in patients with schizophrenia as well as the at-risk population and could constitute an endophenotype of schizophrenia. Subtle sub-clinical striatal DA abnormalities in the at-risk population could be a biomarker of transition from a vulnerability state to the expression of frank psychosis [19]. A significant reduction of ^{18}F-MPPF, a labeled PET ligand for $5-HT_{1A}$ receptors, was found in treated patients with schizophrenia compared to age- and sex-matched healthy subjects. These alterations were mainly localized to the frontal and orbitofrontal cortex and may reflect either the pathophysiology of schizophrenia or medication effects [20]. ^{18}F-FFMZ PET was recently used to measure GABA-A/BZ receptor binding potential. Individuals at ultra-high risk demonstrated significantly reduced binding potential of GABA-A/BZ receptors in the right caudate [21]. PET/SPECT studies testing the effects of NMDA blockade on dopaminergic indices in healthy subjects using ketamine alone found mixed results in the striatum but significant effects in the cortex, consistent with prior rodent data. However, strikingly similar results for amphetamine-induced dopamine release in individuals with schizophrenia and healthy subjects given acute ketamine provide initial support for the glutamate/NMDA hypothesis of schizophrenia. Nevertheless, directly in vivo measurements of glutamatergic indices are necessary to translate preclinical and clinical findings into effective therapies. Although the development of PET/SPECT imaging of the glutamate system has lagged behind that of the dopamine system, MRI-based technologies have been effectively utilized to measure glutamatergic indices in vivo [22].

3.3 Depression

Clinical depression affects 7–18 % of the population on at least one occasion during their life. Major depression is certainly the most prevalent psychiatric disorders and results in the largest number of disability adjusted life years. In contrast to some of the neurodegenerative disorders that mimic depression and are accompanied by decreased frontal lobe metabolism, major depression is associated with elevated metabolism but reduced volume in the subgenual region of the medial frontal lobe. In addition, the activation pattern on fMRI can be used to distinguish these disorders. Orbitofrontal and cingulate activation are greater in patients with depression than in those with AD and healthy controls. Genotypic variants are likely to influence both the likelihood of developing major depression and accompanying imaging findings. For instance, in depression, increased activity of the amygdala in response to negative stimuli appears to be modulated by the 5-HT transporter gene (SLC6A4) promoter polymorphism (5-HTTLPR). Hippocampal volume loss is characteristic of elderly subjects and of patients with chronic illness and depression and may be impacted by the V66M brain-derived neurotrophic factor gene variant and the 5-HTTLPR SLC6A4 polymorphism [16]. 3D-MRI studies reported higher perfusion in the ventral anterior cingulate/basal cingulate of responders compared to non-responders, and perfusion measurements are correlated with changes in the Hamilton depression rating scale [23–25].

PET/SPECT studies have shown an abnormally high serotonergic binding potential in patients with more severe pessimism, suggesting that extracellular serotonin relates to severity of pessimism [26]. Other studies have shown that higher-than-normal dopamine binding potential during depressive episodes worsened in patients with motor slowing, suggesting that dopamine plays a role in motor aspects of depression. These higher binding potentials for serotonin and dopamine are linked to lower extracellular concentration in these neurotransmitters; thus, depression is often said to be due to low serotonin and dopamine levels and treated with medications that inhibit active transport of these neurotransmitters from the extracellular space to intracellular locations, subsequently increasing extracellular levels [27]. PET imaging also provides an important contribution toward understanding the pathophysiology of major depressive disorders (MDDs), identifying endophenotypes and vulnerability traits, as well as assessing therapeutics and identifying new opportunities for prevention. Neuroreceptor PET imaging has associated major depression with decreased 5-HT_{1A} binding potential in the raphe nuclei, medial temporal lobe, and medial prefrontal cortex. Facilitated by the development of suitable radio ligands for monoaminergic receptors such as the 5-HT_{1A}, 5-HT_{2A}, and D2 receptors; reuptake transporters such as the serotonin transporter (SERT/5-HTT), dopamine transporter (DAT), and norepinephrine transporter (NET); and catabolic enzymes (MAO-A and -B), PET imaging has had a considerable impact on the monoamine theory of MDD. Given that MAO-A is an enzyme that metabolizes monoamines, such as serotonin, norepinephrine, and dopamine, elevated MAO-A density is proposed as the primary mechanism of the multiple monoamine reduction observed in MDD. An 80 % occupancy of the 5-HTT by serotonin reuptake inhibitors distinguishes medications from placebo in clinical trials on the treatment of major depressive episode [28]. Low 5-HTT binding activity was found in the dorsolateral prefrontal cortex of healthy twins of patients with mood disorders, indicating a genetic vulnerability that may contribute to the pathophysiology of depression [29]. Moreover, ^{18}F-fluoro-2-deoxy-glucose (FDG) PET imaging showed distinct regional cerebral patterns of glucose metabolism that may be serotonin-sensitive biomarkers of suicide risk [30].

3.4 Anxiety

MRI has been used in studies on anxiety disorders. Relative to controls, patients with generalized anxiety disorder (GAD) have larger volumes of the amygdala and dorsomedial prefrontal cortex (DMPFC). Moreover, patients with GAD showed localized gray matter volume differences in brain regions associated with anticipatory anxiety and emotion regulation [31]. The observation of alterations in pre-frontal regions and reduced activity observed in the striatal and parietal areas have shown that much remains to be investigated within the complexity of social anxiety disorder (SAD). Interestingly, follow-up studies have observed a decrease in perfusion in these same areas after either pharmacological or psychological treatment. The medial prefrontal cortex provides additional support for a cortico-limbic model of SAD pathophysiology, being a promising area of investigation [32]. Although in a fMRI study, patients with SAD showed activation patterns similar to that of the HC group, they showed comparatively decreased activation in the left cerebellum, left precuneus, and bilateral posterior cingulate cortex [33]. DTI can be used to examine the structural integrity of regional white matter and to map white matter tracts. For most anxiety disorders, the results of DTI studies are in line with other structural and fMRI findings and can be interpreted within the frameworks of existing models for the neurocircuitry of various disorders. DTI findings could further enrich neurobiological models for anxiety disorders, although replication is often warranted, and studies in pediatric populations are lagging behind remarkably [34].

In addition, PET/SPECT studies have observed reductions in 5-HT$_{1A}$ availability in anxiety disorders. Interestingly, 5-HTT reductions observed in patients with MDD correlated in magnitude with the severity of co-occurring anxiety, rather than depressive symptoms. A recent meta-analysis found decreased striatal D2 receptor and mesencephalic 5-HTT binding in obsessive compulsive disorder (OCD) and reduced GABA-A receptors in frontocortical regions in panic disorder as well as temporo-cortical areas in generalized anxiety disorder. When all anxiety disorders were pooled, reductions in midbrain 5-HTT and 5-HT$_{1A}$ receptors and striatal D2 and GABA-A receptors were observed, indicating a major role for dopamine, 5-HT, and GABA neurotransmission in anxiety disorders [35].

3.5 Eating Disorders

Eating disorders (EDs) include anorexia nervosa (AN) and bulimia nervosa (BN). Functional brain imaging is commonly performed in conjunction with paradigms and tasks designed to identify areas of brain activation that might be specific for AN pathophysiology. Visual high-calorie presentation elicited high anxiety in individuals with AN, together with left mesial temporal as well as left insular and bilateral anterior cingulate cortex (ACC) activity. The prefrontal cortex could be active to appropriately or inappropriately restrict food, possibly via heightened fear related activation and anxiety followed by related decision making such as food restriction. Heightened brain response to randomly applied pleasant and aversive taste stimuli have been observed in the insula and striatum of recovered individuals with AN, suggesting an overly sensitive taste reward system. Moreover, body image distortion is an integral part of AN pathophysiology and is part of its diagnostic criteria. Perceptual alterations may be related directly to the mechanisms of body image construction. Cingulate and prefrontal activity is frequently different between patients with AN and controls. Those regions may be over-activated when confronted with anxiety-provoking food-related stimuli. Such a heightened vigilance is probably related to anxiety and fear-of-fatness cognitions, followed by actions to avoid weight gain. On the other hand, individuals with AN may respond less to taste and other reward stimuli, which may help to restrict food intake, especially of neurobiologically "rewarding" foods. It further appears that individuals with AN do have altered self-perception-related brain activation and this suggests incorrect processing, and maybe abnormal proprioceptive feedback, which, in turn, may allow over-valued ideas of thinness to control the self-image [36]. In BN, insula activation represents emotional arousal by the image of food, whereas ACC activation acts as a counterbalance to that response, as the ACC is implicated in selection of emotional attention and control of sympathetic autonomic arousal [37, 38]. BN is associated with reduced response in the taste reward circuitry, which may indicate reward pathway desensitization in response to excessive food, possibly similar to that observed in models of substance use. Similarly to AN, BN is associated with reduced lateral fusiform gyrus activation and, compared to AN, high aversion ratings to any body shape. Thus, reduced brain activation in BN may be an aversion-driven restraint in brain response [39].

A ^{18}F-FDG PET study of AN showed hypermetabolism in the frontal lobe, the limbic lobe, lentiform nucleus, left insula, and left subcallosal gyrus. It also showed hypometabolism in the parietal lobe. The hypermetabolism in frontal lobe, hippocampus, and lentiform nucleus decreased after deep brain stimulation [40] (Figs. 3.1 and 3.2). PET studies of monoamine function in AN and BN have focused on 5-HT$_{1A}$ receptor, 5-HT$_{2A}$ receptor, 5-HT transporter (5-HTT), and dopamine. Individuals with AN have a 50–70 % increase in ^{11}C-WAY100635 BP in the subgenual, mesial temporal, orbitofrontal, and raphe brain regions as well as in the prefrontal, lateral temporal, anterior cingulate, and

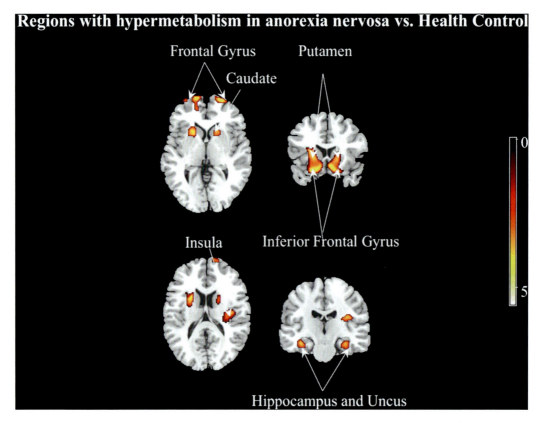

Fig. 3.1 Regions with hypermetabolism in anorexia nervosa patients and controls. The figures were depicted in neurological orientation. The *gray-scale* image was a T1 structural MRI that is representative of MNI space. *Red* areas were where the anorexia nervosa patients exhibit higher relative activity than control subjects

parietal regions. Increased 5-HT$_{1A}$ postsynaptic activity has also been reported in patients with BN. When 5-HT$_{2A}$ receptor binding is compared between subgroups, recovered individuals with ANR and AN-B/P have reductions in the subgenual cingulate, parietal, and occipital cortex. In comparison, only recovered individuals with AN-R have reduced 5-HT$_{2A}$ receptor binding in the mesial temporal region and pregenual cingulate [41]. Patients with BN have been found to have normal 5-HT$_{2A}$ receptor binding. However, PET with ^{18}F-altanserin, a specific 5-HT$_{2A}$ receptor antagonist, showed a significant reduction in bilateral medial orbital frontal cortex 5-HT$_{2A}$ binding in recovered women with BN [36]. A ^{11}C-McN5652 PET study assessing 5-HTT after AN and BN recovery demonstrated that the divergent 5-HTT activity in subtypes of EDs may provide important insights regarding why these subtypes show differences in affective regulation and impulse control [42]. DA dysfunction, particularly in striatal circuits, might contribute to altered reward and affect, decision-making, and executive control, as well as stereotypic motor movements and decreased food ingestion in AN. The DA system is involved in AN, which includes reduced CSF levels of DA metabolites in both ill and recovered individuals with AN, functional DA D2 receptor gene polymorphisms in patients with AN, and impaired visual discrimination learning thought to reflect DA-signaling alteration in AN [36].

Fig. 3.2 Regions with hypometabolisem in anorexia nervosa patients and controls. *Blue* areas were where the anorexia nervosa patients exhibit lower relative activity than control subjects

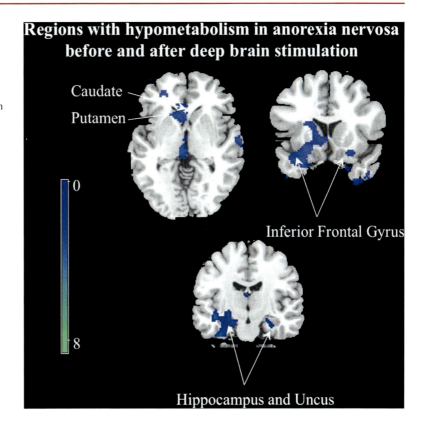

3.6 Obsessive Compulsive Disorder (OCD)

MR-based perfusion imaging in OCD is rare. A study examined the changes in rCBF during symptom provocation and reported most changes in the orbitofrontal-subcortical circuits (i.e., elevated rCBF in the orbitofrontal cortex, caudate nucleus, and thalamus) [43]. Lower CBF in the orbitofrontal cortex and higher rCBF in the posterior cingulate predicted better treatment response. OCD has been more commonly studied using nuclear medicine-based perfusion imaging. Increased perfusion was reported in the right orbitofrontal cortex, bilateral frontal cortex, left premotor cortex, and left precuneus. Based on the findings of perfusion imaging, the orbitofrontal cortex seems to the key region involved in OCD. Therefore, elevated orbitofrontal CBF during symptom provocation may be specific to OCD.

FDG PET is ideally suited to map the dysfunctional cortico-striato-thalamo-cortical circuitry previously reported in OCD. Increased metabolism in the orbital gyrus, caudate nuclei, and cingulate gyrus, suggests dysfunction in these regions in OCD. Stimulation of a ventral striatum/ventral capsule target has been shown to significantly activate the orbitofrontal and anterior cingulate cortices, striatum, globus pallidus, and thalamus [44]. Furthermore, metabolic studies have shown that stimulation of the anterior capsule induced a decrease in prefrontal metabolic activity, especially in the subgenual ACC, which is considered to reflect an interruption of the cortico-thalamo-striato-cortical circuit. In addition, the degree of improvement in OCD inversely correlated with the metabolism of the left ventral striatum, amygdala, and

Fig. 3.3 Brain regions with significant metabolic differences in obsessive compulsive disorder (*OCD*) patients compared with normal subjects. Normalized glucose metabolism in the OCD patients increased (*red*) bilaterally in the orbitofrontal cortex (*OFC*)/ anterior cingulate cortex (*ACC*), inferior frontal gyrus; but decreased (*blue*) bilaterally in the occipital cortex and supplementary motor area relative to the normal controls

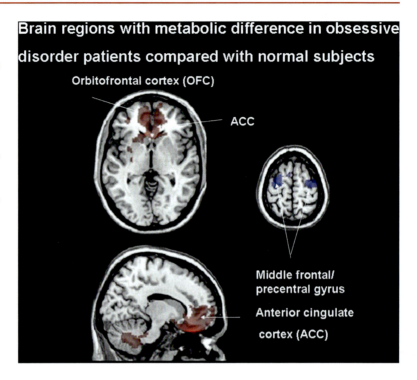

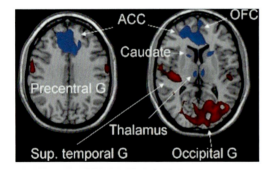

Fig. 3.4 Brain regions with significant metabolic changes in obsessive compulsive disorder (*OCD*) patients after bilateral capsulotomy. Normalized glucose metabolism in the OCD patients decreased (*blue*) bilaterally in the anterior cingulate cortex (*ACC*)/orbitofrontal cortex (*OFC*), caudate and thalamus after the surgery; but increased (*red*) bilaterally in the precentral gyrus, the occipital cortex extending to the cerebellum, and the superior temporal gyrus relative to the preoperative baseline

hippocampus. All these findings support a major role for the dysfunction of the limbic circuits in OCD pathophysiology and show that DBS modulates these pathways [45] (Figs. 3.3 and 3.4).

3.7 Clinical Applications

Neuroimaging is routinely used for workup of patients with psychotic disorders because lesions in the frontal or temporal lobes, most often tumors, can present with psychosis [46]. In older people with cognitive impairment, it may be difficult to differentiate a neurodegenerative disorder from depression. Neuroimaging may be helpful in this situation by revealing characteristic of Alzheimer's disease (AD), diffuse Lewy body disease, or one of the fronto-temporal dementias. Neuroimaging for psychiatric disorders has to contend with the diagnostic issues in psychiatry. The neurobiology of psychiatric disorders is likely to be highly heterogeneous. Thus, the neuroimaging findings in psychiatric disease may lack specificity and often fail to reveal a clear connection to a single neurobiological disturbance. Currently, the neuroimaging pattern determined in a study of a single patient with a psychiatric condition does not allow for an accurate diagnosis. Some characteristic findings, however, have been derived from samples of patients with each of the psychiatric diagnostic groupings [16].

3.8 Drug Discovery and Development

Neuroimaging can be helpful at several levels of drug discovery and development [47]: (1) characterizing preclinical models; (2) conducting early clinical studies to show that target engagement by the new drug induces the biological changes expected to give clinical benefit; (3) evaluating patients in clinical trials to demonstrate proof of concept. In other words, engaging a particular target can be shown to be linked to a meaningful change in a clinical endpoint observable via neuroimaging, thus providing evidence supporting the treatment being studied. Since neuroimaging can likely enable in vivo observation of brain structure and function, it could potentially provide ideal biomarkers for therapeutic intervention development. Considering the definition of biomarker [47], most neuroimaging methods do not meet the biomarker standards for now. However, some methods have the potential to be used as biomarkers or pre-biomarkers because they allow for identification of therapy-relevant characteristics of the disease. For instance, by examining striatal DA D2 receptors in a $[^{11}C]$raclopride PET scan, a link was found between D2 receptor occupancy by a drug and a reduction in the positive symptoms in schizophrenia; ascending doses of up to 80 % receptor occupancy were progressively more effective in relieving delusions and hallucinations [48].

In a conclusion, neuroimaging is being increasingly applied for the development of psychiatric therapies. Neuroimaging is clinically relevant for diagnosis and differential diagnosis. It can yield further insights into the mechanisms of psychiatric diseases. Neuroimaging provides the pre-clinical researcher a relatively easy method to test whether a potential drug target shows an abnormality in a psychiatric disorder and whether, therefore, its correction may be therapeutic. Finally, by identifying the individuals who manifest the expected pharmacological action of the drug, neuroimaging can aid in personalized medicine by selecting individuals most likely to benefit from a particular treatment in a clinical trial.

References

1. Perlini C, Bellani M, Brambilla P. Structural imaging techniques in schizophrenia. Acta Psychiatr Scand. 2012;126(4):235–42.
2. Narayanaswamy JC, Venkatasubramanian G, Gangadhar BN. Neuroimaging studies in schizophrenia: an overview of research from Asia. Int Rev Psychiatry. 2012;24(5):405–16.
3. Sun D, et al. Elucidating a magnetic resonance imaging-based neuroanatomic biomarker for psychosis: classification analysis using probabilistic brain atlas and machine learning algorithms. Biol Psychiatry. 2009;66(11):1055–60.
4. Meisenzahl EM, et al. Structural brain alterations at different stages of schizophrenia: a voxel-based morphometric study. Schizophr Res. 2008;104 (1–3):44–60.
5. Hu M, et al. Decreased left middle temporal gyrus volume in antipsychotic drug-naive, first-episode schizophrenia patients and their healthy unaffected siblings. Schizophr Res. 2013;144(1–3):37–42.
6. Thompson PM, et al. Time-lapse mapping of cortical changes in schizophrenia with different treatments. Cereb Cortex. 2009;19(5):1107–23.
7. Xiao Y, et al. Similar and different gray matter deficits in schizophrenia patients and their unaffected biological relatives. Front Psychiatry. 2013;4:150.
8. Vago DR, et al. Identification of neural targets for the treatment of psychiatric disorders: the role of functional neuroimaging. Neurosurg Clin N Am. 2011;22(2):279–305.
9. Sorg C, et al. Increased intrinsic brain activity in the striatum reflects symptom dimensions in schizophrenia. Schizophr Bull. 2013;39(2):387–95.
10. Ebisch SJ, et al. Altered brain long-range functional interactions underlying the link between aberrant self-experience and self-other relationship in first-episode schizophrenia. Schizophr Bull. 2013.
11. Tu PC, et al. Schizophrenia and the brain's control network: aberrant within- and between-network connectivity of the frontoparietal network in schizophrenia. Schizophr Res. 2013;147(2–3):339–47.
12. Mou X, et al. Voice recognition and altered connectivity in schizophrenic patients with auditory hallucinations. Prog Neuropsychopharmacol Biol Psychiatry. 2013;44:265–70.

13. Zanelli J, et al. Neuropsychological correlates of eye movement abnormalities in schizophrenic patients and their unaffected relatives. Psychiatry Res. 2009;168(3):193–7.
14. Eisenberg DP, et al. Executive function, neural circuitry, and genetic mechanisms in schizophrenia. Neuropsychopharmacology. 2010;35(1):258−77.
15. Blasi G, et al. Nonlinear response of the anterior cingulate and prefrontal cortex in schizophrenia as a function of variable attentional control. Cereb Cortex. 2010;20(4):837−45.
16. Masdeu JC. Neuroimaging in psychiatric disorders. Neurotherapeutics. 2011;8(1):93–102.
17. Fusar-Poli P, Meyer-Lindenberg A. Striatal presynaptic dopamine in schizophrenia, part II: meta-analysis of [(18)F/(11)C]-DOPA PET studies. Schizophr Bull. 2013;39(1):33–42.
18. Fusar-Poli P, Meyer-Lindenberg A. Striatal presynaptic dopamine in schizophrenia, Part I: meta-analysis of dopamine active transporter (DAT) density. Schizophr Bull. 2013;39(1):22–32.
19. Brunelin J, Fecteau S, Suaud-Chagny MF. Abnormal striatal dopamine transmission in schizophrenia. Curr Med Chem. 2013;20(3):397–404.
20. Lerond J, et al. Effects of aripiprazole, risperidone, and olanzapine on 5-HT1A receptors in patients with schizophrenia. J Clin Psychopharmacol. 2013;33 (1):84–9.
21. Kang JI, et al. Reduced binding potential of GABA-A/benzodiazepine receptors in individuals at ultra-high risk for psychosis: an [18F]-fluoroflumazenil positron emission tomography study. Schizophr Bull. 2013.
22. Poels EM, et al. Imaging glutamate in schizophrenia: review of findings and implications for drug discovery. Mol Psychiatry. 2014;19(1):20–9.
23. Clark CP, Frank LR, Brown GG. Sleep deprivation, EEG, and functional MRI in depression: preliminary results. Neuropsychopharmacology. 2001;25(5 Suppl):S79–84.
24. Clark CP, et al. Improved anatomic delineation of the antidepressant response to partial sleep deprivation in medial frontal cortex using perfusion-weighted functional MRI. Psychiatry Res. 2006;146(3):213–22.
25. Clark CP, et al. Does amygdalar perfusion correlate with antidepressant response to partial sleep deprivation in major depression? Psychiatry Res. 2006;146(1):43–51.
26. Meyer JH, et al. Imaging the serotonin transporter during major depressive disorder and antidepressant treatment. J Psychiatry Neurosci. 2007;32:86–102.
27. Theberge J. Perfusion magnetic resonance imaging in psychiatry. Top Magn Reson Imaging. 2008;19 (2):111–30.
28. Meyer JH, et al. Serotonin transporter occupancy of five selective serotonin reuptake inhibitors at different doses: an [11C]DASB positron emission tomography study. Am J Psychiatry. 2004;161(5):826–35.
29. Frokjaer VG, et al. High familial risk for mood disorder is associated with low dorsolateral prefrontal cortex serotonin transporter binding. Neuroimage. 2009;46(2):360–6.
30. Sublette ME, et al. Regional brain glucose uptake distinguishes suicide attempters from non-attempters in major depression. Arch Suicide Res. 2013;17(4):434–47.
31. Schienle A, Ebner F, Schafer A. Localized gray matter volume abnormalities in generalized anxiety disorder. Eur Arch Psychiatry Clin Neurosci. 2011;261(4):303–7.
32. Freitas-Ferrari MC, et al. Neuroimaging in social anxiety disorder: a systematic review of the literature. Prog Neuropsychopharmacol Biol Psychiatry. 2010;34(4):565–80.
33. Nakao T, et al. fMRI of patients with social anxiety disorder during a social situation task. Neurosci Res. 2011;69(1):67–72.
34. Ayling E, et al. Diffusion tensor imaging in anxiety disorders. Curr Psychiatry Rep. 2012;14(3):197–202.
35. Jones T, Rabiner EA. The development, past achievements, and future directions of brain PET. J Cereb Blood Flow Metab. 2012;32(7):1426–54.
36. Frank GK, Kaye WH. Current status of functional imaging in eating disorders. Int J Eat Disord. 2012;45 (6):723–36.
37. Phan KL, et al. Functional neuroanatomy of emotion: a meta-analysis of emotion activation studies in PET and fMRI. Neuroimage. 2002;16(2):331–48.
38. Critchley HD, Mathias CJ, Dolan RJ. Fear conditioning in humans: the influence of awareness and autonomic arousal on functional neuroanatomy. Neuron. 2002;33(4):653–63.
39. Uher R, et al. Functional neuroanatomy of body shape perception in healthy and eating-disordered women. Biol Psychiatry. 2005;58(12):990–7.
40. Zhang HW, et al. Metabolic imaging of deep brain stimulation in anorexia nervosa: a 18F-FDG PET/CT study. Clin Nucl Med. 2013;38(12):943−8.
41. Audenaert K, et al. Decreased 5-HT2a receptor binding in patients with anorexia nervosa. J Nucl Med. 2003;44(2):163–9.
42. Bailer UF, et al. Serotonin transporter binding after recovery from eating disorders. Psychopharmacology. 2007;195(3):315–24.
43. Chen XL, et al. MR perfusion-weighted imaging and quantitative analysis of cerebral hemodynamics with symptom provocation in unmedicated patients with obsessive-compulsive disorder. Neurosci Lett. 2004;370(2–3):206–11.

44. Zuo ct, et al. Metabolic imaging of bilateral anterior capsulotomy in refractory obsessive compulsive disorder: an FDG PET study. J Cereb Blood Flow Metab. 2013;33(6):880−7.
45. Ballanger B, et al. PET functional imaging of deep brain stimulation in movement disorders and psychiatry. J Cereb Blood Flow Metab. 2009;29 (11):1743–54.
46. Bunevicius A, et al. Brain lesions manifesting as psychiatric disorders: eight cases. CNS Spectr. 2008;13(11):950–8.
47. Wong DF, Tauscher J, Grunder G. The role of imaging in proof of concept for CNS drug discovery and development. Neuropsychopharmacology. 2009;34(1):187–203.
48. Grunder G, et al. The striatal and extrastriatal D2/D3 receptor-binding profile of clozapine in patients with schizophrenia. Neuropsychopharmacology. 2006;31 (5):1027–35.

DBS in Psychiatry and the Pendulum of History

4

Marwan I. Hariz

Abstract

Recent published statements on Deep brain stimulation (DBS) by psychiatrists and ethicists claim that DBS was developed first for movement disorders and is now applied in psychiatry; that it was the behavioural and psychiatric side-effects of DBS in subthalamic nucleus (STN) in Parkinsonian patients that prompted investigation of DBS in psychiatry; and that neurosurgeons should not act alone in this field, but should be within multidisciplinary teams in order not to repeat abuses of the past. The present author conducted a review of old literature since the birth of human stereotactic neurosurgery in 1947 and established the following: (1) The first applications of DBS in the early 1950s were in the field of psychiatry, and promoted mainly by neurologists and psychiatrists without involvement of neurosurgeons. (2) Some of these old psychiatric applications of DBS were found to be dubious and precarious even by yesterday's ethical standards. (3) Modern DBS for psychiatric illness started in 1999 on the initiative of neurosurgeons who had involved from the beginning psychiatrists, and it had nothing to do with non-motor side-effects of STN DBS. (4) A recent consensus meeting on psychiatric DBS insisted in its guidelines on multidisciplinarity and included 30 panelists none of whom a neurosurgeon.

Keywords

Deep brain stimulation · Psychosurgery · History · Ethics

M.I. Hariz (✉)
UCL Institute of Neurology, Box 146, Queen
Square, London WC1N 3BG, UK
e-mail: m.hariz@ion.ucl.ac.uk

M.I. Hariz
Department of Clinical Neuroscience, Umeå
University, Umeå, Sweden

B. Sun and A. De Salles (eds.), *Neurosurgical Treatments for Psychiatric Disorders*,
DOI 10.1007/978-94-017-9576-0_4
© Shanghai Jiao Tong University Press, Shanghai and Springer Science+Business Media Dordrecht 2015

> *Hegel remarks somewhere that all great world-historic facts and personages appear, so to speak, twice. He forgot to add: the first time as tragedy, the second time as farce.*

> Karl Marx, 1852: The 18th Brumaire of Louis Bonaparte, (Chap. 1).

4.1 Introduction

Deep brain stimulation (DBS) is an established method for surgical treatments for movement disorders. Today, most of the investigational applications of DBS are in the field of Neuropsychiatry, especially for Obsessive compulsive disorders (OCD), Gilles de la Tourette syndrome and major depressive disorder. It is a common belief that DBS in psychiatry follows upon DBS in movement disorders; for example, Kopell et al. wrote in 2004: "Over the last decade, deep brain stimulation (DBS) has revolutionized the practice of neurosurgery, particularly in the realm of movement disorder. It is no surprise that DBS is now being studied in the treatment of refractory psychiatric diseases" [13]. Also, Stelten et al. [22] wrote: "The DBS procedure was originally introduced for the treatment of movement disorders, but nowadays it is being studied as a possible treatment option for intractable states of neuropsychiatric conditions." It is also common belief that DBS in psychiatry stemmed from observation on psychiatric and behavioural side effects of DBS in the STN in PD patients. Schläpfer and Bewernick [20] wrote: "The observation of induced psychiatric side effects (e.g., changes in mood, hypomania, reduction of anxiety) gave the impulse to try DBS also for psychiatric disorders." Finally, it is assumed that the old stereotactic surgery for psychiatry illness was not enough multidisciplinary with neurosurgeons acting alone, many time without consulting the psychiatrists. As an example of this statement one can read the following written by ethicist Fins et al. in a paper published 2006 in Neurosurgery [9]: "It is ethically untenable for this work to proceed by neurosurgeons in isolation without psychiatrists determining the diagnosis and suitability of patients for treatment. The mere fact that electrodes can be placed is not a moral warrant for their insertion... Such errant behavior is especially inappropriate because it represents a recapitulation of the excesses associated with psychosurgery... If this generation of neuroscientists and practitioners hope to avoid the abuses of that earlier era, and avoid conflation of neuromodulation with psychosurgery, it is critical that neuromodulation be performed in an interdisciplinary and ethically sound fashion" [9].

The aim of the present paper is to scrutinize these statements that are representative of leading opinions in contemporary literature, in the light of available historical literature on the subject.

4.2 Materials and Methods

The author has attempted to trace, through literature search in scientific journals, as well as in published books and proceedings from scientific meetings, the origins of chronic deep brain stimulation to find out which were its first applications in humans, and who were involved in practice of early DBS.

4.3 Results

4.3.1 Origins of DBS

Stereotactic functional neurosurgery started with a co-operation between a neurologist Spiegel, and a neurosurgeon Wycis [21]. They introduced the stereotactic technique in humans with the explicit aim to avoid the side effects of lobotomy by making very focal lesion in pertinent pathways and nuclei in psychiatric patients. Indeed, in their seminal paper published in Science in 1947 [21], they wrote: "This apparatus is being used for psychosurgery... Lesions have been placed in the region of the medial nucleus of the thalamus (medial thalamotomy)…". Soon after, neurophysiologist and neuropsychiatrist José Delgado described in 1952 a technique of implantation of electrodes for chronic recording and stimulation to evaluate its value in psychotic patients [4]. In 1953, in the proceedings of the Mayo Clinic, in an article about depth stimulation of the brain one could read the following [3]: "An observation that may have some practical significance was that several of our psychotic patients seem to improved and become more accessible in the course of stimulation studies lasting several days". The authors thought that a likely explanation for this phenomenon "was that the local stimulation was having a therapeutic effect comparable to that of electroshock". They wrote further: "This aspect of localized stimulation studies requires further investigation since it may lead to a most specific, less damaging, and more therapeutically effective electrostimulation technic than can be achieved by the relatively crude extracranial stimulation methods in use at present" [3]. Meanwhile, Delgado continued to investigate the use of deep brain stimulation and devised a technique of "radio communication with the brain" through chronically implanted electrodes attached to a subcutaneously implanted receiver in the scalp, that he called "stimoceiver", specifically for use in psychosurgical patients [5, 6]. In parallel, a group at Tulane University in New Orleans led by psychiatrist Robert Heath was heavily involved during three decades, starting in the early fifties, in studies of chronic depth stimulation in patients with schizophrenia and in search for the brain's "pleasure center" [1]. Some of Heath's work related to studies of "rewarding" and "aversive" subcortical structures [10], to surgical control of behavior and initiation of heterosexual behavior in a homosexual male [16], and other aspects of modulation of emotion through deep brain stimulation in order to find a treatment for intractable psychiatric illness [12]. The Tulane experience in this field was analysed in 2000 by Alan Baumeister and published in the Journal of the History of the Neurosciences under the title: "The Tulane Electrical Brain Stimulation Program. A historical case study in medical ethics" [1]. Baumeister wrote: "The central conclusion of the present review is that the Tulane electrical brain stimulation experiments had neither a scientific nor a clinical justification… The conclusion is that these experiments were dubious and precarious by yesterday's standards". Long before Baumeister's verdict, neurosurgeon Lauri Laitinen wrote in 1977, in his paper on "Ethical Aspects of Psychiatric Surgery" [14] a comment about one of Heath's papers published in 1972 [11]: "There is no doubt that in this study all standards of ethics had been ignored. The ethical responsibility of the editors who accept reports of this kind for publication should also be discussed" [14].

In view of the above, it is difficult to give any credit to the claim of some ethicists that "It is ethically untenable for this work to proceed by neurosurgeons in isolation" [9], when history shows that when somebody was conducting such work "in isolation", and disclosing such an "inappropriate"… "errant behavior", it was some neuropsychiatrists and not neurosurgeons who were to blame. It is interesting in that context to note the historical ignorance of some of today's psychiatrists who recently published a paper in Advances in Neurology [15] entitled "Behavioral Neurosurgery" and wrote: "One of the most notable surgeons was the American neurosurgeon Walter Freeman… Freeman began to apply his relatively untested procedure, the prefrontal lobotomy, in which he transorbitally inserted an ice pick into the frontal cortex" [15]. In fact Freeman was a neuropsychiatrist and the truth is that he was abandoned by his neurosurgeon James Watts, following Freeman's increasingly uncritical attitude to lobotomy [7]. When neurosurgeons are made scapegoats by some, who remembers that the Norwegian psychiatrist Ornulf Odegård, who was director of Norway's main psychiatrist hospital during more than 30 years, wrote in 1953 in the Norwegian Medical Journal [18]: "Psychosurgery can be easily performed by the psychiatrist himself with the tool he might have in his pocket, and strangely enough it may be harmless and effective."

Coming back to the DBS of the early days, this method continued well into the seventies to be rarely tested primarily for behavioural disorders [8]. Meanwhile, in that same decade, Bechtereva et al. [2] from Leningrad pioneered chronic stimulation of thalamus and basal ganglia in treatment of Parkinson's disease.

4.3.2 "Modern" Applications of DBS in Psychiatry

The first use of modern era DBS in psychiatric disorders had nothing to do with the observation of psychiatric and behavioural side effects of STN DBS, as claimed by some [20]. When Vandewalle et al. [23] pioneered DBS for Tourette, and Nuttin et al. [17] DBS for OCD, both in 1999, these workers were simply targeting the very same brain structures that were stereotactically lesioned in the past for same disorders.

4.4 Discussion

A review of the old scientific literature about DBS bears witness to the inaccuracy of several contemporary statements, in which neurosurgeons are erroneously blamed for (mal)practices of the past, and criticised for neglecting multi-disciplinarity and ethical rules. How ironic and hollow these accusations are is evidenced by a recent publication in the September 2009 issue of the Archive of General Psychiatry entitled "Scientific and Ethical Issues Related to Deep Brain Stimulation for Disorders of Mood, Behavior, and Thoughts" [19]. This paper summarises the results of a 2-day consensus conference held to examine scientific and ethical issues in the application of DBS in psychiatry in order to "establish consensus among participants about the design of future clinical trials of deep brain stimulation for disorders of mood, behavior, and thought" and to "develop standards for the protection of human subjects participating in such studies" [19]. Among the

30 participants at the meeting, 19 of which are authors of the paper, there was not one single neurosurgeon, although the authors insisted on multidisciplinarity in relation to this neurosurgical procedure, but without including a single neurosurgeon on the panel.

4.5 Conclusions

(a) DBS was not "originally introduced for the treatment of movement disorders". DBS started from the very beginning as a tool to study and eventually treat psychiatric illness.

(b) The first application of modern DBS in psychiatric illness tried to mimic lesional surgery by implanting electrodes in the same targets that were lesioned before for the same conditions.

(c) While "It is ethically untenable for this work to proceed by neurosurgeons in isolation without psychiatrists determining the diagnosis and suitability of patients for treatment" [9], it was indeed psychiatrists and neurologists who were working in isolation. Some of today's self-promoted experts in the field need to read history instead of accusing neurosurgeons as scapegoats. It is a scandale that a consensus meeting on DBS in psychiatry with 30 participants insisting on multidisciplinarity did not include a single neurosurgeon.

(d) Multidisciplinarity in functional neurosurgery, including psychosurgery is not new; it has been the rule rather than the exceptions since the very beginning and when there were exceptions to multidisciplinarity it was often the psychiatrists and the neurologists who chose to work alone. This pattern of behavior is unfortunately risking to repeat itself today.

Conflict of Interest Statement The author has occasionally received from Medtronic reimbursement for travel expenses and honoraria for speaking at meetings.

References

1. Baumeister AA. The Tulane Electrical Brain Stimulation Program. A historical case study in medical ethics. J Hist Neurosci. 2000;9:262–78.
2. Bechtereva NP, Kambarova DK, Smirnov VM, Shandurina AN. Using the brain's latent abilities for therapy: chronic intracerebral electrical stimulation. In: Sweet BW, Obrador S, Martín-Rodrígez JG, editors. Neurosurgical treatment in psychiatry, pain and epilepsy. Baltimore: University Park Press; 1977. p. 581–613.
3. Bickford RG, Petersen MC, Dodge HW Jr, Sem-Jacobsen CW. Observations on depth stimulation of the human brain through implanted electrographic leads. Mayo Clin Proc. 1953;28:181–7.
4. Delgado JM, Hamlin H, Chapman WP. Technique of intracranial electrode implacement for recording and stimulation and its possible therapeutic value in psychotic patients. Confin Neurol. 1952;12:315–9.
5. Delgado JM, Mark V, Sweet W, Ervin F, Weiss G, Bach-y-Rita G, Hagiwara R. Intracerebral radio stimulation and recording in completely free patients. J Nerv Ment Dis. 1968;147:329–40.
6. Delgado JMR, Obrador S, Martín-Rodriguez JG. Two-way radio communication with the brain in psychosurgical patients. In: Laitinen LV, Livingstone KE, editors. Surgical approaches in psychiatry. Lancaster: Medical and Technical Publishing Co Ltd; 1973. p. 215–23.
7. El-Hai J. The lobotomist. Hoboken: Wiley; 2005.
8. Escobedo F, Fernández-Guardiola A, Solís G. Chronic stimulation of the cingulum in humans with behaviour disorders. In: Laitinen LV, Livingstone KE, editors. Surgical approaches in psychiatry. Lancaster: Medical and Technical Publishing Co Ltd; 1973. p. 65–8.
9. Fins JJ, Rezai AR, Greenberg BD. Psychosurgery: avoiding an ethical redux while advancing a therapeutic future. Neurosurgery. 2006;59:713–6.
10. Heath RG. Electrical self-stimulation of the brain in Man. Am J Psychiatry. 1963;120:571–7.
11. Heath RG. Pleasure and brain activity in man: deep and surface electroencephalograms during orgasm. J Nerv Ment Dis. 1972;154:3–18.
12. Heath RG. Modulation of emotion with a brain pacemaker. Treatment for intractable psychiatric illness. J Nerv Ment Dis. 1977;165:300–17.
13. Kopell BH, Greenberg B, Rezai AR. Deep brain stimulation for psychiatric disorders. J Clin Neurophysiol. 2004;21:51–67.
14. Laitinen LV. Ethical aspects of psychiatric surgery. In: Sweet WH, Obrador S, Martín-Rodríguez JG, editors. Neurosurgical treatment in psychiatry, pain and epilepsy. Baltimore: University Park Press; 1977. p. 483–8.
15. Malone DA Jr, Pandya MM. Behavioral neurosurgery. Adv Neurol. 2006;99:241–7.
16. Moan CE, Heath RG. Septal stimulation for the initiation of heterosexual behavior in a homosexual male. J Behav Ther Exp Psychiat. 1972;3:23–30.
17. Nuttin B, Cosyns P, Demeulemeester H, Gybels J, Meyerson B. Electrical stimulation in anterior limbs of internal capsules in patients with. Lancet. 1999;354:1526.
18. Odegård O. Nye framsteg i psychiatrien. Tidskrift for den Norske Laegeforening. 1953;123:411–4.
19. Rabins P, Appleby BS, Brandt J, DeLong MR, Dunn LB, Gabriëls L, Greenberg BD, Haber SN, Holtzheimer PE 3rd, Mari Z, Mayberg HS, McCann E, Mink SP, Rasmussen S, Schlaepfer TE, Vawter DE, Vitek JL, Walkup J, Mathews DJ. Scientific and ethical issues related to deep brain stimulation for disorders of mood, behavior, and thought. Arch Gen Psychiatry. 2009;66:931–7.
20. Schläpfer TE, Bewernick BH. Deep brain stimulation for psychiatric disorders—state of the art. Adv Tech Stand Neurosurg. 2009;34:37–57.
21. Spiegel EA, Wycis HT, Marks M, Lee AS. Stereotaxic apparatus for operations on the human brain. Science. 1947;106:349–50.
22. Stelten BM, Noblesse LH, Ackermans L, Temel Y, Visser-Vandewalle V. The neurosurgical treatment of addiction. Neurosurg Focus. 2008;25(1):E5.
23. Vandewalle V, van der Linden C, Groenewegen HJ, Caemaert J. Stereotactic treatment of Gilles de la by high frequency stimulation of thalamus. Lancet. 1999;353:724.

Ablative Surgery for Neuropsychiatric Disorders: Past, Present, Future

5

Yosef Chodakiewitz, John Williams, Jacob Chodakiewitz and Garth Rees Cosgrove

5.1 Historical Perspective

The history of surgical intervention for psychiatric disorders is a long, complex, and controversial one. The original use of surgical methods to treat symptoms of the mind occurred in the prescientific era as far back as antiquity. The ancient practice of trephination involved using a cylindrical saw to perform craniotomy. Literature dating back to 1500 BC can be found describing trephination to relieve psychiatric symptoms, including affective and psychotic disorders [1]. It can further be surmised that surgical trephination was occurring as far back as 5100 BC, based on carbon dating of a trephined skull, which showed evidence of proper healing to suggest a surgical wound origin rather than a traumatic origin, found at the Enshisheim burial site in France [2].

The modern scientific era of psychosurgery can find its origins in the 19th century, when strong correlates between brain and behavior were starting to be drawn. Much of this work was done through clinicopathologic correlates of particular neurological insults leading to particular cognitive dysfunction, as seen in the language aphasias described by Broca and Wernicke

from patient autopsy studies [3, 4]. The case in 1848 of Phineas Gage, a railroad worker who suffered an accident involving a sharp rod piercing his skull and his brain's frontal lobe, is another famous example [5]. In Gage's case, physically, he recovered surprisingly well. However, he was noted by those who knew him to have an undergone an obvious and significant personality change.

It was in this environment of brain-behavior correlative science in the mid-late 1800s that present day psychosurgery came into being, with the Swiss psychiatrist Gottlieb Burckhardt performing the first procedures in 1888. Working to clinically apply the developing theories of neuropsychiatric correlations, he performed bilateral topectomy, which involved selective excision of cortex from multiple foci [1, 6]. These early attempts were not clearly successful, and psychosurgery (a term not yet coined was not particularly accepted by the neuropsychiatric community. Years later in the 1930s, Fulton and Jacobson demonstrated calming behavioral changes, along with some changes in overall cognition, in chimpanzees as a result of surgical bilateral frontal lobe lesions [7, 8]. This work by Fulton and Jacobson particularly influenced the Portuguese neurologist Egas Moniz, who subsequently began proposing the idea that an efficacious psychosurgical procedure to relieve anxiety states in people would involve interruption of afferent and efferent fibers of the frontal lobe [9, 10]. Furthermore, it was in fact Moniz who coined the term "psychosurgery" [10, 11]. Together with his neurosurgical

Y. Chodakiewitz (✉) · J. Williams · G.R. Cosgrove
Department of Neurosurgery, Alpert Medical School, Brown University, Providence, USA

J. Chodakiewitz
Department of Neurosurgery, David Geffen School of Medicine, UCLA, Los Angeles, USA

B. Sun and A. De Salles (eds.), *Neurosurgical Treatments for Psychiatric Disorders*,
DOI 10.1007/978-94-017-9576-0_5
© Shanghai Jiao Tong University Press, Shanghai and Springer Science+Business Media Dordrecht 2015

colleague Almeida Lima, Moniz and Lima developed the procedure that came to be known as the prefrontal leukotomy or lobotomy for psychiatric disease [12].

Moniz' and Lima's original procedure involved the injection of alcohol into frontal lobe white matter to sever connections apparently giving rise to mental illness [13]. Their first patient was a 63 year old woman suffering from paranoid delusions, anxiety and melancholia; the operation was deemed an overall success in terms of ridding the patient of her psychosis and anxiety, though she remained with significant apathy and a blunted affect after the procedure [8, 13]. Moniz and Lima continued to refine their prefrontal leukotomy procedure, devising an instrument known as the leukotome to make their lesions rather than their original use of alcohol injections, which otherwise often required several procedures for repeat injections. The leukotome consisted of a rod with a retractable wire loop that could be inserted into the white matter and rotated to create series of small circular lesions within the frontal lobe white matter tracts [8, 10, 13]. This procedure for psychiatric disease was now becoming much more accepted by the community and resulted in Moniz receiving the Nobel Prize in Medicine/Physiology for this work in 1949 [14].

Starting already in 1936, the neurologist Walter Freeman and the neurosurgeon James Watts began adapting Moniz' and Lima's prefrontal leukotomy in the US. The Freeman-Watts prefrontal lobotomy was performed via bilateral posterior frontal burr holes through which a smooth, blunt, calibrated blade was inserted to the midline and then swept up and down to disconnect the frontal lobes at the level of the genu of the corpus callosum [15].

At the time in the US, there were still no effective psychoactive drugs available and psychiatric disease posed a particularly significant public health problem. In the late 1930s and early 1940s, there were 477 American psychiatric institutions housing over 400,000 patients and treatment of psychiatric illness was costing $1.5 billion annually [16, 17]. It had been argued that more widespread use of prefrontal leukotomies would save American taxpayer $1 million per day, by relieving the heavy costs of funding the asylums [18]. Within this context of the great burden posed to society by mental illness, Freeman further evolved the procedure and fervently promoted it in a mass-market fashion.

By 1948, Freeman began promoting his own modified surgical technique using a transorbital approach [19]. Before this modification, the prefrontal leukotomies had to be carried out by experienced neurosurgeons under operating room conditions to gain appropriate intracranial access; these were conditions not widely available in the psychiatric institutions. Freeman intended his transorbital leukotomy to be simple and quick enough so that the procedure could be performed in the office-setting by non-surgeons. The modified procedure involved using an ice-pick-like instrument, known as an orbitoclast, inserted underneath the upper eye-lid but over the eye globe and then driven by a mallet through the orbital roof to a desired distance of 7 cm into the frontal lobe white matter. At that point, the orbitoclast would be swept side to side with a deft wrist movement to complete the lesion before being removed. The need for an anesthetist was also eliminated, as the procedure was performed on the patient in the immediate post-ictal phase after an electroconvulsive treatment [8, 10, 13, 19]. Freeman fervently popularized this procedure, opening up an infamous chapter in the history of psychosurgery in which his technique was so enthusiastically received that psychosurgery was at times abused and indiscriminately applied. Complications arose related to its practice by unqualified practitioners in unsterile conditions using crude instruments with poor anesthesia care and perioperative monitoring. Furthermore, the morbidity and neurologic sequelae from the procedure became more evident over time, patient selection criteria were questioned, and the procedure's actual efficacy was questioned more criticially.

Freeman's procedure (which also came to be known as "the icepick lobotomy" [20]) quickly fell out of favor with the neurosurgical establishment, including with Watts, leading the two former collaborators to part ways soon thereafter

[13]. Nevertheless, given the public health crisis regarding the mass management of psychiatric illness in the population before the introduction of effective psychotropic medications with chlorpromazine in 1954, the Freeman lobotomy continued to be widely performed, with an estimated 60,000 procedures performed between 1936 and 1956 [15]. However, with the rejection of Freeman's procedure by neurosurgeons, and the continuing social recognition of its excessively exuberant application, along with the availability of effective neuroleptic drugs, the notorious era of the Freeman frontal lobotomy mostly came to an end in the late 1950s [1, 8, 13, 21].

At the same time that Freeman was overzealously promoting his transorbital leukotomy, more responsible practitioners of the day were employing a safer and more restricted approach to psychosurgery [13]. William Beecher Scoville, a neurosurgical contemporary of Freeman, was the first to introduce the concept of minimalism in psychosurgery, which very much diverged from Freeman's industrial scale concept. The idea was to maximize therapeutic efficacy, while minimizing unnecessary morbidity and undesirable sequelae to the patient. In the late 1940s, Scoville developed the technique of orbital undercutting to selectively ablate orbitofrontal cortex in a more anatomically localized manner through bifrontal trephinations [13, 22, 23]. Other more precise open surgical procedures were also described during this time period and included bilateral inferior leucotomy, bimedial frontal leucotomy and anterior cingulectomies, all guided by the most current understanding at that time, of the neuroanatomic pathways underlying psychiatric illness.

The goal of making small, accurate and effective lesions in psychiatric patients without serious mortality and morbidity was the major impetus for the development of stereotactic neurosurgery [10, 13, 20]. All intracranial psychosurgery today stems from the stereotactic school, including both contemporary ablative techniques and deep brain stimulation techniques [20]

In stereotactic neurosurgery, the brain is referenced against a fixed frame of reference, assigning a specific coordinate system to define any point in the brain in Cartesian three dimensional space [24]. Stereotactically guided neurosurgical procedures were first devised for use in humans in 1947 by Ernst Spiegel and Henry Wycis, who designed a stereotactic system referenced by X-ray ventriculography to perform dorsomedial thalamotomy, representing the first attempt at a minimally invasive subcortical ablative procedure [13, 24]. Various other stereotactic systems were developed for clinical use and lesioning of deep brain structures for treatment of psychiatric disease began. Jean Talairach first described ablation in the anterior internal capsule to treat psychiatric disease in 1949 [25, 26], and Leksell began using his stereotactic system to further study and develop methods to perform minimally invasive anterior capsulotomy to treat a variety of psychiatric disorders.

Soon after introducing his stereotactic frame in 1951, Leksell envisioned the concept of radiosurgery to improve upon the minimally invasive nature of stereotactic procedures [25]. Open stereotactic procedures still required a scalp incision, boney access through the cranial vault and a penetrating needle trajectory through the brain paryenchyma to the target, but Leksell imagined that sharply focused radiation beams from external radiation sources could summate at the stereotactic target, to create the desired lesion completely non-invasively. Leksell's concept of stereotactic radiosurgery laid the groundwork for the eventual development of the gamma-knife technology, which became commercially available in the 1980s [13]. In the present day, both "traditional open" stereotactic surgery and minimally invasive stereotactic radiosurgery are pursued as options in psychosurgery. In particular, gamma knife is being investigated for carrying out anterior capsulotomy in a double blind randomized control trial in Brazil, the first study of its kind for a psychiatric lesion procedure [8, 26, 27].

The mortality and morbidity associated with the imprecise methods and risky approaches of the Freeman lobotomy era and other earlier psychosurgical practices were largely erased with the advent of modern stereotactic techniques. A variety of targets were subsequently explored including the anterior cingulate gyrus, anterior limb of the internal capsule and the subcaudate regions. Much of our best contemporary understanding of the neurophysiologic basis of psychiatric disease focuses on the limbic system and its neural circuitry connecting with the frontal lobes and basal ganglia. Consequently, nearly all current psychosurgical interventions place their target in one or more aspect of the limbic system and its connections.

5.2 Relevant Anatomy and Physiology

An understanding of the frontal-subcortical circuitry involved in psychiatric diseases is necessary for understanding target selection in psychosurgical lesioning. Executive dysfunction, apathy, and impulsivity are hallmarks of frontal-subfrontal circuit dysfunction, and the psychiatric illnesses treated by psychosurgery, such as depression and obsessive-compulsive disorder (OCD), are associated with dysfunctional neural substrates in these circuits as well [28].

To understand the importance of the frontal-subcortical circuits of interest, a review of subcortical targets is essential. All three circuits connect through the basal ganglia. The basal ganglia are a group of nuclei situated at the base of the forebrain and include the striatum (caudate nucleus and putamen), the globus pallidus, the substantia nigra, the nucleus accumbens, and the subthalamic nucleus, each with its own complex internal anatomical and neurochemical organization. These nuclei are involved in varied functions, including voluntary motor control, procedural learning, including those involved in behavior and habits, eye movements, as well as cognitive and emotional functions [29]. The most unified, current theory relating the varied nuclei suggests that they are all involved in action selection or the decision of which of several possible behavioral actions to take at any given time [30]. Experimental evidence indicates the basal ganglia inhibit a number of motor systems, wherein discontinuation of this inhibition allows a given motor system to become active. The action selections by the basal ganglia are heavily influenced by input from the prefrontal circuitry described [31, 32]. Lesions in the circuitry connecting the frontal lobes to the basal ganglia can generate disorders closely resembling frontal lobe lesions. These "striatal" syndromes have not been extensively studied, but disinhibition and executive dysfunction are documented consequences [32].

Lesions in basal ganglia structures are implicated as the major substrate for a number of neurological conditions. Movement disorders, including Parkinson's and Huntington's disease, are associated with the degeneration of dopamine-producing cells in the substantia nigra pars compacta and damage to the striatum, respectively [30, 33]. Parkinson's patients exhibit depression, dementia and confusional states. Dysfunction in the basal ganglia are also implicated in disorders of behavior control, including Tourette's syndrome, hemiballismus, and obsessive-compulsive disorder (OCD) [34]. Additionally, positron emission tomography studies of patients with OCD show increased metabolic function in the frontal lobes, cingulum, and caudate nucleus [34].

Arguably, more critical to the success of psychosurgery are the functions and neuroanatomy of the limbic system. The system was named by Paul Broca, with limbic originating from the Latin limbus, meaning "border", as it lies between two functionally different portions of the brain; the neocortex, which mediates external stimuli, and the brainstem, which mediates internal stimuli [35, 36]. The limbic lobe is an intricate set of brain structures, broadly consisting of the arcuate convolution of the cingulate and parahippocampal gyri of the medial aspect of the cerebral hemispheres [37, 38]. These arcuate structures are situated around the thalamus bilaterally, composed of a conglomerate of structures from the telencephalon, diencephalon, and mesencephalon. The limbic system also includes the olfactory bulbs, hippocampus, amygdala, anterior thalamic nuclei, fornix, column of fornix, mammillary body, septum pellucidum, habenular commissure, cingulate gyrus, parahippocampal gyrus, limbic cortex and limbic midbrain regions [39]. These structures have myriad functional capacities, including memory, emotion, behavior, motivation, long-term memory, and olfaction. It is best known as the central system for human emotion and memory formation, and includes the famed Papez circuit [37–39].

The location and role of the limbic system as mediator between internal and external stimuli as reported by the neocortex and primitive brain allow it to regulate the complex processes of subjective, somatic, visceral, and behavioral stimuli integration and modulation necessary for emotional experience. Reciprocal connections converge in the amygdala, symmetric almond shaped nuclei positioned at the anterior end of the hippocampi, which are critically important in emotional processing and memory [40]. Lesions in the amygdala in rhesus monkeys results in the Kluver-Bucy syndrome, characterized by limited emotional arousal regardless of presence or absence of threatening stimuli, hypersexuality, hyperorality, hyperphagia, amnesia and agnosia [41].

The origins of the frontal-subcortical circuits are all located within the frontal lobe. A simplified model of frontal lobe circuitry consists of five major pathways. Two of the pathways are the motor and oculomotor circuits, which originate in the frontal eye fields and drive eye movement, but will not be discussed in detail here. The remaining three circuits are behaviorally relevant with origins in the prefrontal cortex; a dorsolateral prefrontal circuit, which is regarded as the mediator of executive function; the anterior cingulated circuit, which governs motivational functions; and the orbitofrontal circuit, which has two subdivisions: the lateral and medial [28]. All five circuits share common structures and are both parallel and contiguous, yet they are distinctly partitioned anatomically. Brain regions linked by these circuits are functionally related; those governing limbic function synapse heavily with other limbic structures and those related to executive function have diverse connections to higher cortical areas involved in cognition [42–45].

The *dorsolateral prefrontal circuit* begins in the dorsolateral region of the frontal lobe in Broadmann's areas 9 and 10. Neurons from this locus project to the head of the dorsolateral head of the caudate nucleus and medial putamen of the basal ganglia, and the projections communicate information regarding "executive" function [45]. Executive function integrates anticipation, goal selection, planning, observation and incorporation of external and internal feedback in task performance [46]. The clinicopathological correlation between lesions in this circuit and psychiatric illness is elucidated by *dorsolateral prefrontal syndrome*. Individuals affected by this condition have defects in executive function marked by marked perseveration, often measured with the Wisconsin Card Sort Test, designed to gauge test-takers' ability to shift strategies [47]. Other features include impaired verbal and design fluency, memory search strategy, motor programming, and organizational and constructional strategies during learning and copying tasks. As with all frontal circuits, similar syndromic features have been reported with lesions to efferent basal ganglia regions [48, 49]. Psychiatric syndromes including schizophrenia, depression and OCD display impaired executive function, suggesting that this circuit is involved [28].

The *orbitofrontal circuit* consists of the medial and lateral divisions. The lateral division has its origin in the lateral orbital gyrus of Brodmann's area 11 as well as the medial inferior frontal gyrus of areas 10 and 47 [50]. Lateral division projections lead to the ventromedial caudate [51]. The medial division originates in the inferomedial prefrontal cortex in the gyrus rectus and medial orbital gyrus of Brodmann's area 11, projecting to the medial nucleus accumbens [50, 52]. As the orbitofrontal cortex is considered to be the neocortical representation of the limbic system, it functions in calculating appropriate strategy, timing, and place for behavioral responses to environmental stimuli [53]. Thus, lesions in the circuit sever the frontal monitoring and modulation mechanisms necessary to curb impulses from the limbic system, resulting in *orbitofrontal syndrome* with characteristic disinhibition, lability, and irritability [54]. Affected patients appear tactless and may exhibit inappropriate jocularity, improper sexual remarks or gestures. Patients may also display transient irritable outbursts, inattention, distractibility, and increased motor activity along with hypomania or mania [55, 56]. Extreme changes in personality are typically in the setting of bilateral insults to the orbitofrontal regions, however unilateral lesions result in similar changes with lesions to the right hemisphere demonstrating disproportionately greater loss of inhibition [57, 58]. Similarly, patients with lesions to the ventral caudate have been documented exhibiting disinhibition, euphoria, impulsivity, and inappropriate social behaviors, showing the reciprocal relationship between the efferent and afferent ends of the circuit [59].

The *anterior cingulate circuit* originates in the anterior cingulate gyrus (Broadmann's area 24) and projects to the ventral striatum, including the ventromedial caudate, ventral putamen, nucleus accumbens, and olfactory tubercle, all of which are referred to collectively as the limbic striatum [60]. *Anterior cingulate syndrome* at its worst can result in profound apathy and akinetic mutism, a waking state of profound apathy, absence of motor and psychic initiative with a lack of spontaneous movement; indifference to pain, thirst, and hunger; absent verbalization; and failure to respond to commands [61, 62]. This condition has been documented in bilateral lesions to the anterior cingulate cortex and vascular and neoplastic lesions involving the ventral striatum, as well as and obstructive hydrocephalus in the region of the third ventricle and [28, 61]. A less severe form of this condition termed "abulia" involves similar psychomotor qualities, including lack of spontaneity, apathy, and decreased speech and movement. These behavioral syndromes highlight the importance of the frontal lobe pathways in regulating executive and social function as well as mood and motivation [61, 63].

5.3 Contemporary Psychosurgery

5.3.1 Established Psychosurgical Procedures and Indications in the Modern Era

With the application of stereotactic techniques in psychosurgery, several minimally invasive techniques were developed to treat psychiatric illness with impressive results. There are currently four accepted psychosurgical techniques, each with varied targets but all performed bilaterally under stereotactic guidance for optimal precision in targeting. They have evolved to a level of sophistication and critical appraisal far beyond the primitive operations performed by non-expert physicians in the Freeman era of frontal lobotomy.

Anterior Cingulotomy In 1947, Fulton published evidence that stimulating the anterior cingulate in monkeys resulted in significantly less fearful but more aggressive subjects with autonomic responses that mimicked those of heightened emotion [59]. Fulton postulated that modulation of the anterior cingulated cortex could mitigate psychiatric disease, and in the early 1950s, a British group first performed the procedure [64]. The procedure was popularized by the American surgeon Ballantine in the 1960s, who subsequently conducted research over decades [65].

The procedure is currently employed to treat refractory major affective disorder, severe chronic pain, chronic anxiety states and OCD [66]. The cingulate plays a crucial role in the Papez circuit, and OCD studies have shown increased metabolism in the anterior cingulate in individuals affected by the disorder [37, 38, 67]. The procedure is not performed until patients are accepted through a rigorous multidisciplinary screen, after which bilateral stereotactic thermocoagulation lesions are placed bilaterally in the cingulum [68]. Retrospective studies have shown that 25–30 % of medically refractory OCD patients were considered improved post-operatively, where treatment success was considered to be improvement of 35 % or greater on the Yale-Brown OCD Scale [69]. Furthermore, the study highlighted the relative safety of the procedure: no surgery-related deaths were reported, the only complications reported in the post-operative period were seizures responsive to medication. In the first prospective study, a similar success rate of 25–30 % for medically-refractory OCD patients was reported to achieve the same level of improvement [69]. Another prospective study showed 32 % met criteria for response to treatment and an additional 14 % were found to be partial responders at an average of 32 months follow-up. Complications were again limited: one patient reported increased urinary incontinence, one had drug responsive seizures, and one committed suicide. The most recent study of response to anterior cingulotomy by those with medically refractory OCD showed full response (35 % or more severity reduction on the Yale-Brown Scale) rates of 47 % of full response and 22 % partial response (24–35 % reduction on the Yale-Brown Scale) at a mean follow-up of 63.8 months, the most impressive results yet [70]. Additionally, comorbid major depressive disorder severity decreased by 17 % in the same study.

Anterior Capsulotomy This technique was developed by Talairach in France in the 1940s. Indications for this procedure initially included a wide range of conditions, including schizophrenia, depression, chronic anxiety and obsessional neurosis [66]. It uses thermocoagulation or gamma knife to lesion the fronto-limbic fibers that pass between caudate and putamen in the internal capsule of the basal ganglia [71]. When Leksell initially operated on patients with psychiatric disease, he reported a 50 % satisfactory response with "obsessional neurosis" and 48 % with depression, while lower rates of 20 and 14 % satisfactory response were observed with "anxiety neurosis" and schizophrenia, respectively [72]. When compared to anterior cingulotomy, studies have reported a higher index of efficacy with anterior capsulotomy, and success rates as high as 70 % have been published. Unfortunately, the procedure is also associated with the highest frequency of complications and morbidity, most notably weight gain, confusion, nocturnal incontinence and cognitive dysfunction [72].

Subcaudate Tractotomy Designed in England by Geoffrey Knight in 1964, this approach targets fibers from the frontal lobes to subcortical structures in the limbic system, including the amygdala [73]. The procedure was created as a method of reducing the extent of frontal lobe lesioning, and has been more popular in the UK than the US since its advent. Like the anterior cingulotomy, the procedure is indicated for affective and anxiety disorders, including severe, refractory OCD and depression. However, it is not indicated for cognitive disorders. The precise target of the subcaudate tractotomy is the substantia innominata, directly inferior and adjacent to the head of the caudate nucleus [10]. Originally, the procedure involved the placement of radioactive seeds in the frontal lobes, but is currently performed with stereotactic thermocoagulation. In the first major assessment of the efficacy of the procedure in the 1970s, over 60 % of patients with depression or anxiety showed improvement with nearly 50 % of patients affected by obsessive-compulsive disorder showing improvement [74]. A subsequent retrospective study reported a response rate of 34 % in patients undergoing the procedure from 1979 to 1991 [74, 75]. Like the anterior capsulotomy procedure, these high rates of efficacy come at a higher cost than is associated with anterior cingulotomy. Approximately 1.6 % of patients suffered from seizures after surgery, and just under 7 % reported negative personality changes post-operatively [74]. However, a psychometric study performed on 23 patients pre-operatively and at two intervals post-operatively showed no major cognitive deficits [76].

Limbic Leucotomy This technique combines the lesions of the anterior cingulotomy and subcaudate tractotomy, thereby disrupting orbital-frontal-thalamic pathways. The intervention was introduced by a group lead by Kelley and Mitchell-Heggs, and it involves lesioning targets with a cryoprobe or thermocoagulation [77]. That group's first assessment of the procedure was a retrospective follow-up study after 16 months using a 5-point global rating scale. Of 66 patients with a variety of illnesses, 89 % of those with OCD, 66 % of those with chronic anxiety, and 78 % of those with depression reported improvement [77].

The most substantive review of the procedure from the Massachusetts General Hospital reports 36–50 % of patients with refractory OCD and major depressive disorder responded to the treatment [78]. Additionally, 4 of 5 patients treated with limbic leucotomy for medically refractory OCD or schizoaffective disorder who engaged in self-mutilation showed sustained reduction in injurious behavior and 2 of 3 in assaultive behavior after a mean follow-up of 31.5 months [78]. Though the procedure inherently calls for more lesions than either the anterior cingulotomy or subcaudate tractotomy alone, few adverse post-operative effects were reported.

Each of these interventions has shown sufficient evidence for efficacy without significant harm to justify their continued practice despite psychosurgery's sordid past. Any medical treatment that demonstrated the level of efficacy in the treatment of profound, refractory mental illness that these four procedures have, could well be considered a "miracle intervention". However, these studies are largely retrospective, and prospective studies with better efforts to coordinate outcome assessment measures will be necessary to truly establish the success rates of any current or future form of psychiatric neurosurgery along with continued longitudinal follow-up studies to assess long-term outcomes in those that have already undergone existing operations. Efforts to train surgeons outside of major surgical centers will also be necessary to reduce surgical center bias and unify outcome measures to allow for meta-analyses of these procedures.

5.3.2 Future Potential Psychosurgical Indications and Targets

As the field of neuroscience continues to expand, so will theoretical targets for ablation in the treatment of psychiatric illness. President Obama's BRAIN Initiative with its 3 billion dollar budget should provide the awareness and funding to elucidate the circuitry and substrates underlying psychiatric disease on an order never seen before. Furthermore, advances in the understanding of the physiologic alterations underlying the efficacy of deep brain stimulation will provide more insight into the viability of psychosurgical procedures with the same targets as DBS. This evolution will be necessary as pharmacologic treatments advance, making refractory illness more and more challenging to treat.

One of the most promising areas of progress in psychosurgery may be the combination of surgical intervention with electroconvulsive therapeutic techniques. Electroconvulsive therapy (ECT), formerly known as "shock therapy", is another somatic or physical treatment for psychiatric illness. Transcranial magnetic stimulation (TMS) may achieve similar micro-electrical changes as electroconvulsive therapy. TMS involves the placement of a magnetic coil against the scalp, through which pulses of electrical current are sent, generating a magnetic field that can depolarize superficial cortical neurons [79]. Neural responses vary in accordance to the intensity of pulses, regions targeted, and number of sites targeted, and neurochemical changes affected are similar to those found with pharmacologic treatments and ECT [80–82]. Analyses of TCM in depression have been equivocal, but convincing evidence has been accumulating suggesting that 10 Hz rTMS over the left dorsolateral prefrontal cortex can improve depression in a specific subset of patients [83].

ECT and TMS are relatively non-specific in their delivery of electrical pulses to the brain. A combination of electrical stimulation with surgical placement of electrodes for better delivery may have additional benefits. Implantable electrodes have been used widely for focal modulation of the vagal nerve for epilepsy treatment with good results [84, 85]. The vagus nerve is an important conduit for information relay from the body to the brain and serves to cover much of the distance of autonomic feedback loops. The nerve delivers input to the forebrain via the parabrachial nucleus and locus ceruleus, which connect to central structures in the limbic system, such as the amygdala and hypothalamus [86]. Vagal nerve stimulation (VNS) has been explored with increasing reports of long-term success in the treatment for refractory depression [87]. Research has demonstrated VNS has a role in increasing serotonergic and noradrenergic activity in the brain with evidence that it increases perfusion of limbic structures [88, 89]. VNS implantation is relatively minimal in invasiveness with an electrode placed on the nerve in the carotid region of the neck and a battery typically placed subcutaneously over the pectoralis major. Complications in the post-operative period are likely related to intra-vagal cross talk phenomena with primary adverse effects being pain, cough, vocal cord paralysis, hoarseness, nausea, and concerning but transient and rare, reports of asystole and dyspnea [90, 91]. The procedure has been generally well tolerated in epilepsy patients, and there is mounting evidence to suggest that it is a viable extra-cranial surgical intervention that can provide relief for refractory depression without the need for attempts at more invasive procedures.

Advances in genetics and bioengineering have opened an entirely new subfield in the arena of psychosurgery: constructive psychosurgery. Lesioning has been the mainstay of psychosurgery since its advent, and even less destructive manipulations of neural function such as deep brain stimulation (discussed below) are predicated in functional strategies. Psychosurgery, thus far, has been limited to strategies that promote desirable behavior by inhibiting activity that either promotes undesirable behavior or inhibits desirable behavior. With constructive psychosurgery, there is promise for techniques that augment positive function as opposed to ablating the negative. If and when genetic markers for psychiatric illness are elucidated, targeted gene therapy could offer lasting relief. Progress in the understanding of the intersections of infectious, neoplastic, and inflammatory disease processes could shed light on how inflammatory chemical factors modulate electrochemical equilibria in the brain and potentiate psychiatric illness [92]. Evidence is mounting to support the idea that microglia play a significant role in the development of the brain and inflammatory processes that may contribute to the pathogenesis of psychiatric illness [93]. Implanting genetically modified host immune cells to dampen inflammatory processes or using established gene therapy techniques to deliver viral vectors that will alter the genetic expression of inflammatory molecules could be the key therapeutic advances in mental illness [92, 93]. Delivery of cellular products such as stem cells to degenerated or dysregulated parenchyma could enhance regeneration and recovery, promoting healthier behavior and psychiatric states. Stem cell research has already shown success in other neurologic disease and holds great promise in psychiatric disease [94, 95].

5.3.3 Established Ablative Methods in Psychosurgery

In addition to the choosing optimal stereotactic target for specific psychosurgical candidate, the surgeon must decide on the instrument for creating the desired lesion. Methods of stereotactically creating precisely focused CNS lesions continue to be investigated today [96]. Spiegel and Wycis made electrolytic lesions for their original stereotactic procedures [96–98]. Over the years other modalities using focused heat, cold, alcohol, radiofrequency and ultrasound have also been attempted. Various ablating modalities continue to be used today in psychosurgery, and the particular modality used will depend on what has been used historically in the given psychosurgical procedure.

Thermocoagulation for lesioning is an accepted option in several of the traditional psychosurgical procedures, including anterior cingulotomy, limbic leukotomy, and anterior capsulotomy [8, 27, 99]. For anterior capsulotomy, Gamma-knife is another relatively newer accepted modality; it has been used to perform capsulotomy for over 18 years. Gamma-knife anterior capsulotomy appears similar to the efficacy of thermocoagulation [8, 100], while eliminating the need for craniotomy and open surgery. It also produces comparatively smaller lesions and can be performed as an outpatient procedure [27]. However, despite the less invasive nature of gamma-knife radiosurgery over traditional invasive stereotactic surgery, radiosurgery still includes serious side-effects such as radiation-induced edema and necrosis and delayed cyst formation [8].

Gamma-knife anterior capsulotomy for refractory OCD is currently being investigated in a double-blind control study, a first study of this kind for any ablative psychosurgical procedure [8, 26, 27]. In limbic leukotomy, lesions made by freezing with a cryoprobe have also been used as an alternative to thermocoagulation [77, 99].

In stereotactic subcaudate tractotomy, a unique ablative modality was originally used. Small rod-shaped seeds of radioactive yttrium-90 are placed at the stereotactic targets. Beta-radiation emitted from the implanted seeds destroys the surrounding white matter up to 2 mm from the surface of the seed, producing lesion volumes of approximately 2 cm^3 [8, 10, 27, 101, 102]. However, in 1995 yttrium-90 was no longer available and so a modified version of the original procedure now makes the lesion using thermocoagulation instead [8, 103].

5.3.4 Ablation Versus Stimulation

While the practice of psychosurgery has continued to develop and become more refined over the years, it has done so on a much smaller scale in the aftermath of the Freeman lobotomy era of the 1940s and 1950s. While there have been decades of experience and demonstrated efficacy of the ablative psychosurgical procedures described above, the practice of psychosurgery remained limited to very few centers throughout the world. This restricted development is likely largely a result of the notoriety of the Freeman lobotomy, which created a stigma for psychosurgery and its associated methodology of surgical lesioning. However, in recent years, with the demonstrated success of deep brain stimulation technology in the neurosurgical treatment of disorders such as essential tremor and Parkinson's disease, there is

now resurgent enthusiasm in psychosurgery research and practice using DBS for neuromodulation, rather than the historical practice of lesioning in psychosurgery.

From its applications in the treatment of movement disorders, the early experience with DBS suggested that it worked functionally to mimic a lesion, but was reversible. This lesion-mimicry theory was based on the clinical observations that the motor effect of high-frequency stimulation of the subthalamic nucleus (STN) or VIM-Thalamus resembled those following lesions of those nuclei [104]. DBS is thus a more forgiving technology to the neurosurgeon and serves as a more palatable concept for psychosurgical intervention to the general public. In addition, DBS offers particular advantages as an investigational tool: (i) it is amenable to study under blinded placebo-controlled conditions with the ability to turn the stimulator on and off at will, and (ii) its non-destructive and reversible nature facilitates safer and ethical exploration of new brain targets [105]. For these reasons, many assume that DBS is inherently superior to lesioning and argue that the future of psychosurgical practice lies with DBS, while lesioning will be relegated to history. However, DBS is extremely expensive and time intensive requiring continuous programming and replacements. It is important to recognize that the respective roles of both DBS and lesioning in the future of psychosurgery are still being debated, with separate benefits and drawbacks to each modality in their present states. Despite the excitement surrounding DBS in psychosurgery, lesioning still warrants strong consideration for continued study and practice.

Despite the early DBS clinical experience suggesting that DBS functioned in lesion-mimicking fashion, the precise therapeutic mechanism of DBS remains poorly understood to this day. While DBS target selection to date has largely been based on prior lesioning experience [105], it is clear that the previous analogy between DBS and lesioning is overly simplistic. The two modalities are actually quite far from being functionally or clinically equivalent, as their clinical effect can diverge depending on several factors.

Experience from use of DBS in treatment for Parkinson's disease (PD) and essential tremor (ET) showed that, even at the same target nucleus, clinical effects did not always mimic lesions and in fact opposite clinical effects on motor symptoms could be seen depending on stimulation frequency. In PD, high frequency stimulation (>130 Hz) at the STN improved motor symptoms, while some low frequency stimulation levels (10 Hz) actually worsened motor symptoms, as compared to stimulation *off* [104]. Similarly, for ET, thalamic DBS at low frequency (<50 Hz) would fail to suppress tremor and could even be seen to worsen tremor as compared to stimulation *off*, while high frequency stimulation (>90 Hz) did suppress tremor [105].

The functional non-equivalence between DBS and lesioning can also be seen in their differing effects at particular targets. Studies carried out in Parkinsonian monkeys found opposite effects on motor symptoms when comparing GPe lesions and GPe DBS. GPe lesions worsened motor symptoms, while GPe DBS ameliorated motor symptoms [105]. Furthermore, high-frequency stimulation (HFS) generally behaves oppositely depending on whether it is stimulating grey matter or white matter. The effect of HFS can generally be said to be inhibitory and more "lesion-like" on grey matter, while it is generally activating on white matter [106]. The molecular effects and neurophysiologic mechanism of action of DBS is clearly much more complicated than simple lesion-mimicry. While DBS sometimes does appear to mimic lesions clinically, the comparative clinical effects depend on specific target tissues and stimulation frequencies. The mechanism of DBS remains incompletely understood, and it is clear we cannot assume DBS and lesions in general to be clinically equivalent.

With the recognition that DBS and lesioning are neither physiologically nor always clinically equivalent, we ought to also recognize that experience with DBS in psychosurgery is still in its infancy and relatively minimal. In contrast, there is much experience with lesioning, spanning decades, demonstrating its various indications and efficacy, including in the long term.

Therefore, while investigational DBS targets for psychiatric disease are mostly based on the historical lesioning targets, it is not quite the case that DBS has supplanted lesioning techniques in psychosurgery, nor is it obvious that it will do so. More experience with DBS as a psychosurgical intervention will be required before such a judgment can be made.

Beyond recognizing the physiologic and clinical non-equivalence between ablative techniques and DBS, there are practical factors to consider which in the long run may continue to favor ablative methods over DBS in developing psychosurgery as a more standard option in psychiatric treatment. For one, the clinical costs of DBS far outweigh the costs of its ablative counterpart. With DBS, there is ongoing costs stemming from required multiple return follow-ups over the short-term and long-term. These involve follow-ups to adjust stimulation settings, as well as to repair or replace components of the implanted hardware. In particular, given the high-frequency stimulation settings that are generally required to achieve clinical benefit for psychiatric disorders, inevitable battery changes are currently required approximately every 10–18 months [107]. The initial cost to have a DBS system implanted is between $50,000 and $120,000 and the cost to replace a battery is between $10,000 and $25,000 [108–110]. The high cost of DBS systems and the dependence on highly specialized multidisciplinary centers to manage its long-term follow-up care limits use of DBS as a psychosurgical modality to developed nations. Since refractory psychiatric disease is also prevalent in less developed countries, the more economical ablative techniques have a valuable role to play in these countries where DBS will still not be available.

Another disadvantage of DBS systems, in comparison to ablative methods, stems from the very nature of having implanted hardware and the additional possible complications, such as electrode lead fracture, increased risk of infection, and patient compliance issues [105]. Electrode leads can migrate within the parenchyma, distancing them from their intended targets or causing them to become disconnected from their power source. Implanted metal is a contraindication for MRI, meaning patients with DBS implants would have to undergo surgical removal to accurately assess new onset focal neurological deficits related to any etiology. Given the possibility of damaging the implanted hardware, DBS systems may be contraindicated in certain conditions with certain behaviors, such in Tourette's syndrome with head-banging behaviors; if investigations prove there to be a comparatively efficacious target for either ablation or DBS in these types of patients, they therefore may be better served by an ablative option.

A commonly touted feature DBS is the ability to fine-tune stimulation parameters after implantation. Theoretically, this offers an advantage of DBS over lesioning procedures, as it would facilitate maximization of therapeutic benefit of stimulation while minimizing side-effects to the patient over time. While this feature is useful in the movement disorder realm, where the therapeutic effects are objectively observable, it may not be clear how to tune DBS systems when there may be no overt effect of stimulation, as in psychiatric disorders [104]. Therefore, it is not clear that this theoretic of advantage of DBS over ablations is as strong in the psychosurgical realm, as it is in the movement disorder arena.

Finally, a tolerance effect to DBS has been observed to arise in some of the movement disorder patients. In these patients, at given stimulation parameters, therapeutic effectiveness is lost over time. Consequently, such patients may require progressively increasing current output for continued symptomatic control, leading to battery failure and impractical number of battery replacements. In fact, in such cases, the DBS electrodes themselves have sometimes been used to produce therapeutic radiofrequency delivered lesions before surgical removal of hardware [111]. The observed tolerance effect that occurs in some DBS cases may be due to development of true physiologic tolerance or due to loss of earlier placebo effect. If tolerance were to develop in a psychosurgical patient treated with DBS, it is possible such a patient may still benefit from a lesioning procedure. Ablative psychosurgery over the long term has shown increasing rates of successful responses as time goes on after the procedure [70]. This observation from the ablative psychosurgical experience supports its long-term efficacy and argues against any placebo response producing the benefit from this modality.

5.4 Conclusions

Surgical interventions for the treatment of psychiatric disease have a long history. Before the availability of effective psychotropic drugs, the widespread practice of psychosurgery reached a dramatic peak in the mid 20th century, with the notorious era of the Freeman lobotomy. The practice of psychosurgery continued on a much smaller scale for medically-refractory psychiatric patients, continuing to develop with a concept of minimalism out of the school of stereotaxy in neurosurgery. The modern era of psychosurgery has established four procedures with extensive experience supporting their indications and efficacies in properly selected patients. All of modern intracranial psychosurgery is stereotactic in nature, though historically interventions have been lesion-based. More recently, the idea of psychosurgery has been met with renewed enthusiasm, favoring DBS to avoid the historic dependence on lesioning. While there are some advantages to DBS over ablative methods, it is important to keep in mind that the two modalities are neither functionally nor clinically equivalent. Furthermore, while DBS is a new and experimental modality with unproven long-term effects, there is extensive experience with lesioning that supports its benefit for carefully selected psychiatric patients. Furthermore, the theoretical and practical aspects of each modality, warrant continued consideration and research to determine their optimal roles in psychosurgical practice. However, it is clear that ablative methods play an important role in the surgical management of severe, intractable psychiatric disease today and will likely continue to do so in the future.

References

1. Feldman RP, Goodrich JT. Psychosurgery: a historical overview. Neurosurgery. 2001;48(3):647–59.
2. Alt KW, Jeunesse C, Buitrago-Téllez CH, Wächter R, Boës E, Pichler SL. Evidence for stone age cranial surgery. Nature. 1997;387(6631):360.
3. Broca P. Sur le siège de la faculté du langage articulé. Bulletins de la Société d'anthropologie de Paris. 1865;377–93.
4. Wernicke C. Der aphasische Symptomencomplex. 1874.
5. Damasio H, Grabowski T, Frank R, Galaburda AM, Damasio AR. The return of Phineas Gage: clues about the brain from the skull of a famous patient. Science. 1994;264(5162):1102–5.
6. Manjila S, Rengachary S, Xavier AR, Parker B, Guthikonda M. Modern psychosurgery before Egas Moniz: a tribute to Gottlieb Burckhardt. 2008.
7. Fulton J, Jacobsen C. The functions of the frontal lobes: A comparative study in monkeys, chimpanzees and man. Adv Mod Biol. 1935;4:113–25 (Moscow).
8. Patel SR, Aronson JP, Sheth SA, Eskandar EN. Lesion Procedures in psychiatric neurosurgery. World Neurosur. 2013; 80(3–4):S31.e39–S31.e16.
9. Bridges P, Bartlett J. Psychosurgery: yesterday and today. Brit J Psychiatry. 1977;131(3):249–60.
10. Mashour GA, Walker EE, Martuza RL. Psychosurgery: past, present, and future. Brain Res Rev. 2005;48(3):409–19.
11. Kotowicz Z. Gottlieb Burckhardt and Egas Moniz-two beginnings of psychosurgery. Gesnerus. 2005;62(1–2):77–101.
12. Moniz E. Prefrontal leucotomy in the treatment of mental disorders. Am J Psychiatry. 1937;93 (1379–85):1385.
13. Robison RA, Taghva A, Liu CY, Apuzzo ML. Surgery of the mind, mood, and conscious state: an idea in evolution. World Neurosurg. 2013;80(3–4): S2–26.
14. Tierney AJ. Egas Moniz and the origins of psychosurgery: a review commemorating the 50th anniversary of Moniz's Nobel Prize. J Hist Neurosci. 2000;9(1):22–36.
15. Anderson CA, Arciniegas D. Neurosurgical interventions for neuropsychiatric syndromes. Curr Psychiatry Rep. 2004;6(5):355–63.
16. Valenstein ES. Great and desperate cures: the rise and decline of psychosurgery and other radical treatments for mental illness. New York: Basic Books; 1986.
17. Deutsch A. The mentally ill in America. New York City: Columbia University Press; 1949.
18. Fulton J. The frontal lobes: research publication for the association for research in nervous and mental disease. Baltimore: Williams & Wilkins; 1948.
19. Freeman W. Transorbital leucotomy. Lancet. 1948;252(6523):371–3.
20. Lapidus KA, Kopell BH, Ben-Haim S, Rezai AR, Goodman WK. History of psychosurgery: a psychiatrist's perspective. World Neurosurg. 2013; 80(3–4):S27 e21–S27 e16.
21. Heller AC, Amar AP, Liu CY, Apuzzo ML. Surgery of the mind and mood: a mosaic of issues in time and evolution. Neurosurgery. 2006;59(4):720–39.
22. Scoville WB. Selective cortical undercutting as a means of modifying and studying frontal lobe function in man. J Neurosurg. 1949;6(1):65–73.
23. Scoville WB, Wilk EK, Pepe AJ. Selective cortical undercutting results in new method of fractional lobotomy. Am J Psychiatry. 1951;107(10):730–8.
24. Spiegel E, Wycis H, Marks M, Lee A. Stereotaxic apparatus for operations on the human brain. Science. 1947;106(2754):349–50.
25. Leksell L. The stereotaxic method and radiosurgery of the brain. Acta Chir Scand. 1951;102(4):316.
26. Taub A, Lopes A, Fuentes D, et al. Neuropsychological outcome of ventral capsular/ventral striatal gamma capsulotomy for refractory obsessive-compulsive disorder: a pilot study. J Neuropsychiatry Clin Neurosci. 2009;21(4):393–7.
27. Greenberg BD, Rauch SL, Haber SN. Invasive circuitry-based neurotherapeutics: stereotactic ablation and deep brain stimulation for OCD. Neuropsychopharmacology. 2009;35(1):317–36.
28. Bonelli RMCJ. Frontal subcortical circuitry and behavior. Dialogues Clin Neurosci. 2007;9(2):141–51.
29. Chakravarthy VSJD, Bapi RS. What do the basal ganglia do? A modeling perspective. Biol Cybern. 2010;103(3):237–53.
30. Stocco ALC, Anderson JR. Conditional routing of information to the cortex: a model of the basal ganglia's role in cognitive coordination. Psychol Rev. 2010;117(2):541–74.
31. Weyhenmeyer JA. Rapid review of neuroscience. Amsterdam: Mosby Elsevier. 2007.
32. Cameron IGWM, Pari G, Munoz DP. Executive impairment in Parkinson's disease: response automaticity and task switching. Neuropsychologia. 2010;48(7):1948–57.
33. Fix JD. Basal ganglia and the striatal motor system. Neuroanatomy (Board Review Series) 4th ed. Baltimore: Wulters Kluwer & Lippincott Williams & Wilkins; 2007. p. 274–81.
34. Robinson DWH, Munne LA, Ashtari M, Alvir JM, Lerner G, Koreen A, Cole K, Bogerts B. Reduced caudate volume in obsessive compulsive disorder. Arch Gen Psychiatry. 1995;52:393–8.
35. Saunders RCRD. A comparison of efferent's of the amygdala and the hippocampal formation in the rhesus monkey: I. Convergence of the entorhinal, prorhinal, and perirhinal corticies. J Comput Neurol. 1988;271:153–84.
36. Saunders RCRD, Van Hoesen GW. A comparison of efferent's of the amygdala and the hippocampal formation in the rhesus monkey: II. Reciprocal and non-reciprocal connections. J Comput Neurol 1988;271:185–207.
37. Pd M. Psychosomatic disease and the visceral brain: recent developments bearing on the Papez theory of emotion. Psychosom Med. 1949;11:228–353.

38. Jw P. A proposed mechanism of emotion. Arch Neurol Psychiatry. 1937;38:725–43.
39. Sg W. The limbic system. In: Sg W, editor. Clinical neuroanatomy. vol 26. New York: McGraw-Hill; 2010.
40. Dh Z. The human amygdala and the emotional evaluation of sensory stimuli. Brain Res. 2003;41:88–123.
41. Kluver HBP. An analysis of certain effects of bilateral temporal lobectomy in rhesus monkeys. J Psychol. 1938;5:33–54.
42. Groenewegen HJ, Berendse HW. Connections of the subthalamic nucleus with ventral striatopallidal parts of the basal ganglia in the rat. J Comput Neurol. 1990;294:607–22.
43. Parent A. Extrinsic connections of the basal ganglia. Trends Neurosci. 1990;13:254–8.
44. Bonelli RM. KH, Pillay SS., Yurgelun-Todd DA. Basal ganglia volumetric studies in affective disorder: what did we learn in the last 15 years? J Neural Transmitters. 2006;113:255–68.
45. Salmon D. HW, Hamilton JM. Cognitive abilities mediated by frontal-subcortical circuits. In: Lichter DG, Cummings JL, editors. Frontal subcortical circuits in psychiatric and neurological disorders. New York: Guilford Press; 2001. p. 114–50.
46. Alvarez JA, Emory E. Executive function and the frontal lobes: a metaanalytic review. Neuropsychol Rev. 2006;16:17–42.
47. Milner B. Effects of different brain lesions on card sorting. Arch Neurol. 1963;9:90–100.
48. Jl C. Frontal-subcortical circuits and human behavior. Arch Neurol. 1993;50:873–80.
49. Cummings JL, Bogousslavsky J. Emotional consequences of focal brain lesions: an overview. Behavior and mood disorders in focal brain lesions. Cambridge: Cambridge University Press; 2000.
50. Mega MS, Cummings CJ, Salloway S, Malloy P. The limbic system: an anatomic, phylogenetic, and clinical perspective. J Neuropsychiatry Clin Neurosci. 1997;9:315–30.
51. Johnson TN, Rosvold HE. Topographic projections on the globus pallidus and the substantia nigra of selectively placed lesions in the precommissural caudate nucleus and putamen in the monkey. Explor Neurol. 1971;33:584–96.
52. Haber SN. The primate basal ganglia: parallel and integrative networks. J Chem Neuroanat. 2003;26:317–30.
53. Lichter DG, Cummings JL. Introduction and overview. New York: Guilford Press; 2001.
54. Macmillan MLM. Rehabilitating Phineas Gage. Neuropsychologic Rehab. 2010;20(5):641–58.
55. Stuss DT, Gow CA, Hetherington CR. "No longer Gage": frontal lobe dysfunction and emotional changes. J Consult Clin Psychol. 1992;60:349–59.
56. Starkstein SE, Manes F. Mania and manic-like disoders. Cambridge: Cambridge University Press; 2000.
57. Meyers CA, Meyers SA, Scheibel RS, Hayman A. Case report: acquired antisocial personality disorder associated with unilateral left orbital frontal lobe damage. J Psychiatry Neurosci. 1992;17:121–5.
58. Miller BL, Chang L, Mena I, Boone K, Lesser IM. Progressive right frontotemporal degeneration: clinical, neuropsychological and SPECT characteristics. Dement Geriatr Cogn Disord. 1993;4:204–13.
59. Mendez MF, Adams NL, Lewandowski KS. Neurobehavioral changes associated with caudate lesions. Neurology. 1989;39:349–54.
60. Levy R, Dubois B. Apathy and the functional anatomy of the prefrontal cortex-basal ganglia circuits. Cereb Cortex. 2006;16:916–28.
61. Ackermann H, Ziegler W. Akinetischer Mutismus-eine Literaturübersicht. Fortschr Neurologischer Psychiatr. 1995;63:59–67.
62. Mega MS, Cohenour RC. Akinetic mutism: disconnection of frontal-subcortical circuits. Neuropsychiatry Neuropsychol Behav Neurol. 1997;10:254–9.
63. Nielsen JM, Jacobs LL. Bilateral lesions of the anterior cingulate gyri. Bull Los Angeles Neurol Soc. 1951;16:231–34.
64. Whitty CWM, Duffield JE, Tow PM, Cairns H. Anterior cingulectomy in the treatment of mental disease. Lancet. 1952;1:475–81.
65. Ballantine Jr HT, Cassidy WL, Flanagan NB, Marino Jr R. Sterotaxic anterior cingulotomy for neuropsychiatric illness and intractable pain. J Neurosurg. 1967;26:488–95.
66. Hayempour BJ. Psychosurgery: treating neurobiological disorders with neurosurgical intervention. J Neurol Disord. 2013;1(1):1–19.
67. Scarone S, Colombo C, Livian S, Abbruzzese M, Ronchi P, Locatelli M, Smeraldi E. Increased right caudate nucleus size in obsessive compulsive disorder: detection and magnetic resonance imaging. Psychiatry Res. 1992;45:115–21.
68. Martuza RL, Chiocca EA, Jenike MA, Giriunas IE, Ballantine HT. Stereotactic radiofrequency thermal cingulotomy for obsessive compulsive disorder. J Neuropsychiatry Clin Neurosci 1990;2:331–36.
69. Baer L, Rauch SL, Ballantine HT, Martuza R, Cosgrove R, Cassem E, Jenike MA. Cingulotomy for intractable OCD: prospective long-term follow-up of 18 patients. Arch Gen Psychiatry. 1995;52:384–92.
70. Sheth SA, Neal J, Tangherlini F, et al. Limbic system surgery for treatment-refractory obsessive-compulsive disorder: a prospective long-term follow-up of 64 patients: clinical article. J Neurosurg. 2013;118(3):491–7.
71. Leksell LBE. Stereotactic gamma capsulotomy. New York: Elsevier/North Holland Biomedical Press; 1979.
72. Bingley TLL, Meyerson BA, Rylander G. Long-term results of stereotactic capsulotomy in chronic obsessive-compulsive neurosis. Baltimore: University Park Press; 1977.

73. Knight GC. The orbital cortex as an objective in the surgical treatment of mental illness: the development of the stereotactic approach. Brit J Surg. 1964;53:114–24.
74. Göktepe EO, Young LB, Bridges PK. A further review of the results of stereotactice subcaudate tractotomy. Brit J Psychiatry. 1975;126:270–80.
75. Hodgkiss AD, Malizia AL, Bartlett JR, Bridges PK. Outcomes after the psychosurgical operation of stereotactic subcaudate tractotomy. J Neuropsychiatry Clin Neurosci. 1995;7:230–34.
76. Poynton AM, Kartsounis LD, Bridges PK. A prospective clinical study of stereotactic subcaudate tractotomy. Psychol Med. 1995;25:763–70.
77. Mitchell-Heggs N, Kelly D, Richardson A. Stereotactic limbic leucotomy–a follow-up at 16 months. Brit J Psychiatry. 1976;128(3):226–40.
78. Price BH, Baral I, Cosgrove GR, Rauch SL, Nierenberg AA, Jenike MA, Cassem EH. Improvement in severe self mutilation following limbic leucotomy: a series of 5 consecutive cases. J Clin Psychiatry. 2001;62:925–32.
79. Malhi GS, Sachdev P. Novel physical treatments for the management of neuropsychiatric disorders. J Psychosom Res. 2002;53:709–19.
80. Cohen LG, Roth BJ, Nilsson J, Dang N, Panizza M, Bandinelli S, Friauf W, Hallett M. Effects of coil design on delivery of focal magnetic stimulation. Electroencephalogr Clin Neurophysiol. 1990;75:350–57.
81. Ben-Shachar D, Belmaker RH, Grisaru N, Klein E. Transcranial magnetic stimulation induces alterations in brain monoamines. J Neural Transmitters. 1997;104:191–97.
82. Levkovitz Y, Grisaru N, Segal M. Transcranial magnetic stimulation and antidepressive drugs share similar cellular effects in rat hippocampus. Neuropsychopharmacology. 2001;24:608–16.
83. Aleman A. Use of repetitive transcranial magnetic stimulation for treatment in psychiatry. Clin Psychopharmacol Neurosci. 2013;11(2):53–9.
84. Vagus Nerve Stimulation Study Group. A randomized controlled trial of chronic vagus nerve stimulation for treatment of medically intractable seizures. Neurology. 1999;45:224–30.
85. Morris GL, Gloss D, Buchhalter J, Mack KJ, Nickels K, Harden C. Evidence-based guideline update: vagus nerve stimulation for the treatment of epilepsy: report of the Guideline Development Subcommittee of the American Academy of Neurology.
86. Van Bockstaele EJ, Peoples J, Valentino RJ. Anatomic basis for differential regulation of the rostrolateral peri-locus coeruleus region by limbic afferents. Biol Psychiatry. 1999;46:1352–63.
87. Mohr P, Rodriguez M, Slavíčková A, Hanka J. The application of vagus nerve stimulation and deep brain stimulation in depression. Neuropsychobiology. 2011;64(3):170–81.
88. Henry TR, Votaw JR, Pennell PB, Epstein CM, Bakay RAE, FaberTL, Grafton ST, Hoffman JM. Acute blood flow changes and efficacy of vagus nerve stimulation in partial epilepsy. Neurology. 1999;52:1166–73.
89. Jobe PC, Dailey JW, Wernicke JF. A noradrenergic and serotonergic hypothesis of the linkage between epilepsy and affective disorders. Crit Rev Neurobiol. 1999;13:317–56.
90. Charous SJ, Kempster G, Manders E, Ristanovic R. The effect of vagal nerve stimulation on voice. Laryngoscope. 2001;111:2028–31.
91. Schachter SC, Saper CB. Vagus nerve stimulation. Epilepsia. 1998;39:677–86.
92. Kay MA, Glorioso JC, Naldini L. Viral vecotrs for gene therapy: the art of turning infectious agents into vehicles of therapeutics. Nat Med. 2001;7:33–40.
93. Frick LR, Williams K, Pittenger C. Microglial dysregulation in psychiatric disease. Clin Dev Immunol. 2013;2013:1–10.
94. Rossi F, Cattaneo E. Opinion: neural stem cell therapy for neurologic diseases: dreams and reality. Nat Rev Neurosci. 2001;3.
95. Kanno H. Regenerative therapy for neuronal diseases with transplantation of somatic stem cells. World J Stem Cells. 2013;5(4):163–71.
96. Elias WJ, Khaled M, Hilliard JD, et al. A magnetic resonance imaging, histological, and dose modeling comparison of focused ultrasound, radiofrequency, and gamma knife radiosurgery lesions in swine thalamus: laboratory investigation. J Neurosurg. 2013;1–11.
97. Spiegel EA, Wycis HT, Freed H. Stereoencephalotomy in thalamotomy and related procedures. J Am Med Assoc. 1952;148(6):446–51.
98. Spiegel EA, Wycis HT, Marks M, Lee AJ. Stereotaxic apparatus for operations on the human brain. Science. 1947;106(2754):349–50.
99. Hayempour BJ. Psychosurgery: treating neurobiological disorders with neurosurgical intervention. J Neurol Disord. 2013;1(1).
100. Ruck C, Karlsson A, Steele JD, et al. Capsulotomy for obsessive-compulsive disorder: long-term follow-up of 25 patients. Arch Gen Psychiatry. 2008;65(8):914.
101. Binder DK, Iskandar BJ. Modern neurosurgery for psychiatric disorders. Neurosurgery. 2000;47(1):9–21 (discussion 21–23).
102. Newcombe R. The lesion in stereotactic subcaudate tractotomy. Brit J Psychiatry. 1975;126(5):478–81.
103. Malhi GS, Bartlett JR. A new lesion for the psychosurgical operation of stereotactic subcaudate

tractotomy (SST). Brit J Neurosurg. 1998;12(4):335–39.

104. Birdno MJ, Grill WM. Mechanisms of deep brain stimulation in movement disorders as revealed by changes in stimulus frequency. Neurotherapeutics. 2008; 5(1):14–25.

105. Larson PS. Deep brain stimulation for psychiatric disorders. Neurotherapeutics. 2008;5(1):50–8.

106. Bejjani BP, Arnulf I, Houeto JL, Milea D, Demeret S, Pidoux B, Agid Y. Concurrent excitatory and inhibitory effects of high frequency stimulation: an oculomotor study. J Neurol, Neurosurg Psychiatry. 2002;72(4):517–22.

107. Malone DA Jr. Use of deep brain stimulation in treatment-resistant depression. Cleveland Clin J Med. 2010;77(3):S77–80.

108. Yount K. The brain electric: deep brain stimulation for neurologic disorders. DukeMed Magazine. Vol 11. Durham: Duke University Office of Marketing and Communications; p. 28–35.

109. Hall W, Carter A. Science, safety and costs make deep brain stimulation for addiction a low priority: a reply to Vorspan et al. (2011) and Kuhn et al. (2011). Addiction. 2011;106(8):1537–38.

110. McIntosh E, Gray A, Aziz T. Estimating the costs of surgical innovations: the case for subthalamic nucleus stimulation in the treatment of advanced Parkinson's disease. Mov Disord: Off J Mov Disord Soc. 2003;18(9):993–9.

111. Oh MY, Hodaie M, Kim SH, Alkhani A, Lang AE, Lozano AM. Deep brain stimulator electrodes used for lesioning: proof of principle. Neurosurgery. 2001;49(2):363–67 (discussion 367–9).

Legal Issues in Behavioral Surgery

6

Sam Eljamel

Abstract

Surgery for psychiatric illnesses (SPI) is still shrouded by ethical, governance and public concerns because of what happened in the past. There is a need to develop, agree and implement stringent guidelines and protocols to manage patients referred for SPI appropriately. These consensus guidelines are required to safe guard patients and surgeons. Patients considered for SPI must have failed adequate therapies: in obsessive compulsive disorders (OCD) failure of at least three adequate trials of Serotonin reuptake inhibitors (SRIs) including clomipramine and augmentation and behavioural therapies and in depression (MDD) failure of at least four adequate antidepressive therapies including antidepressive medicines, psychotherapy, and electroconvulsive therapy (ECT). Patients should be assessed by psychiatrist-led multidisciplinary team of experienced healthcare professionals, who must confirm the diagnosis, adequacy of previous treatments, and the ability of patients to give informed consent. Ability of patients to give informed consent and the diagnosis must be verified by an independent authority designated for this purpose under jurisdiction of the state where SPI will be carried out, e.g. Mental health welfare commission (MHWC) or Behavioural Surgery Review Boards. The independent body or authority must also decide whether the treating team is adequately trained to perform the procedure and provide aftercare. These procedures should only be performed in adequately resourced centers subject to annual inspections and robust clinical and regulatory governance frameworks. Postoperative assessment should be blinded to avoid placebo effects and biases, i.e. the assessor should be blinded as to what procedure did the patient receive to avoid bias. Adhering to these principles will safe guard the return of SPI and protect those who deliver it to patients.

S. Eljamel (✉)
Department of Neurosurgery, University of Dundee,
Dundee, Scotland, UK
e-mail: sam.eljamel@doctors.org.uk

B. Sun and A. De Salles (eds.), *Neurosurgical Treatments for Psychiatric Disorders*,
DOI 10.1007/978-94-017-9576-0_6
© Shanghai Jiao Tong University Press, Shanghai and Springer Science+Business Media Dordrecht 2015

6.1 Introduction

The majority of patients with psychiatric illnesses can be managed effectively by means of medications and psychotherapy. However, 20–40 % of patients become chronic, refractory to standard therapy or do not tolerate standards therapy because of unacceptable side effects, leading to increased demand on healthcare resources [1, 5, 19]. These patients would be candidates for further therapy such ablative surgery or neurostimulation for psychiatric illnesses [7]. However, such therapeutic options are still shrouded by uncertainties, controversy, skepticism and at times barefaced opposition [7]. The main reason for these attitudes towards such intervention in mental illnesses is that in the 1960s crude ablative surgery was used at times indiscriminately resulting into disrepute and legal ban in some jurisdictions. As a result stringent protocols specifically designed for this area of surgery must be developed and adopted to comply with local ethical and legal requirements. This chapter will explore the ethical and legal issues shrouding surgery for psychiatric illnesses (SPI).

6.2 Issues Leading to the Demise of Psychosurgery

6.2.1 Lack of Scientific Basis

The most important concern that shrouded psychosurgery in the 1960s was lack of scientific evidence to justify targeted brain area and the patient groups treated. The data upon which it was introduced was at most inconclusive and contradictory [3]. Furthermore, psychosurgeons of the past were accused of using vague unverifiable preoperative diagnosis, vague controversial selection criteria, vague or invalid assessment methods, and extreme bias in postoperative outcome reporting. The procedures performed in the past were very crude, imprecise, and inaccurate. Most of the procedures were carried out as part of clinical practice without proper research protocols approved by ethics committees, independent assessments of postoperative outcome, or precise categorization of the psychiatric illness being treated [16]. The practice of psychosurgery in the past was applied to humans after very few animal experiments, which gave unreliable and unpredictable results [18].

6.2.2 Lack of Informed Consent

The second concern-shrouded psychosurgery was informed consent or lack of it. How informed consent was obtained? Did patients understand what they were going to have? Were they aware of potential irreversible risks? Where they told or made aware of alternative management? e.g. Can an appropriate candidate for psychosurgery give valid consent for the procedure or can a third party, family, or society who might benefit from the procedure give consent on behalf of a patient. Some argued that psychosurgery may produce irreversible change in behaviour, self, or mind of the individual on the same bar as body mutilation [3].

6.2.3 Potential Misuse of the Procedure

Opponents and the general public have voiced their concern that psychosurgery had been, may be, or will be used or abused as a social or political tool to control and subdue those who are considered abnormal to justify controlling dissidents, ethnic minorities, political opponents, political opposition leaders or bothersome individuals such prisoners or criminals [3, 7].

6.3 How can These Concerns Be Overcome?

6.3.1 Informed Consent

Current surgical procedures applied to psychiatric illnesses include what is considered "established" techniques: i.e. thermal radiofrequency bilateral anterior capsulotomy (BACA), thermal radiofrequency bilateral anterior cingulotomy (BACI) and left vagus nerve stimulation (VNS). In recent years a number of new techniques and procedures have emerged e.g. deep brain stimulation (DBS) in multiple brain targets: i.e. DBS in the subjenu cingulum, DBS in nucleus accumbens, and other targets. The level of evidence behind these procedures is not robust to alley all criticism and biases, at best the strength of scientific evidence behind "established" procedures is level II. Therefore when consenting patients for such procedures it is very important that patients are made aware of alternative procedures and the degree of evidence behind each procedure, its outcome and potential risks, e.g. in the case of treatment refractory depression (TRMDD) the options would be either to continue with standard therapy, BACI, BACA, VNS or DBS. It is important to be familiar with the evidence base behind each procedure and what is considered accepted procedure in the jurisdiction under which the procedure is being carried out. For example in Belgium BACA is considered "established" ablative procedure for obsessive compulsive disorders (OCD) [13], while in Scotland BACI is considered "established" ablative procedure for TRMDD and OCD [6]. The importance of being familiar with all alternatives is very important for the purpose of informed consent as all neurostimulation procedures apart from VNS for TRMDD are still classified as experimental procedures, though DBS for OCD does have regulatory approval in the USA and Europe. The reason for being familiar with all possible alternative procedures is to give the patient the choice, e.g. if a patient was offered BACI without mentioning any other alternatives e.g. in TRMDD, VNS, and the patient agrees to undergo the procedure, and later on the patient finds out about VNS, the surgeons and psychiatrist might find themselves in an occult situation. Back in 2000, a three arm randomized controlled trial allocating patients with TRMDD to BACI, Cingulate DBS or VNS was designed and approved [6, 7]. When patients were offered the three treatment options or continue as usual, no patient agreed to be randomized as patients choose BACI arguing that if it works, it is one-off treatment, no

hardware and continuous follow up or battery changes and programming. Others however, elected VNS arguing VNS is an extracranial procedure without exposure to risks of surgery on the brain [7]. It is understandable patients' choices might make it hard to recruit patients for newer treatments, but it is essential that patients are give all the information to choose what they think is best for them. Furthermore, what is called "established" procedures for SPI is thermal radiofrequency lesioning with level II scientific evidence. Newer techniques such as stereotactic radiosurgery (SRS) and MRI guided high frequency ultrasound (MgHFUS) do not have this level of evidence behind them [13]. Any "non-established" or unapproved procedures should only be offered within a clinical trial protocol approved by the local ethics committee (LREC), institutional research board (IRB) and local regulatory bodies.

6.3.2 Allaying the Fears of the General Public and Satisfying Regulatory Authorities

Because of the bleak history of surgery for psychiatric illnesses, it is paramount that any programme offering surgery for psychiatric illnesses (SPI) to develop stringent protocols that satisfy and comply with ethical standards and regulatory authorities. For example in Scotland, patients are assessed by a group of specialized psychiatric team to establish the diagnosis, assess adequacy of previous trials of therapies, and assess the capacity of the patient to give informed consent. Patients, who pass these stringent criteria, will then be referred to a Mental Health Welfare Commission (MHWC), an independent authority established by the Scottish Government. The MHWC then visits the patient to confirm the diagnosis, adequacy of previous trials of therapy and assesses the ability of the patient to give informed consent to the proposed procedure. Furthermore, the MHWC or the National Services Division receives six-monthly detailed report about activities, outcomes and morbidity in the centre. Once the patient passes through all these steps, he/she will be admitted for SPI [7]. New procedures, new techniques or new targets must be offered only within the context of well-designed controlled clinical trial that complies with the local ethical and governance standards. There is a need to develop and agree strategies for SPI. These new strategies should include the following points to allay concerns and satisfy ethical and governance requirements:

1. Patients considered for SPI must have failed adequate therapies:
   (a) In OCD failure of at least three adequate trials of SRIs (Serotonin reuptake inhibitors) including clomipramine and augmentation and behavioural therapies.
   (b) In MDD failure of at least four adequate antidepressive therapies including medicines, psychotherapy, and ECT.
2. Patients should be assessed by psychiatrist-led multidisciplinary team of experienced healthcare professionals, who must confirm the diagnosis, adequacy of previous treatments, and the ability of patients to give informed consent. This is very important as the number of patients who might benefit from SPI is relatively very small, comorbid psychiatric illnesses are not uncommon and adequacy of past therapy requires an expert in this field (Fig. 6.1).
3. Ability of patients to give informed consent and the diagnosis must be verified by an independent authority designated for this purpose under jurisdiction of the state where SPI will be carried out, e.g. MHWC or Behavioural Surgery Review Board.
4. The independent body or authority must also decide whether the treating team is adequately trained to perform the procedure and provide aftercare.
5. These procedures should only be performed within adequately resourced centers subject to annual inspections and robust clinical and regulatory governance frameworks.
6. Postoperative assessment should be blinded to avoid placebo effects, i.e. the assessor should be blinded as to what procedure did the patient receive to avoid bias.

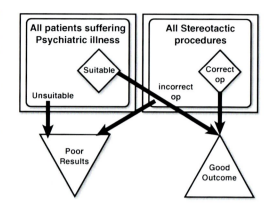

Fig. 6.1 Diagram depicting very small number of patients with psychiatric illnesses who might be candidates for SPI and the number of available SPI procedures and how difficult to match the correct patient to the correct operation particularly early on in a programme due to the very steep learning curve. Established centres should endeavour to support newer ones

There is real danger of implementing new SPI such as DBS without appropriate governance structures in place. Trying this technology in all psychiatric illnesses may lead to similar justifiable reactions and over-reactions from the public, politicians, and lawmakers in this century. There is a real and justifiable fear that SPI can be abused to control dissidents and political opponents or used to subdue those with violent behaviour or rioters. Not long ago (1970), in a book entitled "Violence and the brain," the authors called for the development of an early warning test to detect those with low thresholds for impulsive violence. The authors had also called for better and more effective methods for treating such people once they were identified [8]. Another psychosurgeon was quoted saying, "A person convicted of a violent crime should have the chance for a corrective operation." He went on to say, "Each violent young criminal incarcerated from 20 years to life costs the taxpayers about $100,000. For roughly $6,000, society can provide medical treatment which will transform him into a responsible, well-adjusted citizen" [3]. It is these extreme views that led to psychosurgery disrepute in the past. In reality, SPI is a very expensive and difficult technique to be used to subdue violent behaviour, dissidents, or political opponents. There are much easier, cheaper, and effective ways of mass control, including the use of media, television, medicines, and education systems. Historically, psychosurgery was not based on proper scientific studies; it started by Ego Moniz who turned to psychosurgery as a means to be in the limelight and for fame to obtain a Nobel Prize. Ego Moniz used lobotomy on patients after hearing of Fulton's case report of a single chimpanzee lobotomized by Jacobsen where the agitated chimp became calm [7]. There has been no verification of the exact location of the lesion or report of its potential serious side effects [3]. Almost everyone at the time ignored these important ethical issues because they felt they were morally obliged to help thousands of incarcerated mentally ill patients. They were blinded by the huge unmet need and the greed for wealth and fame. After the introduction of Moniz's lobotomy in the USA, it spread like wildfire and was practiced in smaller and less-equipped hospitals [17]. It was the actions of Walter Freeman, who was neither a neurosurgeon nor a psychiatrist, which brought psychosurgery to disrepute. Recognizing psychosurgery was a "Catch 22" situation; while psychosurgery relieved symptoms of psychosis, it was very costly in terms of loss of affect and creativity. Despite this fact, Walter Freeman continued the procedure and introduced the transorbital lobotomy (today's equivalent of minimally invasive procedure) instead of reflecting and auditing his results [17].

It is comforting to know that the way SPI is practiced today is very different from that of psychosurgery of the past; today's SPI is accurate and precise, and it can allay most of the concerns encountered in the past in this field of neurosurgery. However, a review of the literature on DBS for OCD and MDD uncovers a plethora of articles in recent years; a total of 90 publications during 2009–2011 compared to only 17 articles between 2002 and 2005 [7]. The vast majority of these publications reported unblinded outcomes of small selected study patients with favourable outcome, which was not verified when larger multicentre controlled studies were conducted. My own concern is that many

psychiatric patients are being treated in small groups outside multicenter, controlled, prospective trials. In a survey of North American Functional Neurosurgeons published in 2011, 50 % of the responders were engaged in some sort of SPI, mainly DBS for OCD or MDD, and saw SMI as a growing field of business [9]. Although, DBS and VNS are neither destructive nor irreversible and give sufferers the option to discontinue the stimulation if they wished to do so, these procedures should not be used outside properly designed clinical protocols because of the large placebo effect and inherent biases [7]. Although DBS had Food and Drug Administration (FDA) approval for OCD under Humanitarian Device Exemption (HDE) rules and VNS had FDA approval for MDD, some concerns had been raised regarding their use. These concerns are based on lack of strong scientific evidence on their safety and efficacy in the long run, the numerous conflicts of interests held by investigators such as holding patents for certain procedures, and the ambiguity and lack of transparency of research sponsored by commercial partners [8]. However, recent studies on ablative, VNS-, and DBS-SPI were carried out within stringent protocols that stood the heat of scientific rigor and scrutiny of peer reviewers [4, 6, 10–12, 16]. The outcomes reported in these studies were objective and based on objective assessments. Reduction of YBOCS score of 35 % is considered a clinical response in OCD, while a reduction of 50 % on MADRS or HDRS is considered a worthwhile response in MDD. However, careful observation and further studies of SPI procedures are required to establish their long-term efficacy, longevity, and side effects. Nevertheless, there remain ethical and social challenges facing SPI and consensus guidelines, workshops, and public engagement are just a few things that need to be done to overcome these challenges [2]. SPI must be approached with caution and commitment for long-term care. SPI is complicated by issues such as patient categorization, selection criteria, long-term management of these patients, and the different patterns of potential benefits and burdens [15]. There is a need for stringent ethical, governance, and

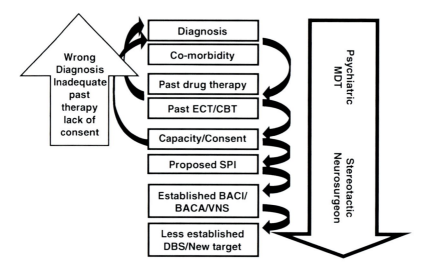

Fig. 6.2 Flow diagram of referral pathways for SPI: *RCT* electroconvulsive therapy, *CBT* cognitive behavioral therapy, *SPI* surgery for psychiatric illness, *BACI* thermal bilateral anterior cingulotomy, *BACA* thermal bilateral anterior capsulotomg, *VNS* left vagus nerve stimulation, *MDT* multidisciplinary team meeting

regulatory frameworks to be put in place in each legal jurisdiction in the world to prevent potential misuse of SPI. In Scotland, the service was centralized at Ninewells Hospital and Medical School. It is regulated by six-monthly review visits from the National Services Division of the Scottish Department of Health. Each patient's diagnosis, suitability for SPI, and his/her ability to give informed consent are determined by independent MHWC. In the state of Victoria, Australia, each request for SPI must be approved at a hearing of an independent Psychosurgery Review Board [14]. The aforementioned are just a few examples of how some jurisdictions around the world ensure the continuation of provision of SPI under stringent regulatory and clinical governance frameworks. Unless similar stringent rules are adopted by other jurisdictions, SPI will face the same fate as its predecessor.

6.4 Flow Chart of SMI

The chart summarizes management of patients referred for SMI (Fig. 6.2).

References

1. Bebbington PE. Epidemiology of obsessive compulsive disorders. Brit J Psychiatry. 1998;2–6.
2. Bell E, Mathieu G, Racine E. Preparing the ethical future of deep brain stimulation. Surg Neurol. 2009;72:577–86.
3. Breggin PH. The return of lobotomy and psychsurgery. Congress Rec (Dly Ed). 1972;13:841–62.
4. Christmas D, Eljamel MS, et al. Long term outcome of thermal anterior capsulotomy for chronic, treatment refractory depression. J Neurol Neurosurg Psychiatry. 2011;82:594–600.
5. Dupont RL, Rice DP, Shiraki S. Economic costs of obsessive compulsive disorders. Med Interface. 1995;8:102–9.
6. Eljamel MS. Ablative neurosurgery for mental disorders: Is there still a role in the 21st century? A personal perspective. Neurosurg Focus. 2008;25:E4.
7. Eljamel S. Strategies fro the return of behavioral surgery. Surg Neurol Int. 2012;3:34–9.
8. Erickson-Davis C. Ethical concerns regarding commercialization of deep brain stimulation for obsessive-compulsive disorder. Bioethics. 2012;8:440–6.
9. Lipsman N, et al. The contemporary practice of psychiatric surgery: Results from a survey of North American functional neurosurgeons. Stereotact Funct Neurosurg. 2011;89:103–10.
10. Meyberg HS, et al. Deep brain stimulation for treatment-resistant depression. Neuron. 2005;45:651–60.

11. Nuttin BJ, et al. Long-term electrical capsular stimulation in patients with obsessive-compulsive disorder. Neurosurgery. 2003;52:1263–74.
12. Nuttin BJ, et al. Long-term electrical capsular stimulation in patients with obsessive-compulsive disorder. Neurosurgery. 2008;62(Suppl 3):966–77.
13. Nuttin B, et al. Consensus on guidelines for stereotactic neurosurgery for psychiatric disorders. J Neurol Neurosurg Psychiatry. 2014;85(9):1003−8. doi: 10.1136/jnnp-2013-306580.
14. Psychosurgery Review Board of State of Victoria, Australia (Home page). http://government-state.goaus.net/melbourne/psychosurgery-review-board-of-victoria/. Accessed 03 Jan 2014.
15. Read CN, et al. Psychiatric neurosurgery 2009; Review and perspective. Semin Neurol. 2009;29:256–65.
16. Steele JD, et al. Anterior cingulotomy for major depression: clinical outcome and relationship to lesion characteristics. Biol Psychiatry. 2008;63:670–7.
17. Sterling P. Ethics and effectiveness of psychosurgery. In: Brady B, editor. Controversy in psychosurgery. Philadelphia: W B Saunders Co.; 1978.
18. Valenstein ES. The practice of psychosurgery: a survey of the literature (1971–1976). Report to National Commission on the Protection of Human Subjects in Biomedical and Behavioural Research. US Dept HEW 1976.
19. World Health Organization (WHO). Chapter 2, Burden of mental and behavioral disorders, in mental health, new understanding, New hope. WHO report 2001.

Preoperative Evaluation and Postoperative Follow-up of Deep Brain Stimulation for Psychiatric Disorders

7

Loes Gabriëls, Hemmings Wu and Bart Nuttin

Abstract

Deep brain stimulation (DBS) is under investigation as a new treatment for an increasing number of psychiatric conditions. Candidates for DBS are treatment refractory, severely incapacitated and have a very low quality of life. Patient selection should identify candidates that obtain and retain the greatest benefit. In psychiatric care, it is evident that a psychiatric disorder does not affect patients alone, but has a profound and devastating impact on those around them. These caregivers cannot be neglected in the follow-up process, since the impact of DBS on the psychiatric symptoms of the patient will reflect on the relationships. After surgery, the search for adequate stimulation parameters and the optimization process with fluctuations in symptom severity may be burdensome. Patients may not be abandoned once the DBS procedure is performed. With improvement of symptoms, patients are less stuck in their chronic psychiatric disorder and may need help in the definition of new goals and new purposes in life.

7.1 Introduction

Despite conscientious compliance and adherence to treatment according to internationally accepted evidence based treatment algorithms, some patients with psychiatric disorders do not respond to pharmacotherapy and psychotherapy treatment. Such patients are treatment refractory and are severely incapacitated and have a very low quality of life.

Deep brain stimulation (DBS) is under investigation as a new treatment for an increasing number of psychiatric conditions. Pilot studies in recent years have begun to demonstrate efficacy of DBS as a possible novel therapeutic modality

L. Gabriëls (✉)
UPC KU Leuven, Herestraat 49, 3000 Leuven, Belgium
e-mail: loes.gabriels@uzleuven.be

H. Wu · B. Nuttin
Laboratory of Experimental Neurosurgery and Neuroanatomy, KU Leuven, Leuven, Belgium

B. Nuttin
University Hospitals Leuven, Leuven, Belgium

for patients suffering from a severe form of these psychiatric disorders.

DBS for psychiatric disorders has evolved from a history of stereotactic ablative neurosurgery. If research of DBS proves non-inferiority in comparison to ablative techniques, DBS may be more acceptable than brain lesioning for patient and general public due to its adjustability and reversibility.

Obsessive compulsive disorder (OCD) was the first psychiatric disorder where the use of DBS was investigated, and sustained beneficial effects were documented by several research groups worldwide [3, 7, 11, 14]. Increasingly, DBS becomes a focus of research for other psychiatric indications such as major depressive disorder [9, 12, 16], addiction [13], eating disorders [8] and impulse control disorders [10].

In this developing domain of DBS for psychiatric disorders, it is of crucial importance to define and accept guidelines that respect the cultural and religious diversity and heterogeneity of healthcare environments of internationally collaborating partners. Such guidelines state a set norms at a given time but can and will evolve in an iterative process, taking into account the evolution of scientific findings, the continuing technical developments and the clinical experience gathered from patients living with DBS. They are meant to guide ethical and effective research and represent an international multidisciplinary consensus on best ethical practices, norms and professional behaviors, both in clinical and research settings [15].

Due to the stringent inclusion criteria, the year prevalence of DBS in psychiatric disorders during the last decade is low [6]. Patients that are candidates for DBS trials have a longstanding course of impairment and are disappointed by many failed treatments.

The DBS process in order to optimize treatment outcome can be divided in sequential phases: ethics of the clinical decision making process, selection procedure of appropriate candidates and preoperative evaluation, surgical intervention, post-surgery treatment and long term follow-up. Problems can emerge at each phase and a patient's progress through this DBS process requires careful monitoring and adequate interventions from multidisciplinary team.

7.2 Ethical Challenges and the Clinical Decision Making Process for DBS in Psychiatric Disorders

According to the World Health Organization [19] it is a patient's right to be offered a treatment that can alleviate suffering and permits improvement in quality of life. If there is enough evidence that DBS can lead to significant relief of symptoms and improvement of quality of life, it seems unethical not to consider the issue of DBS for carefully selected patients.

The protection of the human rights and dignity of psychiatric patients is a major issue and provides the frame to discuss the ethical principles of this ultimate therapeutic approach. Specific normative problems have to be considered such as safety concerns, the best interest of the patient, questions of patient's autonomy and ability to give free informed consent.

The risk/benefit ratio of the surgical intervention should be favorable Expectations and values of the patient and significant others are considered against the potential benefits of the procedure, as established in the context and at the time of the DBS procedure.

The compliance of patients to former treatment plays a role in the decision-making process as a good follow-up after the neurosurgical procedure is a crucial factor. Not only the symptom relief, but transformation of symptom relief into improvement in general wellbeing and amelioration in quality of life depends on this compliance.

The clinical decision making process needs to be considered in the context of a given era and society, with its specific role definitions, customs, moral views and laws. Knowledge of treatment efficacy, risks and alternative treatments and ethical status of DBS may change over time. The perspective of the patient, his/her values, quality of life and consent to treatment need to be taken into account. Regular accurate reviews of available literature on targets, indications, results and adverse events are crucial in this developing field. Honest and solid scientific reporting on the effectiveness and burden of these invasive procedures are an ethical duty of research centers who engage themselves in DBS for psychiatric disorders. To improve benefits and reduce risks, research into the precise definition of the brain target may help. Improvements in the field of technology and biomedical engineering may make interventions less invasive and less destructive. Advances in structural and functional neuroimaging and anatomic and electrophysiological studies, along with microelectrode technology, allow for more precise characterization of the neural pathways involved in certain disease states. However, microelectrode recording may increase the risk for brain haemorrhage, especially when approaching new brain areas via new trajectories, and this increased risk should be weighed against the possible advantage of its use.

DBS influences signal transduction and brain activity. The intention of "ideal" DBS is to normalize pathological brain signals without impact on non-pathological brain activity. The precise neurophysiologic mechanisms of psychiatric disorders and mechanism(s) of action of DBS are not yet fully understood. At the current level of knowledge, we have no strict delineation between pathological and non-pathological brain activity for psychiatric disorders. Knowledge on electrophysiological biomarkers is only very preliminary. DBS is under investigation in several different brain targets and for different psychiatric indications. DBS is not ultimately accurate. It does not only modulate pathological brain circuits. It may also influence other areas which cause unwanted effects. Furthermore, a brain circuit may dysfunction only intermittently. DBS in that circuit may at certain moments be beneficial for the patient, and at other moments have no influence, or even provoke unwanted effects.

The concept of autonomy in this chronically ill, severely impaired patient population needs further development and differentiation [1]. Respect for self-determination is undeniably important, but the intense chronic suffering and vulnerability influence the patients' decision-making process. Some patients want to be fully involved in the deliberative consent process, others defer decision-making to significant others or the physician in charge [18]. A psychiatric disorder does not affect patients alone, but can have a profound and devastating impact on those around them. The involvement of significant others and caregivers in medical decision-making process needs to be acknowledged [2]. Patients depend on these caregivers. Assessment of the expectations and values of both patient and significant others is crucial. Caregivers and patients may have divergent values and priorities, influenced by the burden created by patient's disorder. This can represent an additional, largely unrecognized, source of vulnerability in psychiatric patients. The influence of caregivers or close thirds can potentially translate into taking on additional 'involuntary' risks, including clinical trial enrollment. A dependent relation may result in undesirable pressure on the patient to adopt the caregivers preferences, and their involvement can counter patient autonomy and best interests. An acceptable approach is to consider the psychiatric disorder as a problem of a particular patient as well as to bear in mind the disruptive effects of the patient's psychiatric disorder on significant others. Conceivable secondary gains and expectations from caregivers need clarification before the patient decides to undergo DBS [4]. The effects of DBS reach (indirectly) beyond effects on disease symptoms and not only the patient but also these significant others will have to adapt to a new situation.

Although in psychiatric disorders cognitive distortions and biases may be present, carefully instructed patients (eventually with the aid of a family member, trusted counselor and/or legal guardian) are able to consent to complex, high-risk treatment or research proposals. Patients with treatment refractory psychiatric disorders often initiate the plea for DBS themselves. The very strong and demanding claim for surgery looks in fact closer to a desire than to a statement for informed consent. They may request disproportionate treatments and their desperation may impair their ability to rationally weigh the benefits against the risks. It is this paradoxical ease of securing consent in these patients that requires a higher degree of responsibility from DBS teams in the informed consent process. The patient must fully understand the risks and possible benefits and special attention regarding the concept of therapeutic misconception in the case DBS is required. This concept needs to be actively addressed, without withdrawing every hope the patient has put in the intervention. Furthermore, we want to emphasize the ethical requirement that individuals, participating in trials on DBS for psychiatric disorders, should not be used merely as a mean to increase our scientific knowledge, but always as an entity of their own. The aim of research on therapeutic innovations such as DBS for psychiatric disorders gives priority to the patient, who's safety exceeds the stringent application of the research protocol.

DBS is an intracranial neurosurgical procedure that comes with limited but significant risks. Aside from multidisciplinary assessment to determine suitability for the procedure, the patient must be able to give informed consent. Patients should also be counselled for the possibility that they may derive no benefit from DBS or not tolerate it well, necessitating the devices to be either switched of, or even their complete removal.

Even when a patient is judged to be an appropriate candidate to undergo DBS, the right to decline this treatment proposal remains obvious. The decision to decline can be linked to the psychopathological features of the disorder. Symptoms such as pathological anxiety inherent to anxiety disorders, apathy or indifference or disinterest in mood disorders, contamination fears or obsessive doubting may prevent the patient from making the decision to proceed with the intervention. Regardless the arguments and underpinnings of the patient's refusal, the decision is respected.

7.3 Selection Procedure for Appropriate Candidates and Preoperative Evaluation

Carefully identifying good candidates for DBS for psychiatric disorders is of fundamental importance and must be based on sound ethics and scientific evidence, when available. In the current stage, patients must meet criteria for severity and functional impairment, must demonstrate adequate treatment refractoriness, and must be able to consent to their participation in the research trial. During patient selection doctors should aim to identify candidates who will obtain and retain the greatest benefit from a DBS intervention. Patients must be able to tolerate DBS surgery and participate not only in research protocols, but adhere to the requirements of postoperative care and actively take part in it. Poorly selected patients may obtain less benefit although they are subject to the same risks of the DBS procedure, and thus the risk/benefit ratio in these patients becomes more unfavorable. Presently and under conditions of the investigational status of DBS for psychiatric disorders, there are no standardized criteria for choosing appropriate candidates. Nevertheless establishment of patient eligibility criteria seems of fundamental importance both in optimizing efficacy and safety. Pooling the data of the different research centers is strategically important to discover prognostic factors of poor or good outcome and to incite the continuous optimization of selection criteria.

A formal request for DBS for psychiatric disorders starts with a thorough, scrutinized review of the complete patient file, covering demographic features, family history, present and past illness history and treatment survey. An experienced multidisciplinary DBS team screens potential candidates and each discipline contributes with its specific expertise to the profit of the patient and the whole team. Patients are assessed during several introductory meetings at the outpatient clinic, to complete missing data in the file and to provide general information about DBS. A focus on failing or inadequate information and lacunas in the available records, especially regarding comorbidities or patient compliance is adamant. Comorbid conditions are frequent in psychiatric patients. In this stage, significant others often accompany the patient. The often desperate patients and their equally desperate families may tend to hide facts, in order to get access to DBS, not realizing that this missing information may compromise the outcome. Family support, commitment, and expectation may play an important role in the DBS process ant its outcome and thus it seems wise to assess their role early in the screening process. Individual realistic and unrealistic expectations of both the patient and the caregiver must be considered before including the patient in a study. The use of qualitative data obtained by semi structured or open in-depth interviews of patient and caregiver(s) may be necessary to detect subjective perception and expectations of DBS. Probing the expectations of DBS outcome in both parties enables the clinician to discuss values, to re-explain possible benefits and to correct unrealistic expectations.

7.4 Inclusion Criteria for DBS in Psychiatric Disorders

Applicants for DBS should meet all defined criteria for severity, chronicity, disability, and treatment refractoriness, and must have the ability to give informed consent. The criteria for severity, chronicity and treatment refractoriness will depend on the psychiatric disorder under investigation. Severity can be measured with disease specific, properly validated, standardized outcome scales, and in this stage of research, the threshold for severity may be defined to justify the use of an invasive treatment technique. This limits the number of candidates that participate in research on DBS for the psychiatric disorder under investigation, and restricts the generalizability of the research findings to a restricted group of patients.

Moreover, a quality of life scale and assessment of functioning should be included to quantify the disruption of the psychiatric symptoms in activities in many life domains. For every indication, a proper, state-of-the-art, evidence based treatment algorithm (pharmacologic, psychotherapeutic, less invasive neuromodulation techniques), must be defined to allow for demonstration of treatment refractoriness.

Patients in less severe or earlier stages of the disorder may show a better response to investigational DBS, but in this early phase of research the desire to do no harm justifies restricting this experimental procedure to those with severe psychiatric indication who have failed other forms of treatment. There are no trials conducted in less severe, less chronic, less treatment refractory trial, and until now, reviews and meta-analysis of available data do not demonstrate correlations between specific patient or illness characteristics and outcome, so data to argue for the implementation of DBS in a less severe or earlier stage of the psychiatric disorder are currently lacking.

Participating in DBS research for psychiatric disorders places a high demand on patients and their family or caregivers. They must agree to come frequently to the research center for adequate follow-up and evaluation of specific symptoms of the disorder under investigation, of side effects and adverse events. Moreover there is the follow-up on specific DBS aspects, such as the parameter optimization and replacements of the neurostimulator in case of battery failure. Besides these DBS and research related visits, it is important that patients after surgery remain in follow-up with their treating psychiatrist or psychologist, to guide them through the (sometimes abrupt) changes in symptoms and in many life domains (occupational, social and relational). We tend to discuss this and ask for a formal acceptance on this counseling task.

Patients must be able to understand, comply with instructions and provide their own written informed consent. A significant other is frequently involved in the process of extensive information on available treatment options. Patients and significant others are encouraged to ask questions and clarifications.

7.5 Exclusion Criteria

Exclusion criteria depend again on the psychiatric indication under investigation. Depending on the psychiatric disorder a variety of psychiatric comorbidities may be listed as contraindications. Personality disorders that may increase the risk of impulsive behavior or non-compliance after surgery are evaluated on a case-by-case basis. Surgical contraindications comprehend inability to undergo presurgical MRI (cardiac pacemaker, pregnancy, ...), infection, coagulopathy or, significant cardiac or other medical risk factors for surgery and possibly labeled contraindications for DBS.

While the delineation of disease severity, chronicity and treatment refractoriness is not the major problem for most psychiatric disorders, the toxic effect on the brain of chronic alcohol or drug consumption in addiction, or chronic starvation in the case of anorexia nervosa may challenge another important mandatory aspect of enrolling a patient as a research subject: it may have an important impact on their competence to provide informed consent since altered mental functioning may disrupt their ability to carefully evaluate the risks and benefits of the procedure. Moreover, even in the case of improvement of primary symptoms of the disorder under investigation, irreversible brain damage as a sequel of the psychiatric disorder may become a serious burden for the patient and cause other unwanted cognitive or behavioral challenges.

7.6 Outcome Evaluation

DBS first of all should be effective in reducing the symptoms of the psychiatric disorder in a stable and long-lasting manner. To evaluate this primary outcome, the use of well validated scales, designed specifically for the psychiatric indication under investigation, is indispensable. This does not mean that the aim of DBS is to get full remission of the psychiatric disorder, or that symptoms should be completely suppressed, or the patient completely cured. Many patients continue to live with clinically significantly reduced symptoms, that still may be obviously present.

To provide an actual benefit to the very individual patient, DBS not only has to improve symptoms scores in rating scales, but it also needs to be demonstrated that these reduced scores are associated with an actual improvement for the individual patient. DBS-induced improvement in symptom scores, or in cognitive and physical functions does not necessarily mean that the patient is better off. In other words, statistically significant efficacy is only a necessary, but not a sufficient condition for true effectiveness, and might, in certain cases, present an invalid surrogate parameter for the patient's true well-being [17]. To ascertain that DBS treatment allows the patient to live a more satisfying life, other variables (re-establishing a social life and work, general well-being and multifaceted quality of life) are needed. Assessment of more general psychiatric pathology, neurocognitive status and a comprehensive evaluation of short- and long-term adverse events must complement the primary outcome evaluation. Especially, the incorporation and dependence on the implanted device may not only influence body image, but may be considered as a constant reminder of the continuing psychiatric disorder.

7.7 Surgical Intervention, Post-surgery Treatment and Long Term Follow-up

DBS involves the stereotactic implantation of electrode leads into specific neuroanatomical structures where (in most cases) continuous stimulation is applied. Implanted leads are routed subcutaneously and connected to an implanted neurostimulator fixed onto the pectoral fascia below the clavicle or onto the rectus abdominis fascia in the abdominal region. This neurostimulator delivers electrical pulses through one or several of the four stimulation contacts. Choice of stimulation contacts and other stimulation parameters (amplitude, pulse width, frequency) can be modulated using an external electromagnetic programming device. Multiple adjustments in association with alteration in medical therapy may be required before stable stimulation parameters are achieved. DBS is non-ablative and therefore reversible in the sense that the stimulation can be switched off should the patient want so, or in case of intolerable side effects.

DBS has both acute and long-term effects, and stimulation parameters can and should be adjusted to attain an optimal therapeutic effect in every individual patient. For patients, the stage encompassing the surgical intervention is often marked by emotional instability and insecurity. They go from despair to a state of hope, but at the same time, they react often in a black and white, "now or never" or "all or nothing" manner. The presence of the psychiatrist in the operating theater is not a must, but for patients, this gives rise to trust and reassurance.

Postoperatively, patients must have access to a standardized, frequent follow-up in a multidisciplinary team. A close collaboration within this multidisciplinary team between a psychiatrist with special expertise in the psychiatric disorder under investigation, a neurosurgeon with ample expertise in the field of stereotactic and functional neurosurgery and a neuropsychologist is vital. Moreover, this team must have access to other specialties (neurology, social worker, neuro-imaging specialist, ...) for consultations on an ad hoc basis. Adequate psychiatric and psychotherapeutic post-surgery treatment and follow-up must be available, not only for thorough assessment of research outcome, but also to help patients to resume their lives.

After DBS surgery, there is the time-consuming search for adequate stimulation parameters with sometimes unexpected side-effects and fluctuations in symptom severity. Ultimately the feeling of being dependent on a foreign device may require extra attention from the clinician. The process of programming the leads after DBS surgery is complicated and time/labor-intensive. Nevertheless optimization of possible settings, with thoughtful changes to the configuration of the active electrodes, pulse widths, frequencies, amplitudes and configuration of anodes and cathodes, is critical for therapeutic success or failure. Acute stimulation effects are sometimes disturbing for the patients and may fade away after some days. They are not always predictive for the long-term outcome. The time involved to observe clinical effects after a programming change is sometimes very short (seconds to minutes), and the changes may appear very abrupt, but it often takes longer to obtain a stable symptom reduction. This contributes to the many months, with several sessions of optimization of stimulation parameters, necessary to obtain the full clinical benefit from DBS. The person who programs must know the patient well enough to read changes in symptoms associated with changes in parameters. The use of standardized self-rated and observer-rated instruments and blinded DBS adjustments is only a partial aid.

Patients may not be abandoned or left without professional after-care once the DBS procedure is performed. With improvement of symptoms, patients are less stuck in their chronic psychiatric disorder and sometimes need help in the definition of new goals and new purposes in life and with the development of new intentions and new plans. They often go through a mourning process for the years and life options lost in the disorder due to the formerly severe psychiatric symptoms. In the follow-up period, guidance should focus on the development of new abilities in the event of major therapeutic benefits, and on the acceptance of limitations if residual symptoms remain. Over the extended period of follow-up, significant others are interested in providing the best guidance, but they require instruction in their expectations as well [5]. Patient and families often have a lot of questions about living with DBS. Since DBS gives mostly symptomatic relief, they feel dependent on the optimal functioning of the hardware and dread a malfunction.

Patients may need help to adjust to their greater degree of independence and autonomy. Moreover, postoperative psychiatric and psychotherapeutic care are important since sometimes postoperative psychiatric problems may be related to emergence of previously existing disorders that had not been noted preoperatively, or were covered by the very severe primary psychiatric disorder for which DBS was indicated.

When patients change as a consequence of symptom reduction, meaningful relationships with caregivers may need redefinition. Patients may become less dependent or even independent on their caregivers. Partners need to switch from the role of a caregiver to more equality in the relationship. They may need help to cope with the changed balance, and sometimes partners need training in coping and communication skills. Moreover, patients and caregivers need to learn to live with the technical aspects of DBS and need close monitoring for re-appearance of psychiatric symptoms due to battery depletion or accidental deactivation.

Since one of the purposes of current research on DBS for psychiatric disorders is to test efficacy, patients need to be aware that there is a certain possibility of failure, hitherto unknown adverse events and an insufficient understanding of the reasons why some patients respond well to DBS treatment and others don't. If the patient expects full remission of the psychiatric symptoms in the context of a trial, but turns out to be either a partial responder or non-responder, the resulting disappointment needs to be dealt with. Occasionally, although the multidisciplinary DBS team may be satisfied with the outcome of DBS treatment, patient or family do not necessarily share this opinion. In optimal circumstances adequate pre-operative education regarding reasonable and unreasonable expectations would have prevented such discrepancy, but patients may still fail to appreciate the complexity of symptom relief on the one hand and satisfaction and general quality of life on the other. Patients may show dissatisfaction with symptom control, or with the emergence of new or worsening symptoms and adverse effects. Often, the residual symptoms they complain about include both symptoms of the psychiatric disorder that were expected to benefit from DBS as well as symptoms for which DBS was not intended in the first place (e.g. they want more energy, a better relationship, less headache, …), but hoped to obtain. The need of repetitive pre-operative education to reinforce realistic expectations is once-more crucial to prevent disappointment with the outcome.

References

1. Agich GJ. Reassessing autonomy in long-term care. Hastings Cent Rep. 1990;20:12–7.
2. Anita H. Relational autonomy or undue pressure? Family's role in medical decision-making. Scand J Caring Sci. 2008;22:128–35.
3. Denys D, Mantione M, Figee M, et al. Deep brain stimulation of the nucleus accumbens for treatment-refractory obsessive-compulsive disorder. Arch Gen Psychiatry. 2010;67:1061–8.
4. Donchin A. Understanding autonomy relationally: toward a reconfiguration of bioethical principles. J Med Philos. 2001;26:365–86.
5. Gabriëls L, Cosyns P, Nuttin B. Clinical guidance in neuromodulation: keeping track of the process and the patient. Neuromodulation. 2007;10(2):179–80.
6. Gabriëls L, Nuttin B, Cosyns P. Applicants for stereotactic neurosurgery for psychiatric disorders: role of the Flemish advisory board. Acta Psychiatr Scand. 2008;117(5):381–9.
7. Greenberg B, Gabriels L, Malone DA Jr, et al. Deep brain stimulation of the ventral internal capsule/ventral striatum for obsessive-compulsive disorder: worldwide experience. Mol Psychiatry. 2008;15(1):64–79.
8. Israël M, Steiger H, Kolivakis T, et al. Deep brain stimulation in the subgenual cingulate cortex for an intractable eating disorder. Biol Psychiatry. 2010;67 (9):e53–4.
9. Lozano AM, Mayberg HS, Giacobbe P, et al. Subcallosal cingulate gyrus deep brain stimulation for treatment-resistant depression. Biol Psychiatry. 2008;64(6):461–7.
10. Maley JH, Jorge E, Alvernia JE, et al. Deep brain stimulation of the orbitofrontal projections for the treatment of intermittent explosive disorder. Neurosurg Focus. 2010;29(2):E11.
11. Mallet L, Polosan M, Jaafari N, et al. Subthalamic nucleus stimulation in severe obsessive-compulsive disorder. N Engl J Med 2008;359(20):2121–34.
12. Malone DA Jr, Dougherty DD, Rezai AR, et al. Deep brain stimulation of the ventral capsule/ventral striatum for treatment-resistant depression. Biol Psychiatry. 2009;65(4):267–75.
13. Müller UJ, Sturm V, Voges J, et al. Successful treatment of chronic resistant alcoholism by deep brain stimulation of nucleus accumbens: first experience with three cases. Pharmacopsychiatry. 2009;42:288–92.

14. Nuttin B, Gabriëls L, Cosyns P, et al. Long-term electrical capsular stimulation in patients with obsessive-compulsive disorder. Neurosurgery. 2003;52(6):1263–74.
15. Nuttin B, Wu H, Mayberg H, et al. Consensus on guidelines for stereotactic neurosurgery for psychiatric disorders. J Neurol Neurosurg Psychiatry. 2014. doi:10.1136/jnnp-2013-306580.
16. Schlaepfer TE, Cohen MX, Frick C, et al. Deep brain stimulation to reward circuitry alleviates anhedonia in refractory major depression. Neuropsychopharmacology. 2008;33(2):368–77.
17. Synofzik M, Schlaepfer TE. Electrodes in the brain—ethical criteria for research and treatment with deep brain stimulation for neuropsychiatric disorders. Brain Stimul. 2011;4(1):7–16.
18. Waterworth S, Luker KA. Reluctant collaborators: do patients want to be involved in decisions concerning care? J Adv Nurs. 1990;15:971–6.
19. World Health Organization: Health for all by the year 2000: strategies. Geneva, Switzerland, 1980. WHO official document 173.

Ablative Surgery for Depression

8

Sam Eljamel

Abstract

Treatment refractory depression (TRMDD) is not uncommon despite adequate anti-depressive treatment trials. Patients who failed adequate trials of anti-depressive therapy including electroconvulsive therapy (ECT) are candidates for stereotactic surgery for mental illnesses. Ablative neurosurgery for TRMDD is performed in 21st century in highly specialized centers, where stereotactic surgeons teamed up with specialized psychiatrists working within stringent governance and ethical guidelines specifically designed for this purpose. The most commonly used procedures today are stereotactic bilateral anterior cingulotomy (BACI) or capsulotomy (BACA). Both thermal coagulation and stereotactic radiosurgery are used to ablate the desired targets. These procedures are safe with good track record. Forty to sixty percent of carefully selected patients with TRMDD are expected to respond or remit within a year of follow up. Response is defined as at least 50 % improvement on validated depression scales, while remission is defined as returning to normal mood and behavior.

8.1 Introduction

The World Mental Health Survey conducted in 17 countries found that on average about one in twenty people reported having an episode of depression [17], with a lifelong prevalence of major depression disorder (MDD) of 6.7 % [28]. Up to 20 % of MDD becomes chronic lasting more than two years and treatment resistant [14]. The management of patients with treatment resistant MDD (TRMDD) is very challenging with only 13 % or less remit after four adequate antidepressant trials [22].

Ablative surgery was first used to treat chronic neuropathic pain and during surgery some patients reported changes in mood during the procedures, particularly in patients with co-morbid symptoms of depression or anxiety leading to its use in TRMDD for several decades. Foltz and White described cingulotomy in 1962 [6], while stereotactic anterior capsulotomy was described by Leksell in 1978 [16]. Several other targets in the limbic system circuits were used to treat TRMDD. This chapter summarizes the different ablative surgery for TRMDD.

S. Eljamel (✉)
Department of Neurosurgery, University of Dundee, Dundee, Scotland, UK
e-mail: sam.eljamel@doctors.org.uk

B. Sun and A. De Salles (eds.), *Neurosurgical Treatments for Psychiatric Disorders*,
DOI 10.1007/978-94-017-9576-0_8
© Shanghai Jiao Tong University Press, Shanghai and Springer Science+Business Media Dordrecht 2015

8.2 Mechanism of Action

The exact mechanism by which ablative surgery exerts its effects in TRMDD is not fully understood. However neuroimaging, studies have shed some light on how these surgical lesions might influence mood, e.g. the anterior limb of the internal capsule connects areas of the brain thought to form part of the frontal-striatal-pallidothalamic network implicated in the symptom generation and pathology of depression [23]. Furthermore, Positron emission tomography (PET) scan demonstrated reduced cerebral blood flow (CBF) in prefrontal, premotor, and anterior insula cortex, and dorsal-anterior cingulate gyrus and elevated CBF in the subjenu cingulate gyrus in MDD [18].

8.3 Targets Used in Ablative Surgery for TRMDD

Several targets were used over the years to treat TRMDD using ablative techniques as follows.

8.3.1 Bilateral Anterior Cingulotomy (BACI)

BACI was first suggested as a treatment target for psychiatric disorders by Fulton in 1947, on the basis that electric stimulation of the anterior cingulum in monkeys produced changes associated with emotions and lesions in the same region produced less fearful and less aggressive animals [29]. Flotz first used BACI to treat chronic refractory neuropathic pain in 1962 [6]. During this procedure stereotactic lesions of about 8 mm in diameter and 12 mm in length are made centered around a point 20 mm posterior to the tip of the frontal horn of the lateral ventricle on each side, 7 mm from the midline, and just above the roof of the third ventricle avoiding any vessels nearby. Recent neuroimaging analysis of target location of BACI suggested that more anterior location was more effective [25], but this finding is by no means confirmed. The aim of BACI is to disrupt the cingulate bundle

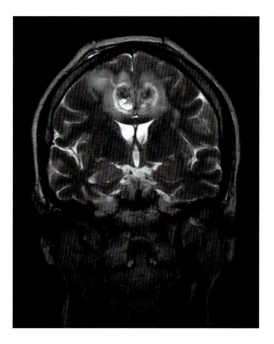

Fig. 8.1 Coronal T2-weighted MRI image of a patient who had TRMDD treated with BACI, the scan was performed within 72 h after BACI. Note the symmetrical position of the BACI lesions and surrounding oedema

connecting the anterior thalamus to the prefrontal and striatal areas and the limbic system, however lesion in the bundle is by no means essential to gain clinical benefits of BACI [24]. Figure 8.1 demonstrates BACI in intractable TRMDD

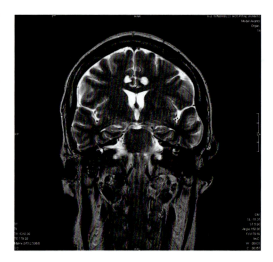

Fig. 8.2 Coronal T2-weighted MRI image 12 months after BACI, when the patient was in remission from TRMDD

8 Ablative Surgery for Depression

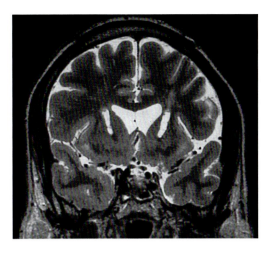

Fig. 8.3 Coronal T2-weighted MRI scan demonstrating BACA a year after the lesions were made in TRMDD

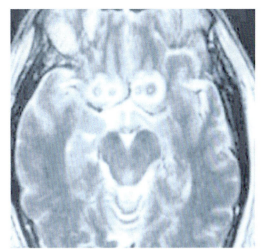

Fig. 8.4 Axial T2-weighted MRI scan image depicting BSCT

obtained in 72 h of surgery and Fig. 8.2 depicts the same 12 months after surgery.

Some authors reported making two further lesions in the same region on either side, what is called the six-pack BACI, however there is no strong scientific evidence to suggest that six-pack BACI is better or worse than single BACI of adequate size and precise locations.

8.3.2 Bilateral Anterior Capsulotomy (BACA)

BACA involved making lesions in the most anterior part of the anterior limb of the internal capsule on either side. The principles of BACA was first described by Talairach et al. [26] and developed as stereotactic procedure by Lars Leksell [16]. The white matter fibers connecting the frontal cortex and anterior cingulate to the thalamus, hippocampus, and amygdala are targeted during BACA by making lesions about 12 mm long as shown in Fig. 8.3.

8.3.3 Bilateral Subcaudate Tractotomy (BSCT)

Geoffrey Knight performed BSCT in 1964 [7], which involved stereotactic insertion of a row of radioactive yttrium (^{90}Y) seeds to destroy tissue below the head of the caudate nuclei in the frontal lobes. These lesions disconnect the subfontal and prefrontal cortex to the thalamus, hippocampus and amygdala. Figure 8.4 depicts BSCT.

8.3.4 Bilateral Limbic Leukotomy (BLL)

BLL is essentially a combined procedure consisting of BACI and BSCT on the assumption that a combined procedure has a better chance of

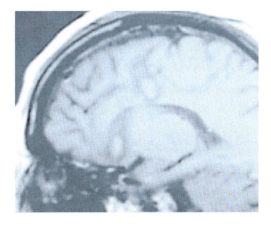

Fig. 8.5 Sagittal T1-weighted MRI image depicting BACI + BSCT = BLL

success than BACI or BSCT alone. This procedure was introduced in 1973 by Kelly et al. [13]. Figure 8.5 shows an MRI of BLL.

8.4 Techniques to Perform Ablative Surgery for TRMDD

Creation of a lesion at a target in the brain such as BACI, BACA, or BSCT is performed using any stereotactic frame (e.g. Cosman-Robertson-Wells (CRW), ZD or Leksell frame) and MRI or merged MRI and CT images, using stereotactic software (Fig. 8.6).

Tissue ablation can be achieved by several methods as follows.

8.4.1 Radiofrequency Thermocoagulation

Radiofrequency thermocoagulation has been used for several decades to generate lesions in the treatment of intractable pain, movement disorders and psychiatric disorders. This is the main technique I have used to generate BACI and BACA in our cohort of TRMDD. A radiofrequency electrode with 3 mm exposed tip, 3 mm in diameter was used in BACI and 6 mm exposed tip, 3 mm in diameter was used in BACA. The aim of the ablative procedure was to generate a lesion of at least 8 mm wide and 12 mm long using a lesion generator (Radionics, Boston, MA, USA). The temperature was raised to 70° for 90 s twice at the target point followed by extension along the track trajectory to cover 12 mm in length. The advantage of stereotactic thermocoagulation is its portability, immediate lesion generation, no ionizing radiation and low cost. However, there is no real time feedback regarding the location or size of the lesion, but this can be overcome by performing immediate MRI scan to assess the exact location and size of the lesion.

8.4.2 Stereotactic Radiosurgery (SRS)

Lars Leksell first suggested SRS in 1978, where gamma rays were focused stereotactically to generate tissue damage at the target area. The main advantage of this technique is non-invasiveness, however, it does take some time for the lesions to generate and it does not have real time monitoring

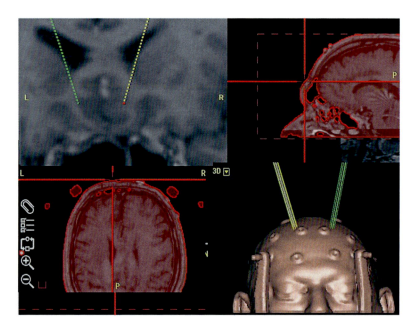

Fig. 8.6 Screen shot of stereotactic plan for subgenu cingulum (*top left*), fused MRI and CT (*top right* and *bottom left*) and 3D image of the plan (*bottom right*)

of the location or size of the lesions. Although the cost of a gamma unit is prohibitive if the gamma unit is only used for low volume of surgical procedures such as BACI or BACA, most gamma units however are currently available in major centers to perform other procedures and therefore it might be more economic to use these units to perform ablative surgery for psychiatric illnesses.

8.4.3 MRI Guided High Frequency Focused Ultrasound (MgHFU)

MgHFU is an emerging technology using MRI scan for guidance and intraoperative monitoring and use high frequency focused ultrasound to create lesions in the brain. The main advantages are the non-invasiveness, no ionizing radiation, real time monitoring of the location and size of the lesions and the immediate formation of the desired lesions. However, the system is costly, not widely available and requires total head shave.

8.4.4 Stereotactic Implantation of Radioisotopes

Stereotactic implantation of radioisotopes can be used to generate lesions in the brain e.g. the use of radioactive yttrium in BSCT, however the use of radioisotopes to generate brain lesions have disappeared in recent decades because SRS is more user friendly and less invasive technology than implanting radioisotopes.

8.5 Outcome of Ablative Surgery for TRMDD

In general published data suggest that ablative stereotactic surgery for TRMDD results into 40–60 % response rate. Response is defined as 50 % or more improvement on a validated depression scoring system such as Hamilton Rating Scale for Depression (HRSD) [8], or the Montgomery-Asberg Depression rating Scale (MADRS) [20].

An early report of the results of BACI was reported in 1973, where the authors classified 85 % as a "success" [1]. Another study included 198 patients with major affective disorders was reported in 1987 with a follow up average of 8.6 years. 62 % of the patients demonstrated long-term improvements [2]. Furthermore, there were no deaths and very low morbidity in this series; 1 % developed seizures, 0.3 % hemiplegia and 9 % suicide rate. All patients who committed suicide after surgery had suicidal ideation before surgery with more than 72 % had attempted suicide before surgery. Furthermore, subsequent neuropsychological assessment of a cohort of these patients found to have no diminution of intellectual function or emotional tone and no evidence of neurological or behavioral deficits except a decline in Taylor Complex Figure task [27]. A more recent study reported 53 % response rate [24]. In my own experience the response rate in patients with treatment refractory major depression that failed on average 4.6 adequate treatment trials of anti-depressive therapies including ECT (Table 8.1) 60 % responded and 40 % remitted after BACI at 12 months follow up.

In 78 patients treated for depression out of 208 patients who had BSCT for psychiatric illness, 68 % of patients with depression had no or minimal symptoms at 2 years mean follow up [7]. However, in another study reported in 1995, 34 % had improved out of 63 patients with MDD of a total of 183 patients who had BSCT for psychiatric disorders [11].

In 1973 it was reported that 61 % of 40 patients with TRMDD have improved following BLL [13], while two out of five were classified as responders in a more recent report in 2002 after BLL [21].

In the long term follow up of 30 patients after BACA, 50 % were responders and 40 % were in remission (Table 8.1) [5].

In another study published in September 2002, five out of seven patients with MDD were responders based on 50 % or more improvements in their scores at 12 months after BSCT, and the overall HDRS score improved from an average of 28.5–16.5. The total number of patients in this

Table 8.1 Clinical characteristics of TRMDD treated at the Scottish National Centre of NMD

Parameter	BACI		BACA	
	Response	Remission	Response	Remission
Mean age	43 years SD 9.79 years			
Gender	73.3 % females and 26.7 % males			
Employment	100 % unemployed		100 % unemployed	
Duration	Duration of current episode of MDD was 353.1 weeks			
Treatments	4.6 adequate trials including ECT and SD 1.1			
Outcome at 12 months (%)	60	20	25	10
Outcome at long term (%)	40	40	50	40

Response was defined as improvement by at least 50 % in HRSD or MADRS scores and remission was defined as a score of 7 or less on HRSD or a score of 10 or less on MADRS

series of all pathologies was 21 [15]. There was no morbidity reported in this series except transient urinary incontinence.

Another report on long term outcome after a mean follow up of 7 years (SD 3.4 years) following BACA have shown 50 % response rate and 40 % remission rate. 55 % were classified as improved, 35 % were unchanged and 10 % deteriorated. There were no deaths, neuropsychological testing demonstrated no changes and there were some improvements in executive functions [4].

8.6 Safety Record of Ablative Surgery in Psychiatric Illness

In our own modern series one patient developed urinary urgency and one weight gain after BACI, one patient developed nocturia and one memory problems after BACA. Assessment of cognitive functions in our cohort demonstrated more than 10 % improvements in verbal fluency, and problem solving ability. There was however decline in block design by 5–10 %. Table 8.2

Table 8.2 Safety data of ablative surgery in psychiatric illnesses

Authors	Side effect	BACI	BACA	BSCT	BLL
Hemmer [10]	Epilepsy 3.4 %, incontinence, weight gain		116 patients 33 % MDD		
Kelly et al. [13]	Confusion, lethargy, transient incontinence				40 patients
Goktepe et al. [7]	Epilepsy 2.2 %, personality change 7 %			139 patients	
Mitchell-Heggs et al. [19]	Confusion, lethargy, incontinence				66 patients
Ballantine et al. [2]	Seizures 1 %, hemiplegia 0.3 %, suicide 9 %	198 patients			
Jenike et al. [12]	Seizures 9 %, transient mania 6 %	33 OCD			
Hay et al. [9]	Epilepsy 10 %, personality change 10 %				26 OCD
Bridges et al. [3]	Confusion, seizures 1.6 %, suicide 1 %			249 mixed	
Sprangler et al. [24]	Seizures 6 %	34 patients			

summarizes the safety record of ablative surgery in psychiatric illnesses.

In summary ablative surgery fro TRMDD is safe, the risk of seizures is the same as any other stereotactic procedure 1–2 %, which can be abolished by using non-invasive techniques to preform the lesions e.g. SRS or MgHFUS. Transient confusion or transient incontinence are not common and they resolve within days to weeks, and the risk of permanent neurological deficit is less than 1 %.

8.7 Conclusions

The most commonly used ablative procedures for TRMDD in the 21st century are BACI and BACA, they carry very low risk of seizures or permanent neurological deficit. 40–60 % of TRMDD respond to ablative surgery. These procedures however, should only be performed under stringent protocols by qualified multidisciplinary teams consisting of a stereotactic neurosurgeon, specialized psychiatrists, specialized neuropsychologists, specialist psychiatric nurses and supportive staff.

References

1. Bailey H, Dowling J, Davies E. Studies in depression III. Med J Aus. 1973;2:366–71.
2. Ballantine HT, et al. Treatment of psychiatric illness by stereotactic cingulotomy. Biol Psychiatry. 1987;22:807–19.
3. Bridges PK, et al. Psychsurgery: stereotactic subcaudate tractotomy, an indispensible treatment. Brit J Psychiatry. 1994;165:599–613.
4. Christmas D, Eljamel S, et al. Long term outcome of thermal anterior capsulotomy for chronic treatment refractory depression. JNNP. 2011;82:594–600.
5. Eljamel S. Strategies fro the return of behavioral surgery. Surg Neurol Int. 2012;3:34–9.
6. Foltz EL, White LE. Pain relief by frontal cingulotomy. J Neurosurg. 1962;19:89–94.
7. Goktepe EO, Young LB, Bridges PK. A further review of the results of stereotactic subcaudate tractotomy. Brit J Psychiatry. 1975;128:270–80.

8. Hamilton A. A rating scale for depression. JNNP. 1960;23:56–63.
9. Hay P, et al. Treatment of obsessive compulsive disorder by psychosurgery. Acta Psychiatr Scand. 1995;87:197–207.
10. Hemmer T. Treatment of mental disorders with frontal stereotactic thermo-lesions: a follow up of 116 cases. Acta Psychiatr Scand. 1961;153:36.
11. Hopkins AD, et al. Outcome after the psychosurgical operation of stereotactic subcaudate tractotomy 1979–1991. J Neuropsychiatry Clin Neurosci. 1995;7:230–4.
12. Jenike MA, et al. Cingulotomy for refractory obsessive compulsive disorder: a long term follow up in 33 patients. Arch Gen Psychiatry. 1991;48:548–55.
13. Kelly D, et al. Stereotactic limbic leucotomy: a preliminary report on forty patients. Brit J Psychiatry. 1973;123:141–8.
14. Kennedy N, et al. Remission and recurrence of depression in the maintenance era: long term outcome in a Cambridge cohort. Psychol Med. 2003;33:927–38.
15. Kim M-C, Lee T-K, Choi C-R. Review of long term results of stereotactic psychosurgery. Neurol Med Chir (Tokyo). 2002;42:365–71.
16. Leksell L, et al. Radiosurgical capusolotomy—a closed surgical method for psychiatric surgery. Lakartidningen. 1978;75:546–7.
17. Marcus M, et al. Depression: a global public health concern. http://www.who.int/mental_health/management/depression/who_paper_depression_wfmh_2012.pdf. Accessed on 29 Dec 2013.
18. Meyberg HS, et al. Deep brain stimulation for treatment resistant depression. Neuron. 2005;45:651–60.
19. Mitchell-Heggs N, Kelly D, Richardson A. Stereotactic limbic leucotomy: a follow up at 16 months. Brit J Psychiatry. 1976;128:226–40.
20. Montgomery SA, Asberg M. A new depression scale designed to be sensitive to change. Brit J Psychiatry. 1979;134:382–9.
21. Montoya A, et al. Magnetic resonance imaging guided stereotactic limbic leucotomy for treatment of intractable psychiatric disease. Neurosurg. 2002;50:1043–52.
22. Rush AJ, et al. Acute and longer-term outcomes in depressed patients requiring one or several treatment steps. Am J Psychiatry. 2006;163:1905–17.
23. Siminowicz DA, et al. Limbic-frontal circuitry in major depression, a path modeling metanlysis. Neuroimage. 2004;22:409–18.
24. Spangler WJ, et al. Magnetic resonance image-guided stereotactic cingulotomy for intractable psychiatric disease. Neurosurgery. 1996;38:1071–6.
25. Steele JD, et al. Anterior cingulotomy for major depression: clinical outcome and relationship to

lesion characteristics. Biol Psychiatry. 2008;63: 670–7.

26. Talairach J, et al. Lobotomie prefontale limitee par electrocoagulation des fibres thalamo-frontalis emergence du bras anterior de la capsule interne. Proceedings of the 4th Congress Neurologique Internationale. 1949;41.

27. Teuber HL, Corkin SH, Twitchell TE. Study of cingultomy in man. In: Sweet WH, Obradar S, Martin-Rodriguez JG, editors. Neurosurgical treatment in psychiatry, pain and epilepsy. Baltimore: University Park Press; 1977. p. 355–62.

28. Waraich P, et al. Prevalence and incidence studies of mood disorders, a systematic review of the literature. Can J Psychiatry. 2004;124:0706–7437.

29. Ward AA. The cingular gyrus, area 24. J Neurophysiol. 1948;11:13–23.

Deep Brain Stimulation for the Management of Treatment-Refractory Major Depressive Disorder

9

Nir Lipsman, Peter Giacobbe and Andres M. Lozano

Abstract

Major Depressive Disorder (MDD) is among the most common psychiatric conditions, and is responsible for substantial human morbidity worldwide. The last two decades have seen significant progress in our understanding of the neural circuits driving MDD, which is now increasingly understood as a disorder of neural circuitry. The success of deep brain stimulation (DBS) as a modulator of circuit dysfunction in motor disorders such as Parkinson's Disease has generated interest in it's use in other circuit-based conditions, including MDD. The result has been resurgence in interest in surgery for refractory mood disorders, where advances in functional imaging have helped identify key anatomic targets as critical notes in the circuit. This chapter reviews the history of surgery for major depression, the rationale for focal neuromodulation in the condition, and provides a summary of the clinical experience of DBS in MDD to date.

9.1 Background

Major Depressive Disorder (MDD) is among the most common psychiatric conditions, with a population lifetime prevalence of 14–17 % [1–3]. The costs of MDD are substantial, and represent one of society's most significant sources of lost wages and productivity [4]. Other costs are more difficult to measure, and relate to the human suffering wrought by an illness that has challenged clinicians for centuries [5]. The last two decades, however, have seen much progress in elucidating the brain circuits driving depressed mood, and offer hope that a better understanding of the illness may lead to new and improved therapeutic options.

MDD is highly heterogeneous. Although sadness is a defining feature, other brain systems such as reward, cognition, and vegetative functions, are involved, suggesting a more complex picture of disease etiology and maintenance. For example, patients with MDD report high degrees of anhedonia, or lack of pleasure with previously pleasurable activities, which implicates dysfunction in reward circuitry. Basal vegetative functions, such as sleep, sexual arousal and appetite,

N. Lipsman (✉) · A.M. Lozano
Division of Neurosurgery, Toronto Western
Hospital, University Health Network, University of
Toronto, Toronto, Canada

P. Giacobbe
Department of Psychiatry, Toronto General Hospital,
University Health Network, University of Toronto,
Toronto, Canada

B. Sun and A. De Salles (eds.), *Neurosurgical Treatments for Psychiatric Disorders*,
DOI 10.1007/978-94-017-9576-0_9
© Shanghai Jiao Tong University Press, Shanghai and Springer Science+Business Media Dordrecht 2015

are often disturbed, implicating dysfunction in autonomic and regulatory circuits. Further, symptoms such as rumination, agitation, pathologic crying, and suicidality, all support the notion that MDD is more than merely a 'deficit' state [6]. MDD, therefore, cannot be ascribed to a single anatomic structure or circuit, and is likely a manifestation of network wide dysfunction affecting multiple circuits and involving multiple neurotransmitter systems.

The mainstays of treatment for MDD are psychopharmacologic and psychotherapeutic, and are most effective when used in tandem. Medical treatments are aimed at restoring concentrations of key neurotransmitters, most notably serotonin, dopamine and norepinephrine, while psychosocial treatments attempt to identify and correct maladaptive cognitive biases influencing behavior. A large study in nearly 3,000 patients with MDD found that response and remission rates with a single serotonin-reuptake inhibitor (SRI) were 47 and 28 %, respectively [7]. Subsequent studies found that even after continued dose and drug escalations remission rates improved to only 60 % [8, 9]. Such results show that despite optimal medical management, at least one-third of MDD patients remain symptomatic. For these patients neuromodulation options are available [8].

Neuromodulation for MDD can be divided into non-invasive and invasive. The advantages of non-invasive approaches, such as electroconvulsive therapy (ECT) and repetitive transcranial magnetic stimulation (rTMS), are the absence of surgical risk as well as their relatively low-cost and widespread availability. Although effective in some patients, it may be difficult to maintain efficacy in long-term follow-up, and in some instances, such as with ECT, repeated use may be associated with deleterious effects on cognitive functioning [10]. Nevertheless, ECT is highly effective in the management of some types of refractory MDD, and remains the 'gold-standard' for neuromodulation in this patient group [8]. Invasive approaches are typically reserved for patients who have failed non-invasive attempts, and provide a permanent or chronic means of adjusting dysfunctional neural circuitry. Next, we review the rationale and experience for invasive neuromodulation in MDD, focusing specifically on the development of DBS.

9.2 Rationale for DBS in Major Depression

Several factors led to the investigation of DBS for MDD. First, was the establishment of DBS as a safe and effective procedure for a range of neurologic, typically motor, diseases [11–14]. As a result, over 100,000 patients world-wide have undergone DBS, most commonly for Parkinson's Disease, essential tremor, and dystonia [11]. This ability to focally modulate neural circuits motivated the investigation of DBS in other circuit-based disorders, including psychiatric conditions. An additional development has been structural and functional imaging, which have helped identify key nodes in limbic circuitry driving pathologic mood. fMRI and PET helped establish hypothesis-driven models of neural circuit dysfunction, and suggested anatomic targets for DBS procedures. Finally, the existence of a core group of patients, up to a third with MDD, who have no available treatment options, has spurred clinicians to search for novel, safe and effective treatment options (Fig. 9.1).

9.2.1 Neurosurgery for Depression

Surgery for depression is among the oldest procedures in neurosurgery, with reports of limbic leucotomy, and prefrontal lobotomy, extending back to the early 1940s [15–17]. Early attempts, however, were crude with targeting aided only by surface landmarks, and involving broad disconnections of frontal white matter tracts [16–18]. The introduction of stereotactic techniques, whereby lesions could be generated anywhere in the brain with millimeter-scale accuracy, led to the development of cingulotomy and capsulotomy, which specifically tackled disorders of mood. Cingulotomy involves bilaterally lesioning the anterior cingulate cortex

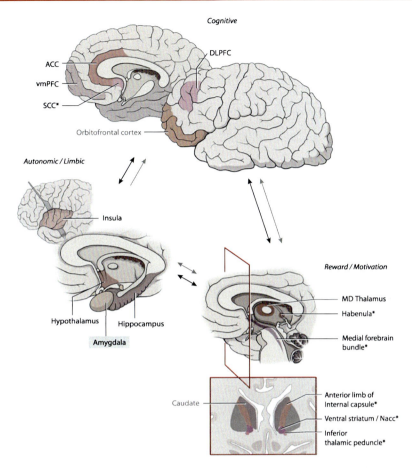

Fig. 9.1 Circuitry of mood and affective regulation. Structures marked with an asterisk have been investigated in DBS trials for major depression. *ACC* Anterior cingulate cortex, *vmPFC* ventromedial prefrontal cortex, *SCC* Subcallosal cingulate cortex, *DLPFC* dorsolateral prefrontal cortex, *MD* mediodorsal. Modified with permission from Lozano and Lipsman [11]

approximately 2 cm posterior to the front of the corpus callosum. The procedure is generally well-tolerated and very safe, with several prospective and retrospective studies describing few adverse effects [19, 20]. A large proportion of patients also derive a significant clinical benefit, with rates of response (defined as a significant reduction in a depression ratings scale and improvements in overall functioning) ranging from 38 to 75 % [20–22]. Capsulotomy involves a lesion in the anterior limb of the internal capsule and is designed to influence fronto-subcortical circuits involved in affective regulation. In one recent paper, 8 patients with refractory MDD underwent bilateral capsulotomy, with 4 of them classified as treatment responders at 2–3 years follow-up [23]. Similar results were reported in a prospective case series of 20 patients, wherein 40 % were in remission and 50 % treatment responders, at a mean follow-up of 7 years [24].

Fifty years of clinical experience with lesions in psychiatric disorders have shown that: (1) Lesions in limbic circuits can be performed accurately and safely; and, (2) Such lesions can effectively influence pathological mood circuits, yielding positive effects in about half of otherwise refractory patients. The disadvantage of lesions, however, remains their permanence. One cannot titrate the clinical effect, 'escalate' or 'reduce' the dose, or change the location of the lesion once performed. Repeat procedures, particularly with cingulotomy, are routinely done but expose patients to additional surgical risk.

9.2.2 Neurocircuitry of MDD

Several structures have been implicated in circuit models of MDD, including the medial and dorsolateral prefrontal cortex (mPFC; DLPFC), anterior cingulate cortex (ACC), nucleus accumbens/ventral striatum (NAcc/VS), as well as the amygdala. Neuroimaging has been the primer driver of progress in the investigation of mood circuitry, and both structural and functional abnormalities have been found in MDD patients. For example, ACC and hippocampal volumes are both diminished in patients with acute depression, with additional studies finding diffuse gray matter volume reductions. Pre-clinical models have further established a direct link between activity in the nucleus accumbens and both the enjoyment of reward ("liking") as well as it's pursuit ("wanting") [25–27]. Imaging studies have linked activity in reward pathways to both the mPFC and the ventral tegmental area (VTA), a key brainstem dopaminergic center. The ability of VTA to influence both 'top-down' cortical centers, via mesocortical pathways, and 'bottom-up' regulatory centers, via mesolimbic pathways, has been proposed as a key maintenance system for depressed mood, and anhedonia specifically. For example, dysfunction in both or either mesolimbic or mesocortical systems can result in failure to anticipate or expect a rewarding outcome. Hypoactivation of NAcc in response to otherwise rewarding stimuli has been shown in conditions where reward deficits are well established, such as anorexia nervosa, further linking activity of this structure to affect-laden decisions [28, 29].

Studies performed in healthy subjects and unmedicated MDD patients have shown that activity in the ventral PFC, and subcallosal cingulate (SCC) specifically, is increased in response to sad stimuli in the former, and in the resting state in the latter [30]. This activity is attenuated with medical treatment of depression as well as with DBS in otherwise refractory patients [31, 32]. This has been found in both patients with unipolar depression as well as those with anorexia nervosa with comorbid MDD [33]. Such results have suggested that depression may be linked to a functional 'decoupling' of cortical-amygdalar projections, whereby increased activity in both regions leads to a failure of brain homeostatic control over affect [6]. Neurophysiological studies involving recordings directly from neurons are also informing the mechanisms of mood disturbance and the function of key limbic regions. For example, our group has shown using microelectrode recordings from single neurons in the SCC, that neurons in this region fire preferentially to negative pictures compared to neutral or positive ones [34]. Additional work in bipolar depression patients found that SCC neuronal populations undergo synchronization of firing immediately prior to making an emotional decision [35]. These results suggest that this region may be 'programmed' to respond to sad and depression-maintaining stimuli.

9.3 Clinical Experience of MDD DBS to Date

Several targets are currently under investigation for DBS in major depression (Table 9.1). These include structures involved in reward (nucleus accumbens/ventral striatum), affective regulation (subcallosal cingulate), and pathways that bridge top-down and bottom-up mood processing (medial forebrain bundle, inferior thalamic peduncle, habenula). Although the global experience with DBS for MDD is growing, all of these trials remain investigational. Below we review the rationale and results to date with the most commonly investigated DBS targets.

9.3.1 Subcallosal Cingulate (SCC)

The target with the most experience to date is the subcallosal cingulate cortex (SCC). The SCC is a

Table 9.1 Studies of deep brain stimulation for major depressive disorder, by anatomic target

Study	Number of patients	Outcome
Subcallosal Cingulate		
Mayberg et al. [32]	6	Follow-up 6 months. 4/6 responders, 2/6 remission as measured by HDRS
Kennedy et al. [52]	20	At last follow-up (3–6 years following implantation, mean = 3.5), response rate = 64.3 % and remission rate = 42.9 % (by HDRS). Considerable improvement in social functioning: 65 % of patients engaged in work-related activity at last follow-up compared to 10 % prior to DBS
Puigdemont et al. [40]	8	Response and remission at 1 year, 62.5 and 50 %, respectively
Holtzheimer et al. [53]	17 (10 MDD, 7 with bipolar II)	At one year follow-up, remission and response rate of 36 %. At 2 years, remission rate of 58 % and response rate of 92 %. Remission and response rates based on Hamilton Depression Rating Scale (HDRS). Efficacy similar for MDD and bipolar patients
Lozano et al. [39]	20	At 6 months follow-up, response rate of 48 %; at one-year follow-up, response rate of 29 %. Response measured by HDRS
Nucleus Accumbens/Ventral Striatum		
Schlaepfer et al. [54]	3	Double-blind changes to stimulation parameters and assessment. HDRS scores decreased with stimulation and increased with stimulation off
Malone et al. [44]	15	Follow-up from 6–51 months. 8/15 responders and 6/15 in remission at last follow-up measured by Montgomery-Asberg Depression Scale (MADRS)
Bewernick et al. [41]	10	At 12 months, 5/10 had achieved >50 % reduction in HDRS scores (i.e., responders). Antidepressant, antianhedonic, and antianxiety effects observed
Inferior Thalamic Peduncle		
Jimenez et al. [50, 51]	1	Double-blind assessment protocol following initial period of 8 months with "on" stimulation. No relapse of depressive symptoms with DBS turned off for 12 months. Sustained remission at 24 months with DBS on
Habenula		
Sartorius et al. [49]	1	Remission of MDD following stimulation of the lateral habenula
Medial Forebrain Bundle		
Schlaepfer et al. [47]	7	>50 % reduction in depression scores in most patients by day 7 post-op, at 12–33 weeks 6/7 responders, 4/7 in remission

MDD Major depressive disorder, *HDRS* Hamilton Depression Rating Scale

key node in the affective circuit, receiving inputs from a diverse range of structures including the medial prefrontal cortex, orbitofrontal cortex, anterior cingulate, nucleus accumbens and insula [36, 37]. Additional projections between the SCC and amygdala underscore the relationship, described above, between mood and it's subcortical regulation by autonomic circuits [6, 36]. Functional imaging studies have shown that the SCC is closely involved in regulating emotions, and in particular negative emotions in both healthy subjects and patients. SCC activity has been linked to the degree of depression, and neurophysiologic studies have confirmed the preferential response of SCC neurons to negative stimuli and decision-making. As a result, the SCC has been proposed as an important node in mood circuitry and the first study of SCC DBS for refractory MDD was performed in 2005. This study included 6 patients and found that at 6-months follow-up, 4 were in remission, and that SCC perfusion, measured using PET, was significantly lower compared to baseline [32]. A larger study, published in 2008 in 20 patients followed to 1-year, found a 50 % response rate [defined as a >50 % reduction in Hamilton Depression Rating (HAMD) Scale scores] [38]. A multicenter study utilizing the same target found a more modest response rate of 29 % at 1-year, which increased to 62 % if treatment response was defined as an improvement in the HAMD by at least 40 % [39]. These results indicated that the majority of patients were either full or partial responders. Similar results were obtained by another group who reported a 50 % response rate with SCC DBS in otherwise refractory patients [40].

9.3.2 Nucleus Accumbens/Ventral Striatum (NAcc/VS)

Given the prominence of anhedonia and deficits in reward processing, there is much interest in modulating reward circuits in MDD. The nucleus accumbens exists at the interface between the striatum and caudate at it's infero-lateral border. There is a robust pre-clinical and human literature linking activity within the NAcc to virtually every element of the reward experience, from anticipation to enjoyment [25–27]. Dopaminergic pathways predominate in the NAcc and it's key mesolimbic afferent projections, namely from the ventral tegmental area, via the medial forebrain bundle (MFB). Modulating these pathways to address pathological anhedonia is the goal of NAcc and ventral striatum (VS) DBS. In one early report, authors found a 50 % response rate following DBS when patients were followed to 1-year, with key metabolic changes in the brain mirroring those detected with SCC DBS [41, 42]. Whether DBS at reward pathways has an influence on dopaminergic transmission

remains to be seen and investigated, although such a symptom-based approached to MDD management could be promising.

An additional target that has been explored is the ventral caudate/ventral striatum, a region that is sometimes used interchangeably with NAcc, given the anatomic location of the latter. VC/VS has previously shown promise as a target in refractory OCD, and further allows the DBS electrode to influence regions close to the anterior limb of the internal capsule, which is the traditional capsulotomy target [43]. In open-label studies to date, results from VC/VS stimulation have been positive, with rates of response and remission at 6-months of 53 and 20 %, respectively [44]. Results from a placebo-controlled, randomized trial of VC/VS DBS in MDD have not yet been published.

9.3.3 Medial Forebrain Bundle (MFB)

Another DBS target in the reward system is the medial forebrain bundle (MFB). The MFB contains both ascending and descending fibers and is a prominent component of the mesolimbic pathway connecting brainstem dopaminergic centers, such as the VTA, with limbic basal ganglia structures, such as NAcc [45]. In animal models, the MFB is most closely associated with the septal nuclei, which were the subject of classic experiments by Olds and Milner, who demonstrated the rewarding effects of intracranial self-stimulation of these structures in rats [46]. One recent paper investigated MFB stimulation in 7 patients with severe, long-standing MDD, and found rapid anti-depressant effects with stimulation [47]. Within 7 days of stimulation onset, 6 patients were treatment responders. This work is currently being expanded to a larger patient cohort, but such results are nevertheless promising and suggest a potentially different anti-depressant mechanism than either SCC or NAcc stimulation, where treatment response is expected to take weeks to months.

9.3.4 Habenula (Hab) and Inferior Thalamic Peduncle (ITP)

Other targets that have been investigated include the habenula and the inferior thalamic peduncle, both components of the brain's reward system. The habenula is a collection of cells in the pineal region divided into medial and lateral components. The lateral habenula has generally been associated with reward processing and receives hippocampal as well as thalamic and Nacc projections [48]. Accordingly, the lateral habenula has been proposed as a DBS target for depression, with at least one case report showing significant improvements in mood following DBS at this target [48, 49].

The inferior thalamic peduncle (ITP), similar to MFB is a reward pathway, suggested to have an important role in both mood and anxiety disorders, such as OCD. The ITP is closely associated with the mediodorsal thalamus, with projections to orbitofrontal regions as well as the amygdala. The first report of ITP DBS in a patient with MDD was published in 2007, and described significant clinical benefit in one patient [50]. An additional paper described results in a mixed population of OCD and MDD patients, and found significant effects on both refractory anxiety and mood, with the MDD patient experiencing a clinical remission [51].

9.4 Future Directions

Results of DBS studies for depression have thus far been promising, but the field's enthusiasm should be tempered by the limited amount of available data and the lack of published blinded, randomized trials. Several of these are currently in progress, and may yet shed light on the role that DBS may play, if any, in the management of the severely depressed patient. There remain, further, many open questions regarding the mechanisms of DBS in MDD, as well which types of patients would benefit from the procedure. Work is currently ongoing to identify biomarkers of depression, whether radiologic, serologic or genetic, that may portend more or less favourable outcomes with neuromodulation. Further, it may be that different regions of the brain may be influencing the same anatomic circuit, supported by the roughly similar rates of response in trials at different targets. Alternatively, it may be that stimulation of some regions, even within the same structure, may yield differential effects, as it is still unclear which stimulation parameters are optimal for which patient.

The future of DBS for MDD will see both technical and conceptual advances. Technical advances will see a miniaturization of the technology, improved battery life, and more streamlined programming, which may make the procedure more efficient, and hence, more attractive for clinicians and patients. Emerging technologies such as optogenetics, nanomedicine and focused ultrasound may further offer alternative means of modulating mood circuits. Conceptual advances will see an improved characterization of the clinical response such that the procedure can be tailored to the patient's clinical picture and anatomy. Such work will help improve the safety and tolerability of DBS, enhance patient outcomes, and provide a clearer picture of the circuitry of major depression.

References

1. Bromet E, Andrade LH, Hwang I, Sampson NA, Alonso J, de Girolamo G, de Graaf R, Demyttenaere K, Hu C, Iwata N, Karam AN, Kaur J, Kostyuchenko S, Lepine JP, Levinson D, Matschinger H, Mora ME, Browne MO, Posada-Villa J, Viana MC, Williams DR, Kessler RC. Cross-national epidemiology of DSM-IV major depressive episode. BMC Med. 2011;9:90. doi:10.1186/1741-7015-9-90.
2. Kessler RC, Berglund P, Demler O, Jin R, Koretz D, Merikangas KR, Rush AJ, Walters EE, Wang PS. The epidemiology of major depressive disorder: results from the National Comorbidity Survey Replication (NCS-R). J Am Med Assoc. 2003;289(23):3095–105. doi:10.1001/jama.289.23.3095.
3. Kessler RC, Petukhova M, Sampson NA, Zaslavsky AM, Wittchen HU. Twelve-month and lifetime prevalence and lifetime morbid risk of anxiety and mood disorders in the United States. Int J Methods Psychiatric Res. 2012;21(3):169–84. doi:10.1002/mpr.1359.

4. Sobocki P, Lekander I, Borgstrom F, Strom O, Runeson B. The economic burden of depression in Sweden from 1997 to 2005. Eur Psychiatry: J Assoc Eur Psychiatrists. 2007;22(3):146–52. doi:10.1016/j.eurpsy.2006.10.006.

5. Berrios GE. Melancholia and depression during the 19th century: a conceptual history. Brit J Psychiatry: J Mental Sci. 1988;153:298–304.

6. Giacobbe P, Mayberg HS, Lozano AM. Treatment resistant depression as a failure of brain homeostatic mechanisms: implications for deep brain stimulation. Exp Neurol. 2009;219(1):44–52. doi:10.1016/j.expneurol.2009.04.028.

7. Trivedi MH, Rush AJ, Wisniewski SR, Nierenberg AA, Warden D, Ritz L, Norquist G, Howland RH, Lebowitz B, McGrath PJ, Shores-Wilson K, Biggs MM, Balasubramani GK, Fava M. Evaluation of outcomes with citalopram for depression using measurement-based care in STAR*D: implications for clinical practice. Am J Psychiatry. 2006;163(1):28–40. doi:10.1176/appi.ajp.163.1.28.

8. Lipsman N, Sankar T, Downar J, Kennedy SH, Lozano AM, Giacobbe P. Neuromodulation for treatment-refractory major depressive disorder. Can Med Assoc J. 2013. doi:10.1503/cmaj.121317.

9. McGrath PJ, Stewart JW, Fava M, Trivedi MH, Wisniewski SR, Nierenberg AA, Thase ME, Davis L, Biggs MM, Shores-Wilson K, Luther JF, Niederehe G, Warden D, Rush AJ. Tranylcypromine versus venlafaxine plus mirtazapine following three failed antidepressant medication trials for depression: a STAR*D report. Am J Psychiatry. 2006;163(9):1531–41 (quiz 1666). doi:10.1176/appi.ajp.163.9.1531.

10. Sackeim HA, Prudic J, Fuller R, Keilp J, Lavori PW, Olfson M. The cognitive effects of electroconvulsive therapy in community settings. Neuropsychopharmacology. Off Publ Am Coll Neuropsychopharmacol. 2007;32 (1):244–54.

11. Lozano AM, Lipsman N. Probing and regulating dysfunctional circuits using deep brain stimulation. Neuron. 2013;77(3):406–24. doi:10.1016/j.neuron.2013.01.020.

12. Deuschl G, Schupbach M, Knudsen K, Pinsker MO, Cornu P, Rau J, Agid Y, Schade-Brittinger C. Stimulation of the subthalamic nucleus at an earlier disease stage of Parkinson's disease: concept and standards of the EARLYSTIM-study. Parkinsonism Relat Disord. 2013;19(1):56–61. doi:10.1016/j.parkreldis.2012.07.004.

13. Follett KA, Weaver FM, Stern M, Hur K, Harris CL, Luo P, Marks WJ Jr, Rothlind J, Sagher O, Moy C, Pahwa R, Burchiel K, Hogarth P, Lai EC, Duda JE, Holloway K, Samii A, Horn S, Bronstein JM, Stoner G, Starr PA, Simpson R, Baltuch G, De Salles A, Huang GD, Reda DJ. Pallidal versus subthalamic deep-brain stimulation for Parkinson's disease. N Engl J Med. 2010;362(22):2077–91. doi:10.1056/NEJMoa0907083.

14. Weaver F, Follett K, Hur K, Ippolito D, Stern M. Deep brain stimulation in Parkinson disease: a metaanalysis of patient outcomes. J Neurosurg. 2005;103(6):956–67. doi:10.3171/jns.2005.103.6.0956.

15. Birley JL. Modified frontal leucotomy: a review of 106 cases. Brit J Psychiatry: J Mental Sci. 1964;110:211–21.

16. Freeman W, Watts JW. Prefrontal lobotomy: the surgical relief of mental pain. Bull NY Acad Med. 1942;18(12):794–812.

17. Freeman W, Watts JW. Psychosurgery. Progress Neurol Psychiatry. 1946;1:649–61.

18. Freeman W, Watts JW. Prefrontal lobotomy; survey of 331 cases. Am J Med Sci. 1946;211:1–8.

19. Cosgrove GR, Rauch SL. Stereotactic cingulotomy. Neurosurg Clin N Am. 2003;14(2):225–35.

20. Spangler WJ, Cosgrove GR, Ballantine HT, Jr, Cassem EH, Rauch SL, Nierenberg A, Price BH. Magnetic resonance image-guided stereotactic cingulotomy for intractable psychiatric disease. Neurosurgery. 1996;38(6):1071–76 (discussion 1076–1078).

21. Shields DC, Asaad W, Eskandar EN, Jain FA, Cosgrove GR, Flaherty AW, Cassem EH, Price BH, Rauch SL, Dougherty DD. Prospective assessment of stereotactic ablative surgery for intractable major depression. Biol Psychiatry. 2008;64(6):449–54. doi:10.1016/j.biopsych.2008.04.009.

22. Steele JD, Christmas D, Eljamel MS, Matthews K. Anterior cingulotomy for major depression: clinical outcome and relationship to lesion characteristics. Biol Psychiatry. 2008;63(7):670–7. doi:10.1016/j.biopsych.2007.07.019.

23. Hurwitz TA, Honey CR, Allen J, Gosselin C, Hewko R, Martzke J, Bogod N, Taylor P. Bilateral anterior capsulotomy for intractable depression. J Neuropsychiatry Clin Neurosci. 2012;24(2):176–82. doi:10.1176/appi.neuropsych.11080191.

24. Christmas D, Eljamel MS, Butler S, Hazari H, MacVicar R, Steele JD, Livingstone A, Matthews K. Long term outcome of thermal anterior capsulotomy for chronic, treatment refractory depression. J Neurol Neurosurg Psychiatry. 2011;82(6):594–600. doi:10.1136/jnnp.2010.217901.

25. Carelli RM. Nucleus accumbens cell firing and rapid dopamine signaling during goal-directed behaviors in rats. Neuropharmacology. 2004;47(1):180–9. doi:10.1016/j.neuropharm.2004.07.017.

26. Martin PD, Ono T. Effects of reward anticipation, reward presentation, and spatial parameters on the firing of single neurons recorded in the subiculum and nucleus accumbens of freely moving rats. Behav Brain Res. 2000;116(1):23–38.

27. Nicola SM, Yun IA, Wakabayashi KT, Fields HL. Firing of nucleus accumbens neurons during the consummatory phase of a discriminative stimulus task depends on previous reward predictive cues. J Neurophysiol. 2004;91(4):1866–82. doi:10.1152/jn.00658.2003.

28. Frank GK, Bailer UF, Henry SE, Drevets W, Meltzer CC, Price JC, Mathis CA, Wagner A, Hoge J, Ziolko S, Barbarich-Marsteller N, Weissfeld L, Kaye WH. Increased dopamine D2/D3 receptor binding after recovery from anorexia nervosa measured by positron emission tomography and [11c]raclopride. Biol Psychiatry. 2005;58(11):908–12. doi:10.1016/j.biopsych.2005.05.003.

29. Kaye WH, Wierenga CE, Bailer UF, Simmons AN, Bischoff-Grethe A. Nothing tastes as good as skinny feels: the neurobiology of anorexia nervosa. Trends Neurosci. 2013;36(2):110–20. doi:10.1016/j.tins.2013.01.003.

30. Mayberg HS. Limbic-cortical dysregulation: a proposed model of depression. J Neuropsychiatry Clin Neurosci. 1997;9(3):471–81.

31. Kennedy SH, Konarski JZ, Segal ZV, Lau MA, Bieling PJ, McIntyre RS, Mayberg HS. Differences in brain glucose metabolism between responders to CBT and venlafaxine in a 16-week randomized controlled trial. Am J Psychiatry. 2007;164(5):778–88. doi:10.1176/appi.ajp.164.5.778.

32. Mayberg HS, Lozano AM, Voon V, McNeely HE, Seminowicz D, Hamani C, Schwalb JM, Kennedy SH. Deep brain stimulation for treatment-resistant depression. Neuron. 2005;45(5):651–60. doi:10.1016/j.neuron.2005.02.014.

33. Lipsman N, Woodside DB, Giacobbe P, Hamani C, Carter JC, Norwood SJ, Sutandar K, Staab R, Elias G, Lyman CH, Smith GS, Lozano AM. Subcallosal cingulate deep brain stimulation for treatment-refractory anorexia nervosa: a phase 1 pilot trial. Lancet. 2013. doi:10.1016/S0140-6736(12)62188-6.

34. Laxton AW, Neimat JS, Davis KD, Womelsdorf T, Hutchison WD, Dostrovsky JO, Hamani C, Mayberg HS, Lozano AM. Neuronal coding of implicit emotion categories in the subcallosal cortex in patients with depression. Biol Psychiatry. 2013. doi:10.1016/j.biopsych.2013.03.029.

35. Lipsman N, Kaping D, Westendorff S, Sankar T, Lozano AM, Womelsdorf T. Beta coherence within human ventromedial prefrontal cortex precedes affective value choices. Neuroimage. 2013. doi:10.1016/j.neuroimage.2013.05.104.

36. Hamani C, Mayberg H, Stone S, Laxton A, Haber S, Lozano AM. The subcallosal cingulate gyrus in the context of major depression. Biol Psychiatry. 2011;69(4):301–8. doi:10.1016/j.biopsych.2010.09.034.

37. Price JL, Drevets WC. Neurocircuitry of mood disorders. Neuropsychopharmacol: Off Publ Am Coll Neuropsychopharmacol. 2010;35(1):192–216. doi:10.1038/npp.2009.104.

38. Lozano AM, Mayberg HS, Giacobbe P, Hamani C, Craddock RC, Kennedy SH. Subcallosal cingulate gyrus deep brain stimulation for treatment-resistant depression. Biol Psychiatry. 2008;64(6):461–7, doi:10.1016/j.biopsych.2008.05.034.

39. Lozano AM, Giacobbe P, Hamani C, Rizvi SJ, Kennedy SH, Kolivakis TT, Debonnel G, Sadikot AF, Lam RW, Howard AK, Ilcewicz-Klimek M, Honey CR, Mayberg HS. A multicenter pilot study of subcallosal cingulate area deep brain stimulation for treatment-resistant depression. J Neurosurg. 2012;116(2):315–22. doi:10.3171/2011.10.JNS102122.

40. Puigdemont D, Perez-Egea R, Portella MJ, Molet J, de Diego-Adelino J, Gironell A, Radua J, Gomez-Anson B, Rodriguez R, Serra M, de Quintana C, Artigas F, Alvarez E, Perez V. Deep brain stimulation of the subcallosal cingulate gyrus: further evidence in treatment-resistant major depression. Int J Neuropsychopharmacol. 2011;1–13. doi:10.1017/S1461145711001088.

41. Bewernick BH, Hurlemann R, Matusch A, Kayser S, Grubert C, Hadrysiewicz B, Axmacher N, Lemke M, Cooper-Mahkorn D, Cohen MX, Brockmann H, Lenartz D, Sturm V, Schlaepfer TE. Nucleus accumbens deep brain stimulation decreases ratings of depression and anxiety in treatment-resistant depression. Biol Psychiatry. 2010;67(2):110–6. doi:10.1016/j.biopsych.2009.09.013.

42. Bewernick BH, Kayser S, Sturm V, Schlaepfer TE. Long-term effects of nucleus accumbens deep brain stimulation in treatment-resistant depression: evidence for sustained efficacy. Neuropsychopharmacol: Off Publ Am Coll Neuropsychopharmacol. 2012;37(9):1975–85. doi:10.1038/npp.2012.44.

43. Aouizerate B, Cuny E, Martin-Guehl C, Guehl D, Amieva H, Benazzouz A, Fabrigoule C, Allard M, Rougier A, Bioulac B, Tignol J, Burbaud P. Deep brain stimulation of the ventral caudate nucleus in the treatment of obsessive-compulsive disorder and major depression. Case report. J Neurosurg. 2004;101(4):682–6. doi:10.3171/jns.2004.101.4.0682.

44. Malone DA Jr, Dougherty DD, Rezai AR, Carpenter LL, Friehs GM, Eskandar EN, Rauch SL, Rasmussen SA, Machado AG, Kubu CS, Tyrka AR, Price LH, Stypulkowski PH, Giftakis JE, Rise MT, Malloy PF, Salloway SP, Greenberg BD. Deep brain stimulation of the ventral capsule/ventral striatum for treatment-resistant depression. Biol Psychiatry. 2009;65(4):267–75. doi:10.1016/j.biopsych.2008.08.029.

45. Coenen VA, Honey CR, Hurwitz T, Rahman AA, McMaster J, Burgel U, Madler B. Medial forebrain bundle stimulation as a pathophysiological mechanism for hypomania in subthalamic nucleus deep brain stimulation for Parkinson's disease. Neurosurgery. 2009;64(6):1106–14 (discussion 1114–1105). doi:10.1227/01.NEU.0000345631.54446.06.

46. Olds J, Milner P. Positive reinforcement produced by electrical stimulation of septal area and other regions of rat brain. J Comp Physiol Psychol. 1954;47(6):419–27.

47. Schlaepfer TE, Bewernick BH, Kayser S, Madler B, Coenen VA. Rapid effects of deep brain stimulation for treatment-resistant major depression. Biol Psychiatry. 2013;73(12):1204–12. doi:10.1016/j.biopsych.2013.01.034.

48. Sartorius A, Henn FA. Deep brain stimulation of the lateral habenula in treatment resistant major depression. Med Hypotheses. 2007;69(6):1305–8. doi:10.1016/j.mehy.2007.03.021.

49. Sartorius A, Kiening KL, Kirsch P, von Gall CC, Haberkorn U, Unterberg AW, Henn FA, Meyer-Lindenberg A. Remission of major depression under deep brain stimulation of the lateral habenula in a therapy-refractory patient. Biol Psychiatry. 2010;67 (2):e9–11. doi:10.1016/j.biopsych.2009.08.027.

50. Jimenez F, Velasco F, Salin-Pascual R, Velasco M, Nicolini H, Velasco AL, Castro G. Neuromodulation of the inferior thalamic peduncle for major depression and obsessive compulsive disorder. Acta Neurochir Suppl. 2007;97(Pt 2):393–8.

51. Jimenez F, Nicolini H, Lozano AM, Piedimonte F, Salin R, Velasco F. Electrical stimulation of the inferior thalamic peduncle in the treatment of major depression and obsessive compulsive disorders. World Neurosurg. 2012. doi:10.1016/j.wneu.2012.07.010.

52. Kennedy SH, Giacobbe P, Rizvi SJ, Placenza FM, Nishikawa Y, Mayberg HS, Lozano AM. Deep brain stimulation for treatment-resistant depression: follow-up after 3 to 6 years. Am J Psychiatry. 2011;168 (5):502–10. doi:10.1176/appi.ajp.2010.10081187.

53. Holtzheimer PE, Kelley ME, Gross RE, Filkowski MM, Garlow SJ, Barrocas A, Wint D, Craighead MC, Kozarsky J, Chismar R, Moreines JL, Mewes K, Posse PR, Gutman DA, Mayberg HS. Subcallosal cingulate deep brain stimulation for treatment-resistant unipolar and bipolar depression. Arch Gen Psychiatry. 2012;69(2):150–8. doi:10.1001/archgenpsychiatry.2011.1456.

54. Schlaepfer TE, Cohen MX, Frick C, Kosel M, Brodesser D, Axmacher N, Joe AY, Kreft M, Lenartz D, Sturm V. Deep brain stimulation to reward circuitry alleviates anhedonia in refractory major depression. Neuropsychopharmacol: Off Publ Am Coll Neuropsychopharmacol. 2008;33 (2):368–77. doi:10.1038/sj.npp.1301408.

Ablative Surgery for Obsessive-Compulsive Disorders

10

Roberto Martinez-Alvarez

Abstract

Intractable OCD and depression cause tremendous suffering. An estimated 20 % of patients remain severely affected in spite of the best available medication and behavioural therapies. Existing data suggest that lesion procedures can benefit a large proportion (ranging from about 60 to 80 %) of patients with medically intractable OCD. Long-term serious adverse events are very infrequent. Functional neuroimaging studies play an extremely important role in understanding the mechanisms of disease development and therapeutic action. Our experience over the past 10 years provides evidence that the most recent lesion procedures are even safer, alleviate suffering, and improve the quality of life of patients with these disabling disorders.

10.1 Introduction

Obsessive-compulsive disorder (OCD) affects 2–3 % of the population; there are some six million patients in the United States alone [36]. Prevalence is similar in other countries and cultures [39]. Features of the disorder are recurring notions, termed "obsessions", that are a source of distress and can result in patients' being unable to function; "compulsions", described as the ineluctable need to carry out actions that gratify the obsessions, commonly associated with guilt and anxiety; and "rituals", i.e., performing repetitive, mechanical actions likewise related to the obsessions. Onset of this disorder takes place in the first few decades of life, commonly starting in adolescence. Symptoms gradually increase and can prevent patients from being able to carry out activity of any kind at all [1]. In the past 20 years OCD has been the tenth cause of disability worldwide, according to statistics released by the World Health Organization. There is a genetic component to the disorder, with the likelihood that a first-degree relative of a patient will have the disorder being three times greater than the reported incidence [12].

Current behavioural and pharmacological therapies are far from universally effective. Selective serotonin reuptake inhibitors (SSRIs) are the mainstays of pharmacological treatment. Clo mipramine, a tricyclic antidepressant and a potent but non-serotonin reuptake inhibitor, is a second-line agent. Typical and atypical neuroleptics have

R. Martinez-Alvarez (✉)
Functional Neurosurgery and Radiosurgery Department, Ruber International Hospital, Madrid, Spain
e-mail: rob.martinez@telefonica.net

B. Sun and A. De Salles (eds.), *Neurosurgical Treatments for Psychiatric Disorders*,
DOI 10.1007/978-94-017-9576-0_10
© Shanghai Jiao Tong University Press, Shanghai and Springer Science+Business Media Dordrecht 2015

been effective in controlled studies but impose the additional burden of unwanted secondary effects. Even when effective, undesirable effects may substantially limit the treatment compliance usually required for ongoing relief of symptoms. An estimated 20 % of patients remain severely affected, even when the best available medication and behavioural therapies are brought to bear [16, 17, 38]. This group suffers from intractable OCD, a source of tremendous suffering [1] and overall functional impairment. For this group, surgical treatment is the next step.

10.2 Historical Background

Surgical techniques for treating psychiatric illnesses by creating lesions in the frontal lobes have been around since the 1930s. These lesions produced in patients a certain disconnect from their milieu and their inhibitions, typical of large frontal lobe lesions. Dr. António Egas Moniz was awarded the Nobel Prize for developing the "frontal leucotomy" procedure [5]. In the 1940s various groups of neurosurgeons and psychiatrists developed more refined methods of producing lesions at different sites in the frontal lobe. Specifically, Freeman and Watts launched a "crusade" advocating Freeman's leucotomy procedure, with dire consequences that still haunt the memories of some psychiatrists even today [14]. At the present time these procedures have been abandoned, and they are unrelated to the treatments discussed in this chapter.

10.3 Current Concepts

The purpose of neurosurgical procedures used to treat psychiatric disorders is to improve a series of specific symptoms caused by mental illnesses, the same purpose that informs their use in treatments in response to other functional disorders, such as pain and abnormal movements. This type of surgery involves making specific lesions to disconnect the limbic system circuits related to the different psychiatric disorders [13, 18]. Blocking certain interconnecting pathways enhances brain function, with patients experiencing relief of certain symptoms without undergoing alterations in their personalities, and their cognitive functions ordinarily improve [6, 37].

10.3.1 Neuroanatomy, Brain Connectivity, and Neurosurgical Techniques

Functional neuroimaging findings relating to OCD have laid the theoretical foundation for surgical procedures intended to alleviate OCD. These studies constitute the groundwork for the now well-established identification of anatomical projections reaching into the caudate nucleus from the orbitofrontal cortex and the cingulum [4, 44]. Patients in a resting state examined using PET and SPECT show heightened metabolic activity in the orbitofrontal cortex, cingulate cortex, and caudate nucleus. Furthermore, metabolic activity in these regions has been observed to return to normal levels in patients who improve in response to pharmacological or behavioural therapy.

Functional MR neuroimaging has also revealed hyperactivity in the cortical-striatal-thalamic circuit, including the orbitofrontal cortex and caudate nucleus [8]. These findings indicate that the basal ganglia are not functioning properly, giving rise to changes in other structures. Combining neuropsychology and functional MRI has improved our understanding of these alterations and allows us to select the most suitable targets for surgery [32].

Modern procedures enabling functional MRI and tractography guided stereotactic ablation and the use of special computer software for guidance make it possible to create lesions in the pathways interconnecting the limbic system with ever greater precision and safety (Fig. 10.1) [15, 18]. The lesions currently effected by our team, which has gained extensive experience over the past 20 years, are:

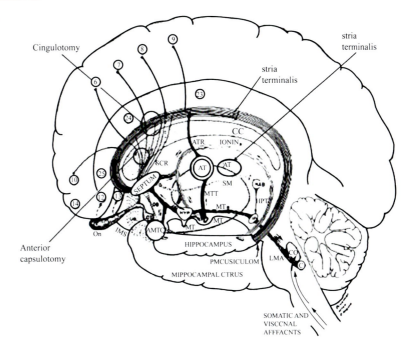

Fig. 10.1 Diagram of the brain through the midsagittal plane showing the locations of capsulotomy (*cap*), cingulotomy (*c*), and stria terminalis (*ST*) lesioning

10.3.1.1 Anterior Capsulotomy

A lesion is created in the anterior limb of the internal capsule starting at the frontal horn of the lateral ventricle along the head of the caudate nucleus (Fig. 10.2). The genu of the capsule stands out clearly in sagittal views, and the lesion is made in this region. We tend to start the lesions in the posterior part of the limb at the level of the anterior commissure, moving in an anterior direction at higher levels. Bilateral lesions are produced, in most cases by performing two overlapping thermocoagulations on each side, using an electrode 4 mm long and 2 mm in diameter (Elekta Instruments®).

10.3.1.2 Anterior Cingulotomy

Lesions are effected in the anterior cingulum adjacent to Brodman areas 24 and 32 (Fig. 10.1) and may be unilateral or bilateral [2, 20, 25]. We currently use tractography to locate the cingulum and to verify the degree of disconnection achieved. Thermal lesions are made using an

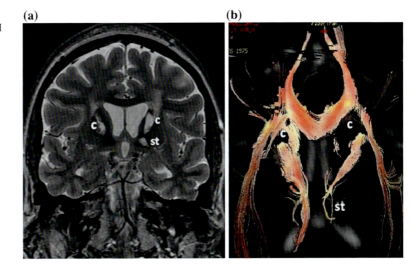

Fig. 10.2 Coronal MRI (**a**) and an overlay of MRI and tractography in the axial projection (**b**) after bilateral anterior capsulotomy (*c*) and stria terminalis (*st*) lesioning

electrode 4 mm long and 2 mm in diameter. The lesions we make are smaller than those previously described and are restricted exclusively to the cingulum.

10.3.1.3 Stria Terminalis Lesioning

This procedure was described in the 1970s and has been developed by Dr. Juan Burzaco, with good results [32]. The stria in the external, posterior part of the frontal horn 2 mm lateral, 1 mm anterior, and 1 mm superior to the anterior commissure is located (Fig. 10.2). This procedure is useful in alleviating the aggressive behaviour and depression that is sometimes associated with obsessions. Lesioning is ordinarily carried out in the tract on the left side. In contrast to the two previous procedures, simultaneous bilateral lesioning may give rise to such adverse secondary effects as hyperthermia, confusion, and persistent nausea-vomiting lasting up to a week. An electrode 4 mm long and 1 mm in diameter (Elekta Instruments®) is used.

10.3.1.4 Combined Lesioning

Unlike neurostimulation, stereotactic ablative surgery allows various lesion procedures to be combined in a single intervention. In cases of OCD associated with depression or anxiety, we perform bilateral anterior capsulotomy together with bilateral anterior cingulotomy. If compulsions and aggression are also a major component, left stria terminalis lesioning is added to the other two procedures.

Other teams have used two additional lesion procedures:

10.3.1.5 Subcaudate Tractotomy

Neurosurgical lesions are produced in the *substantia innominata*, an area ventral to the caudate nucleus, containing neuronal cell bodies with connections similar to those in the ventral portions of the striatum and the *globus pallidus*. Lesions are created in the fibres that connect the thalamus to the orbitofrontal cortex and cingulated gyrus [7, 27, 46].

10.3.1.6 Limbic Leucotomy

This procedure combines subcaudate tractotomy and anterior cingulotomy [21].

10.3.2 Gamma Knife Radiosurgery

We have performed capsulotomies and cingulotomies using Gamma Knife radiosurgery (Elekta Instruments®). With our equipment, 192 beams of gamma radiation emitted by Cobalt-60 sources are focused on the target to be treated, the lesions can be located in the posteriormost areas of the anterior limb of the internal capsule (Fig. 10.3) or in the cingulum (Fig. 10.4) [23, 33]. The radiation dose of the individual beams is low, but focusing 192 beams with high precision so that they converge on a single point for exposure times of several hours subjects the selected anatomical site to doses equal to or greater than 120 Gy, producing a lesion at the desired point while at the same time achieving low adjacent radiation exposure. The primary advantage of this technique is that it obviates having to make any incisions in the skull.

Fig. 10.3 Axial (**a**) and coronal (**b**) MRI 18 months after bilateral anterior capsulotomy performed by Gamma knife radiosurgery

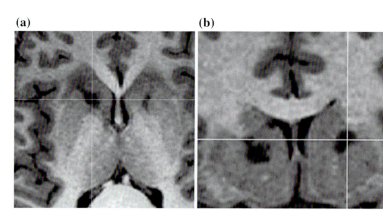

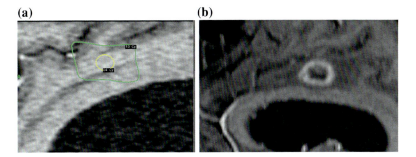

Fig. 10.4 Cingulotomy performed by gamma knife radiosurgery: dose planning (**a**) and MRI follow-up one year later (**b**)

10.4 Clinical Course and Procedure Results

Results are to be assessed at least six months after surgery, and changes in patient condition take place up to two years after the procedure [34]. There are scales for rating OCD symptoms, the most common being the Yale-Brown obsessive compulsive scale (Y-BOCS). The Beck and Hamilton scales are also used, to rate anxiety, along with scales to rate quality of life, Lehman's quality of life (QOL) scale being the one most commonly employed.

10.4.1 Anterior Capsulotomy

Initial results reported by Dr. L. Leksell yielded favourable responses in 50 % of OCD cases [19, 29]. Later series of patients treated from the 1970s to 1990s achieved improvement in 70 % of OCD patients undergoing the procedure [35, 40, 45]. Results for recent series have been consistent with these latter success rates, with fewer adverse effects [30, 41]. Outcomes for patients treated by Gamma Knife radiosurgery reported by the Karolinska Institute team have been similar [23].

Immediate undesirable secondary effects associated with this procedure are transient, lasting three to six months, and include headache, transient urinary incontinence, impaired cognitive function, especially memory, and confusion. Focal neurological deficits associated with haemorrhage and tardive epileptic seizures have been observed in 3 % of cases [10, 35].

10.4.2 Subcaudate Tractotomy

Series published from the 1970s to the 1990s yielded a significant percentage improvement in around 50 % of OCD cases, with good results in 40 % of patients suffering from anxiety. Epileptic seizures in 2 % of cases were the most frequent adverse effect apart from initial, transient symptoms similar to those reported for capsulotomy [27].

10.4.3 Anterior Cingulotomy

Large series have been reported over the past 40 years, with improvement rates in OCD patients ranging between 56 and 36 % of cases [3, 20]. For the most recent published series there were complete long-term responses in 47 % of cases and partial responses in 22 % [11]. Anxiety improved to a large extent, specifically in 43 % of cases in the most recent series [26, 43]. Immediate, transient symptoms have included headache, confusion, and urinary incontinence. Tardive epileptic seizures have affected up to 9 % of cases in some series. With modern targeting procedures this unwanted effect has now decreased considerably.

10.4.4 Limbic Leucotomy

Initial results were extremely encouraging, with 89 % of OCD patients improving [22]. In more recent studies the improvement rate for OCD patients has reached 80 % [9, 24]. Adverse effects include drowsiness for variable lengths of

10.5 Our Results

Over the past 10 years our team has operated on 100 OCD patients with suitable follow-up of cases; current mean follow-up is six years. Obsessions and compulsions underwent significant improvement in 71 % of the OCD cases treated. Improvement was evidenced by a sustained decrease of more than 50 % in the Y-BOCS score. Overall, quality of life in these patients improved in 75 % of cases as measured by Lehman's quality of life (QOL) scale in late follow-up, with scores increasing by 50 % or more [32].

Transient symptoms observed for time periods of between two and six months have included confusion, some degree of cognitive impairment, urinary incontinence, fever of central origin, nausea-vomiting, hallucinations, heightened response to psychotropic medication, and tardive depression. Haemorrhagic lesions were observed in 5 % of cases, requiring intervention in two cases (40 % of the patients with bleeding), infections were recorded in 2 % of cases, and epileptic seizures were observed in 4 % of formerly seizure-free patients.

Results are attained gradually over the course of the two years following surgery, as confusion and cognitive impairment improve. In 30 % of cases patient condition worsened, making a second surgery necessary. In the cases that underwent a second surgical intervention, improvement was similar to the rate achieved after the first procedure.

10.6 Gamma Knife Radiosurgery

10.6.1 Bilateral Anterior Capsulotomy

There have been few published series since the 1960s [23, 28, 29, 31, 33, 42]. With improvements in imaging definition, the precision of lesion localization has increased, with less damage to more posterior areas of the thalamus. Symptoms improve without collateral effects to the extent that surgery succeeds in cutting off only the anterior limb of the internal capsule by locating the target in the area that includes the medial connections of the internal capsule between the thalamus and the basal frontal region visualized by functional MRI. For cases with the proper indications, outcomes are similar to those attained using open ablative procedures, that is, significant improvement in 70 % of cases. Changes appear in patients from between six months to a year after treatment, and our team has not observed any adverse effects, though cognitive impairment and other disorders such as apathy (indifference towards one's surroundings) have been reported in a significant number of cases in earlier series with long-term follow-up [9]. These effects have been related to the presence of lesions in the posterior and basal regions of the thalamus.

Our series includes five patients suffering from OCD treated by capsulotomies carried out using a Gamma Knife and followed up for from one to six years. We observed better than 50 % improvement in the Y-BOCS score in all cases one year after the procedure without adverse effects, while follow-up MRI visualized the lesions without disclosing any damage to peripheral structures. Our team stands out for its use of a maximum dose (120 Gy) lower than previously reported doses and for employing tractography in the planning stage in all cases [33].

10.7 Conclusions and Future Outlook

Optimum indications for performing these procedures are conditions suitable for the creation of localized lesions capable of disconnecting the limbic system circuits related to a variety of psychiatric disorders. We have made appreciable progress along this path, and both stimulation of different brain centres and disconnection of the pathways interconnecting them hold out the potential of solving a significant proportion of psychiatric illnesses that do not respond to pharmacological therapy. Specifically, for OCD there is sufficient evidence to support the view that stereotactic surgery using ablation or radiosurgery is a safe, efficacious option for treating cases refractory to medication and cognitive therapy.

As is the case with other surgical procedures, adverse effects and complications have been gradually decreasing, and these lesioning techniques are gaining increasing acceptance by the psychiatric profession. The outcomes achieved, in particular the improved quality of life of patients, have amazed recent cohorts of psychiatrists.

The objective of our work is to unsettle psychiatrists, psychologists, neurophysiologists, and radiologists more and more and thereby to encourage them to form multidisciplinary teams that will work together to make this type of surgery progressively more efficacious, safe, well known, and commonplace in all sectors of the psychiatric profession.

References

1. Alonso P, Segalas C, Real E, Pertusa A, Labad J, Jiménez-Murcia S, Jaurrieta N, Bueno B, Vallejo J, Menchón JM. Suicide in patients treated for obsessive-compulsive disorder: a prospective follow-up study. J Affect Disord. 2010;124:300–8.
2. Ballantine HT. Stereotactic anterior cingulotomy for neuropsychiatric illness and intractable pain. J Neurosurg. 1967;26:488–95.
3. Ballantine HT Jr, Bouckoms AJ, Thomas EK, Giriunas IE. Treatment of psychiatric illness by stereotactic cingulotomy. Biol Psychiatry. 1987;22:807–19.
4. Baxter LR Jr, Schwartz JM, Bergman KS, Szuba MP, Guze BH, Mazziotta JC, Alazraki A, Selin CE, Huan-Kwang F, Munford P, Michael P. Caudate glucose metabolic rate changes with both drug and behavior therapy for obsessivecompulsive disorder. Arch Gen Psychiatry. 1992;49:681–9.
5. Berrios GE. The origins of psychosurgery: Shaw, Burckhardt and Moniz. Hist Psychiatr. 1997;8:61–81.
6. Binder DK, Iskandar BJ. Modern neurosurgery for psychiatric disorders. Neurosurgery. 2000;47:9–21.
7. Bridges PK, Bartlett JR, Hale AS, Poynton AM, Malizia AL, Hodgkiss AD. Psychosurgery:

stereotactic subcaudate tractomy. An indispensable treatment. Brit J Psychiatry. 1994;165:599–611.
8. Cannistraro PA, Makris N, Howard JD, Wedig MM, Hodge SM, Wilhelm S, Kennedy DN, Rauch SL. A diffusion tensor imaging study of white matter in obsessive-compulsive disorder. Depress Anxiety. 2007;24:440–6.
9. Cho DY, Lee WY, Chen CC. Limbic leukotomy for intractable major affective disorders: a 7-year follow-up study using nine comprehensive psychiatric test evaluations. J Clin Neurosci. 2008;15:138–42.
10. D'Astous M, Cottin S, Roy M, Picard C, Cantin L. Bilateral stereotactic anterior capsulotomy for obsessive-compulsive disorder: long-term follow-up. J Neurol Neurosurg Psychiatry. 2013;84:1208–13.
11. Dougherty DD, Baer L, Cosgrove GR, Cassem EH, Price BH, Nierenberg AA, Jenike MA, Rauch SL. Prospective long-term follow-up of 44 patients who received cingulotomy for treatment-refractory obsessive-compulsive disorder. Am J Psychiatry. 2002;159:269–75.
12. Eisen JL, Goodman WK, Keller MB, Warshaw MG, DeMarco LM, Luce DD, Rasmussen SA. Patterns of remission and relapse in obsessive-compulsive disorder: a 2 year prospective study. J Clin Psychiatry. 1999;60:346–52.
13. Feldman RP, Alterman RL, Goodrich JT. Contemporary psychosurgery and a look to the future. J Neurosurg. 2001;95:944–56.
14. Freeman W, Watts J, Hunt TC. Psychosurgery: intelligence, emotion and social behavior following prefontal lobotomy for mental disorders. Springfield: Bailliére, Tindall & Cox; 1942.
15. Gaviria M, Ade B. What functional neurosurgery can offer to psychiatric patients: a neuropsychiatric perspective. Surg Neurol. 2009;71:337–43.
16. Greenberg BD, Price LH, Rauch SL, Friehs G, Noren G, Malone D, Carpenter LL, Rezai AR, Rasmussen SA. Neurosurgery for intractable obsessive-compulsive disorder and depression: critical issues. Neurosurg Clin N Am. 2003;14:199–212.
17. Greenberg BD, Rauch SL, Haber SN. Invasive circuitry-based neurotherapeutics: stereotactic ablation and deep brain stimulation for OCD. Neuropsychopharmacology. 2010;35:317–36.
18. Heller AC, Amar AP, Liu ChY, Apuzzo ML. Surgery of the mind and mood: a mosaic of issues in time and evolution. Neurosurgery. 2006;59:720–39.
19. Herner T. Treatment of mental disorders with frontal stereotactic thermolesions: a follow-up of 116 cases. Acta Psychiatrica Scand. 1961;58(36):1–140.
20. Jenike MA, Baer L, Ballantine T, Martuza RL, Tynes S, Giriunas I, Buttolph ML, Cassem NH. Cingulotomy for refractory obsessive-compulsive disorder. A long-term follow-up of 33 patients. Arch Gen Psychiatry. 1991;48:548–55.
21. Kelly D, Richardson A, Mitchell-Heggs N. Stereotactic limbic leucotomy: neurophysiological aspects and operative technique. Brit J Psychiatry. 1973;123:133–40.

22. Kelly D, Richardson A, Mitchell-Heggs N, Greenup J, Chen C, Hafner RJ. Stereotactic limbic leucotomy: a preliminary report on forty patients. Brit J Psychiatry. 1973;123:141–8.
23. Kihlström L, Hindmarsh T, Lax I, Lippitz B, Mindus P, Lindquist C. Radiosurgical lesions in the normal human brain 17 years after gamma knife capsulotomy. Neurosurgery. 1997;41(2):396–401.
24. Kim MC, Lee TK, Choi CR. Review of long-term results of stereotactic psychosurgery. Neurol Med Chir (Tokyo). 2002;42:365–71.
25. Kim CH, Chang JW, Koo MS, Kim JW, Suh HS, Park IH, Lee HS. Anterior cingulotomy for refractory obsessive-compulsive disorder. Acta Psychiatrica Scand. 2003;07:283–90.
26. Kim MC, Lee TK. Stereotactic lesioning for mental illness. Acta Neurochir Suppl. 2008;101:39–43.
27. Knight G. Further observations from an experience of 660 cases of stereotactic tractotomy. Postgrad Med J. 1973;49:845–54.
28. Kondziolka D, Flickinger JC, Hudak R. Results following gamma knife radiosurgical anterior capsulotomies for Obsessive Compulsive Disorder. Neurosurgery. 2011;68:28–33.
29. Leksell L. Modern concepts in pshchiatric surgery. Amsterdam: Elsevier; 1979.
30. Liu K, Zhang H, Liu Ch, Guan Y, Lang L, Cheng Y, Sun B, Wang H, Zuo Ch, Pan L, Xu H, Li S, Shi L, Qian J, Yang Y. Stereotactic treatment of refractory obsessive compulsive disorder by bilateral capsulotomy with 3 years follow-up. J Clin Neuros. 2008;15:622–9.
31. Lopes AC, Greenberg B, Norén G, Montes Canteras M, Busatto G, Mathis ME, Taub A, Chaubet C, Queiroz M, Sauerbronn F, Cecconi J, Gentil A, Arzeno Y, Fuentes D, Campi de Castro C, Leite C, Salvajoli J, Duran F, Rasmussen S. Treatment of resistant obsessive-compulsive disorder with ventral capsular/ventral striatal gamma capsulotomy: a pilot prospective study. J Neuropsychiatry Clin Neurosci. 2009;21:381–92.
32. Martínez R. Psicocirugía ablativa. In: García de Sola R, García Navarrete E, editors. Neurocirugia Funcional y Estereotáctica. Viguera, Barcelona; 2011.
33. Martínez R, Cruz MA. Radiocirugía en trastornos psiquiátricos In: Samblas J, Sallabanda K, Martinez R, Calvo FA, editors. Radiocirugia: Fundamentos, avances tecnológicos, indicaciones y resultados. Aran, Madrid; 2012.
34. Mindus P, Rasmussen SA, Lindquist C. Neurosurgical treatment for refractory obsessive-compulsive disorder: implications for understanding frontal lobe function. J Neuropsychiatry Clin Neurosci. 1994;6:467–77.
35. Mindus P, Meyerson BA. In: Schmideck HH, Sweet WH, editors. Operative neurosurgical tecniques. Indications, methods and results, 3rd edn. WB Saunders: Philadelphia; 1995. p. 1443–54.
36. Narrow WE. Revised prevalence estimates of mental disorders in the United States: using a clinical significance criterion to reconcile surveys stimates. Arch Gen Psychiatry. 2002;59:115–23.
37. Nyman H, Andreewitch S, Lundback E, Mindus P. Executive and cognitive functions in patients with extreme obsessive-compulsive disorder treated by capsulotomy. Appl Neuropsychol. 2001;8:91–8.
38. Pallanti S, Quercioli L. Treatment-refractory obsessive-compulsive disorder: methodological issues, operational definitions and therapeutic lines. Prog Neuropsychopharmacol Biol Psychiatry. 2006;30:400–12.
39. Rasmussen SA, Eisen JL. The epidemiology and clinical features of obsessive compulsive disorder. Psychiatr Clin North Am. 1992;15:743–58.
40. Rück C, Karlsson A, Steele JD, Edman G, Meyerson BA, Ericson K, Nyman H, Asberg M, Svanborg P. Capsulotomy for obsessive-compulsive disorder: long-term follow-up of 25 patients. Arch Gen Psychiatry. 2008;65:914–22.
41. Ruck C, Larsson KJ, Mataix-Cols D. Predictors of medium and long-term outcome following capsulotomy for obsessive-compulsive disorder: one site may not fit all. Eur Neuropsychopharmacol. 2012;22:406–14.
42. Sheehan JP, Patterson G, Schlesinger D, Xu Z. Gamma knife surgery anterior capsulotomy for severe and refractory obsessive-compulsive disorder. J Neurosurg. 2013;119(5):1112–8.
43. Sheth SA, Neal J, Tangherlini F, Mian MK, Gentil A, Cosgrove GR, Eskandar EN, Dougherty DD. Limbic system surgery for treatment-refractory obsessive-compulsive disorder: a prospective long-term follow-up of 64 patients. J Neurosurg. 2013;118:491–7.
44. Vago DR, Epstein J, Catenaccio E, Stern E. Identification of neural targets for the treatment of psychiatric disorders: the role of functional neuroimaging. Neurosurg Clin N Am. 2011; 22:279–305.
45. Waziri R. Psychosurgery for anxiety and obsessive-compulsive disorders. In: Burrows GD, Noyes Jr R, Roth M, editors. Handbook of anxiety: the treatment of anxiety. Amsterdam: Elsevier;1990. p. 519–35.
46. Woerdeman PA, Willems PW, Noordmans HJ, Berkelbach van der Sprenkel JW, van Rijen PC. Frameless stereotactic subcaudate tractotomy for intractable obsessive-compulsive disorder. Acta Neurochir (Wien). 2006;148:633–7.

DBS for Obsessive-Compulsive Disorder

11

Mayur Sharma, Emam Saleh, Milind Deogaonkar and Ali Rezai

Keywords

Neuromodulation · Deep brain stimulation · Obsessive-compulsive disorder · Psychosurgery

Abbreviations

DBS	Deep brain stimulation
OCD	Obsessive-compulsive disorder
Y-BOCS	Yale-Brown obsessive compulsive scale
fMRI	Functional magnetic resonance imaging
PET	Positron emission tomography
NAcc	Nucleus accumbens
STN	Subthalamic nucleus
ALIC	Anterior limb of internal capsule
Vc/Vs	Ventral capsule and ventral striatum
ITP	Inferior thalamic peduncle
Gpi	Globus pallidus internus

M. Sharma
Center of Neuromodulation, Wexner Medical Center, The Ohio State University, 410 W 10th Ave, Room 1047, Columbus, OH 43210, USA
e-mail: Mayur.Sharma@osumc.edu

E. Saleh · M. Deogaonkar
Department of Neurosurgery, Center of Neuromodulation, Wexner Medical Center, The Ohio State University, 480 Medical Center Drive, Columbus, OH 43210, USA
e-mail: Emam.saleh@osumc.edu

M. Deogaonkar
e-mail: Milind.deogaonkar@osumc.edu

A. Rezai (✉)
Neuroscience Program and Center for Neuromodulation, Wexner Medical Center, The Ohio State University, 480 Medical Center Drive, Columbus, OH 43210, USA
e-mail: Ali.Rezai@osumc.edu

11.1 Introduction

According to Diagnostic and Statistical Manual of Mental disorders, fifth edition (DSM-V), Obsessive compulsive disorder (OCD) is characterized by persistent obsessions with intrusive thoughts leading to severe generalized anxiety and/or compulsions in the form of repetitive tasks to relieve this distress. OCD is often associated with depression and other co-morbidities [1]. There is also an increase in the incidence of suicidal ideation and suicide among patients with OCD [2, 3]. OCD is a chronic and severe disabling heterogeneous disorder that has a significant impact on the life of patients and their families with public health consequences. It affects approximately 2–3 % of population in the United States and worldwide and is the 10th

B. Sun and A. De Salles (eds.), *Neurosurgical Treatments for Psychiatric Disorders*,
DOI 10.1007/978-94-017-9576-0_11
© Shanghai Jiao Tong University Press, Shanghai and Springer Science+Business Media Dordrecht 2015

leading cause of disability worldwide [1, 4–8]. OCD affects both genders equally [7, 8]. Pharmacological [Selective Serotonin reuptake inhibitors (SSRIs)] and non-pharmacological therapies such as cognitive behavior therapy (CBT) are the first line treatment options in patients with medical refractory OCD [9, 10]. These modalities are effective in approximately 50 % of patients with 40–60 % reduction in OCD symptoms [6, 11]. However, 10–25 % of these refractory patients have persistent OCD symptoms despite aggressive pharmacotherapy and behavior therapy [5, 9, 12, 13].

Neurosurgical management of various psychiatric disorders including OCD can be dated back to the origin of this specialty. However, availability of effective pharmacotherapy with a higher incidence of surgical morbidity/mortality and limited understanding of the pathophysiology of these disorders, led to the rapid fall of psychoneurosurgery. Technological advances and evolution of neuroimaging techniques revived interest in the neurosurgical management of patients with medical refractory psychiatric disorders. Integration of stereotaxis, neuroimaging and electrophysiology not only improved our understanding of OCD pathophysiology but also made it possible to aim different target or targets with submillimetric accuracy. Ablative (capsulotomy, cingulotomy, subcaudate tractotomy and limbic leucotomy) or neuromodulation (DBS) techniques have been utilized in the surgical management of patients with refractory OCD with varied success. Reversibility, adjustability, adaptability and ability to blind the stimulation for research studies are the advantages of DBS therapy over ablative surgeries. Till now over 100 patients underwent DBS implantation surgery for medical refractory OCD and DBS for OCD has been granted a humanitarian device exemption (HDE) status by FDA in 2009 [14–17]. In this chapter, we have focused on the DBS therapy for OCD, historical aspects of psychoneurosurgery, pathophysiology and involved circuits, surgical techniques, different anatomical targets for OCD and ethical consideration with an overview of the pertinent literature.

11.2 Deep Brain Stimulation (DBS) for OCD

DBS is a reversible, adjustable and a well-accepted surgical therapy for patients with medical refractory movement disorders. The success of DBS therapy in movement disorders with over 100,000 implants in the last couple of decades led clinicians to explore this treatment option for patients with medical refractory OCD. Psychosurgery has evolved over the years following a torment past. Surgery for psychiatric disorders was first presented in a scientific meeting in 1889. Talairach first presented the stereotactic guided targeting of the frontothalamic fibers in the internal capsule at the 4th international neurology congress in Paris in 1943. In 1950s, various researchers performed experimental DBS in patients with refractory psychiatric disorders with an intent to reduce the severity of clinical symptoms [18, 19]. Stimulation of the area near the parafascicular complex and cerebellar vermis has been shown to ameliorate OCD symptoms by targeting neural circuits in patients with refractory OCD [16, 20]. These initial studies fostered with advances in imaging and technology pushed the frontiers of psychosurgery. Subsequently in 2009, DBS for OCD has been granted a humanitarian device exemption status by FDA [14–17]. The advantages of DBS in terms of reversibility, adjustability as per patient's requirements, excellent safety profile and ability to enroll patients in cross over blinded research studies to determine the efficacy of DBS, made neurostimulation surgery an attractive treatment option for patients with severe medical refractory OCD. Till date, over 100 patients underwent DBS implantation surgery for OCD. However, results from these studies need to be cautiously interpreted due to challenges such as heterogeneous cohort of patients with medical refractory OCD, non-uniform assessment criterion, prolonged titration intervals and practical implication for patients travelling from far-off places for titration.

The exact mechanism of action of DBS therapy is still elusive. It is widely believed that DBS therapy works similar to ablation therapy by inducing neuronal inhibition by depolarizing neurons in the vicinity of a stimulating electrode [21]. Contrary to this, recent studies supported that high frequency stimulation results in axonal excitation which subsequently blocks the pathological bursting and oscillatory activity [21]. Synaptic inhibition, synaptic depression, depolarization blockade and stimulation-induced modulation of pathological network activity are the putative mechanisms underlying the efficacy of DBS [22, 23]. DBS therapy has also been shown to improve the fidelity of thalamocortical neurons and to modulate the pathological cognitive-behavior-emotional circuit [24].

Advances in neuroimaging, Neuronavigation techniques coupled with improved understanding of the intricate neural circuits implicated in the pathophysiology of OCD, enabled neurosurgeons to target various nodal points to modulate these pathological neural circuits. Anterior limb of internal capsule (ALIC), Ventral Capsule/Ventral striatum (Vc/Vs), Nucleus accumbens (Nu Acc), subthalamic nucleus (STN) and Inferior thalamic peduncle have been investigated as potential DBS targets in various research studies to benefit patients with medical refractory OCD.

11.2.1 Anterior Limb of Internal Capsule (ALIC)

Based on the beneficial effects of anterior capsulotomy in patients with refractory OCD, ALIC was the first target to be selected for DBS therapy [25, 26]. The fibers connecting the orbitofrontal, subgenual anterior cingulate cortex, medial dorsomedial and anterior thalamic nuclei courses through the anterior limb of the internal capsule and therefore ALIC could be a potential surgical node to modulate this neural circuit. This target was first explored by Nuttin et al. [25] in 1999 in 4 patients with medical refractory OCD with the target coordinates similar to that used for capsulotomies. In this controlled study, 75 % of patients (3 out of 4) experienced reduction in their obsessive compulsive symptoms. However, this improvement was not quantified using clinical scales and 1 patient experienced 90 %

improvement in her OCD symptoms following 2 weeks of stimulation in this study. In 2003 and 2008, same group published significant improvement in Y-BOCS and GAF scales in 6 patients with medical refractory OCD who underwent bilateral ALIC-DBS [27, 28]. In this double blind controlled study, >35 % reduction in Y-BOCS score compared to baseline was considered as a "responder" criterion. 3 of 4 patients who entered the assessment phase in this study, reported significant improvement in mean Y-BOCS (DBS off: 32.2; on: 19.8) and clinical global severity scores (DBS off: 5; on: 3.3) following DBS stimulation which worsened in the DBS "off" state [27, 28]. This reduction in core OCD symptoms following DBS was observed 21 months after surgery in patients with medical refractory OCD. Of note, DBS electrode contacts 0 was located in the nucleus accumbens, contacts 1 and 2 in the anterior limb of the internal capsule and contact 3 was located dorsal to the internal capsule. This study also reported increased metabolism in pons on fMRI and decreased metabolism in the frontal lobe on PET scans following 10 days and 3 months of continuous bilateral stimulation [27]. Mild cognitive and behavior disinhibition was noted at higher voltages in this study, which improved with changes in programming parameters. No significant complications related to the DBS implantation surgery was reported in this study [27]. Abelson et al. [29] in a double blind controlled study reported 19.8 % decrease in Y-BOCS score in DBS "ON" state following bilateral ALIC DBS in 4 patients with medical refractory OCD. In the blind phase of the study, 1 patient experienced >35 % improvement in Y-BOCS score, another one reported 17 % reduction in Y-BOCS score and other 2 patients had no impact on their OCD symptoms following DBS stimulation. During the open phase of the study, 2 out of 4 patients (50 %) reported >35 % reduction in Y-BOCS score following stimulation [29]. Another study reported a 27 point decrease in Y-BOCS score following bilateral ALIC-DBS stimulation at 10 months in an isolated patient with medical refractory OCD [30].

11.2.2 Ventral Capsule and Ventral Striatum (Vc/Vs)

The ventral portion of the caudate nucleus and nucleus accumbens together forms the ventral striatum and are considered to be the reward centers of the brain [31, 32]. Following the success of both ablative and DBS surgeries involving the anterior limb of anterior capsule, ventral striatum in combination with ventral capsule was explored as the potential DBS target in patients with medical refractory OCD [33]. Greenberg et al. [34] reported complete (>35 % reduction in Y-BOCS score) and partial (25–35 % reduction in Y-BOCS scores) response in 40 and 20 % of patients respectively, following bilateral Vc/Vs DBS in 10 patients with medical refractory OCD. In this uncontrolled study, there was 12.3 points decrease in Y-BOCS score with improvement in symptoms such as anxiety, depression, independent living and self-care at 36 months of DBS stimulation as compared to baseline [34]. Asymptomatic hemorrhage, seizure, superficial infection, hypomania and worsening of depression were reported in this study [34]. In 2010, Greenberg et al. [35] reported a response rate of 62 % following bilateral ALIC-Vc/Vs DBS in 26 patients with medical refractory OCD across three centers in United States (Butler Hospital/Brown Medical School, Cleveland Clinic and University of Florida) and one center in Europe (Leuven/ Antwerp). This open study over 8 years reported a 13.1 points decrease in Y-BOCS score following neurostimulation as compared to baseline at 3–36 months follow up [35]. They also noted increased responsiveness on stimulating DBS electrode contacts closer to the ventral caudate or nucleus accumbens than otherwise. A total of 23 adverse events in 11 patients related to DBS implantation surgery (asymptomatic intracerebral hemorrhage in 2 patients, seizure in 1 patient, superficial wound infection in one case and one case each of stimulating lead and extension wire breakage) and 9 adverse events (increased depression in 4 patients, three events of increased OCD symptoms, one case of hypomania and one report of domestic problems/irritability) related

to stimulation was reported in this study [35]. Goodman et al. [36] in a randomized controlled study reported response rate of 67 % following bilateral Vc/Vs DBS in 6 patients with refractory OCD at 1 year follow up. There was 15.7 points decrease in Y-BOCS score following bilateral Vc/Vs DBS as compared to baseline in this study [36]. No significant adverse effects related to implantation and hypomania in 4 of 6 patients related to chronic stimulation was reported in this study [36]. Tsai et al. [37] investigated the relationship between stimulation induced smile/ laughter and long term DBS outcome in 4 patients, who underwent bilateral Vc/Vs DBS for medical refractory OCD. They reported that acute Vc/Vs DBS was associated with mood changes, hemodynamic, sensory, or motor effects that were transient and tend to adapt over time [37]. In this study, they noticed that the stimulation induced smile/laughter was significantly correlated with the reduction in Y-BOCS score at 15 months of stimulation [37].

11.2.3 Nucleus Accumbens (NAc)

Nucleus accumbens is one of the components of ventral striatum located at the junction of the end of the anterior limb of the internal capsule, head of caudate nucleus and anterior portion of putamen. NAc is considered the "reward center" of brain [38, 39]. In 2003, Sturm et al. [40] reported a response rate of 75 % (3 of 4 patients) following DBS implantation in the shell region of right NAc in patients with medical refractory OCD and anxiety disorders at 24–30 months follow up. In this study, PET imaging performed in one of the patients during stimulation also supported the role of nucleus accumbens in modulating the limbic loop [40]. However, clinical assessment tools such as Y-BOCS or other scoring systems were not used to quantify post-operative improvement in this study. Another study reported remission of OCD (Y-BOCS < 16) with 13 points decrease in Y-BOCS score compared to baseline following DBS of the ventral caudate nucleus in an isolated patient with intractable severe OCD and associated

11 DBS for Obsessive-Compulsive Disorder

depression at 12–15 months [41]. Similarly, another study reported sustained improvement of OCD symptoms in an isolated patient with residual schizophrenia following right ALIC-NAc DBS at 24 months [42]. This patient did not meet the criteria for "responder" (>35 % reduction in Y-BOCS scale) in this study [42]. In 2010, an open study reported a response rate of 50 % (1 of 2 patients) with a 13 point decrease in Y-BOCS score compared to baseline following bilateral NAc DBS in patients with medical refractory OCD at 24–27 months follow up [43]. In 2010, Huff et al. [44] in a double blind controlled study reported that 10 % of patients (n = 10) were complete responders (>35 % reduction in Y-BOCS score) and 50 % were partial responders (>25 % reduction in Y-BOCS score) following right NAc-DBS for medical refractory OCD. The mean Y-BOCS score decreased from 32.2 at baseline to 25.4 following DBS with alleviation in depression, global functioning, quality of life and no changes in anxiety, global symptom severity and cognitive function at 12 months [44]. Implantation related mild adverse effects such as dysesthesia in the subclavicular region in 1 patient with no other significant adverse events reported in this study [44]. Stimulation related side effects such as hypomania, agitation/anxiety, weight gain, concentration difficulties with failing memory, suicidal thoughts, headache, and insomnia were reported following stimulation [44]. Denys et al. [45] reported >35 % reduction in Y-BOCS score in 9 out of 16 patients (56 % responders) following bilateral NAc-DBS for medical refractory OCD at 21 months follow up. Overall, there was 17.5 points decrease in Y-BOCS score following stimulation with a difference of 8.3 points between 2 weeks DBS On and 2 weeks DBS off phases [45]. In addition, there was significant improvement in symptoms such as depression and anxiety following stimulation in this study. Mild side effects related to implantation and stimulation such as superficial wound infection, numbness at the incision site, feeling of extension leads, word finding problems, mild forgetfulness, hypomania, were reported in this study [45].

11.2.4 Subthalamic Nucleus (STN)

STN is one of the preferred targets to ameliorate motor symptoms in patients with Parkinson's disease. Researchers have noticed improvement in mood, anxiety and other neuropsychological symptoms in patients who underwent STN DBS for PD [46–51]. In addition, psychological symptoms such as transient acute depression, episodes of hypomania/mania or mirthful laughter following STN stimulation at supra threshold levels have been reported in literature [51–54]. STN is one of the components of dorsolateral prefrontal, orbitofrontal and limbic neural circuits and thus can be modulated to improve symptoms in patients with medical refractory OCD. Specifically, medial/ventromedial portions of STN and structures in close proximity to STN such as lateral hypothalamus, ventral tegmental area, substantia nigra and zona incerta have been implicated in the neuropsychological effects of STN stimulation. An uncontrolled study reported >35 % reduction in Y-BOCS score in 2 patients with PD and severe OCD who underwent bilateral STN DBS at 6 months of stimulation [49]. In this study, electrodes were implanted either in the anteromedial portion of STN, between anteromedial portions of STN/zona incerta, or in the anterior portion of zona incerta and reported 20 points decrease in Y-BOCS score compared to baseline following stimulation [49]. In 2004, Fontaine et al. [55] reported a 31 points decrease in Y-BOCS score compared to baseline following bilateral STN-DBS in an isolated patient with refractory OCD at 12 months. Subsequently, in a randomized multicenter controlled study, Mallet et al. [56] reported a response rate of 75 % (12 of 16 patients) with >25 % reduction in Y-BOCS score compared to baseline following bilateral STN DBS for refractory OCD. Overall, there was an improvement in global assessment of function scale with no effect on neuropsychological parameters such as depression or anxiety following stimulation in this study. Adverse events such as intracerebral hemorrhage (n = 1), and serious infections leading to explantation of hardware (n = 2) were reported in this study.

Chabardes et al. [57] reported >70 % reduction in Y-BOCS score in 3 out of 4 patients (75 % response rate) who underwent bilateral STN DBS for refractory OCD at 6 months.

11.2.5 Inferior Thalamic Peduncle (ITP)

There is only one open study investigating the efficacy of inferior thalamic peduncle as a potential DBS target to alleviate symptoms in patients with medical refractory OCD. ITP provides a route to the white fibers connecting thalamus to the orbitofrontal cortex and therefore ITP can be explored as a potential nodal point for neuromodulation [58]. In 2009, Jimenez-Ponce et al. [59] reported a significant response (>35 % reduction in Y-BOCS score) in all 5 patients (100 % responders) who underwent bilateral ITP DBS for medical refractory OCD. In this open study, there was 17.2 points decrease in Y-BOCS score following stimulation at 12 months follow up compared to base line. The mean global assessment of functioning scale (GAF) improved from 20 to 70 % following stimulation in this study [59]. Neither significant adverse effect related to implantation surgery/chronic stimulation or changes in neuropsychological functions following stimulation reported in this study [59]. Although the results of this study are instigating, randomized controlled studies are needed to substantiate the efficacy of ITP as potential DBS target in patients with medical refractory OCD.

11.2.6 Globus Pallidus Internus (Gpi)

In 2013, Nair et al. [60] reported 100 and 85 % improvement in Obsessive-compulsive inventory scale (OCI) in 2 patients each following bilateral anteromedial (limbic) globus pallidus internus (Gpi) DBS for Tourette's syndrome and severe OCD at 3–26 months follow up. In this study, bilateral Gpi was targeted to mitigate the motor symptoms associated with Tourette's syndrome and they noted that this target also alleviated the symptoms associated with OCD [60]. Therefore, Gpi can be explored as a potential DBS target for medical refractory OCD and necessitates further controlled studies to validate its efficacy.

11.3 Patient Selection, Team Approach and Ethics in Psychosurgery

In 1977, the National Commission for the Protection of Human subjects was formed under the national research act to avoid indiscriminate use of psychosurgery in patients with psychiatric disorders in both clinical and research settings [61]. According to the guidelines laid down by this commission, patients who are being considered for psychosurgery, should meet the criterion for chronic and medical refractory OCD [Diagnostic and Statistical Manual V (DSM-5)] [62]. The team involved in care of these patients consists of psychiatrist, neurologist, functional neurosurgeon, neuropsychologist, bioethicist and lay personnel to ensure appropriate selection of surgical candidates. Patients should be educated and counselled regarding surgery, possible risks involved and expected benefits. Patients should also be able to understand the procedure and have the ability to take decisions including opting out of the study. A written informed valid consent is then obtained from the patient or patient's legal guardian. Quantitative scales such as Yale-Brown obsessive-compulsive scale (Y-BOCS) or obsessive-compulsive inventory (OCI) must be used by an experienced psychiatrist to quantify the severity of disease before and after the procedure as well as to ensure uniformity across different research studies. Following approval of the study protocol and procedure by the Institutional review board (IRB), the procedure is carried out by an experienced team of functional neurosurgeons, psychiatrists and neurologists [15]. It is crucial to follow a series of protocols, safety measures and ethical considerations to avoid mimicking the torment history of psychosurgery and to help patients with these complex disorders [63]. Furthermore, psychosurgery should not be used in pediatric patients, to enhance memory functions, to modify one's behavior/identity or enforced by legal or political causes [15, 64]. With appropriate patient selection, strict adherence to safety protocols and consideration to ethical issues, we are likely to push the frontiers of psychosurgery and to benefit patients with this clinical conundrum.

11.4 Surgical Techniques of DBS Implantation

Operative set up and technique of DBS lead placement for OCD is similar to that established for movement disorders. An outline of the procedure as it is performed in our institution is described below. The procedure is usually performed in two stages 7–10 days apart.

Stage 1: Involves stereotactic guided implantation of DBS electrode into deep anatomical targets. The procedure is done according to the following steps:

(a) Frame placement: Patient's head is shaved and stereotactic Leksell frame (Elekta Inc., Atlanta, GA) is attached to the patient's head under sedation and local anesthesia. This is followed by head CT scan using stealth protocol (1-mm contiguous cuts). These stealth images are then exported to the stealth station and fused to the stealth CT scan to acquire the coordinates of the target. The target is localized using either indirect targeting method in reference to the coordinates of mid-commissural point or by direct visualization of the nucleus on T-2 weighted MRI. A safe surgical trajectory to the target avoiding the cortical sulci, intracranial vessels and ventricular walls is planned on the stealth station.

(b) Neurophysiological mapping using microelectrodes: On the day of Stage 1 surgery, the location of the

burr hole is defined by the Leksell frame coordinates acquired from the stealth station and the surgical site is prepared and draped in a standard manner. With the patient in supine position, a burr hole is made at the predetermined location according to the Leksell coordinates. Following burr hole, the Navigus Stimloc™ Burr Hole Cover system (Medtronic, Minneapolis, MN, USA) is attached over the burr hole and fixed to the skull with screws, to secure the DBS lead following implantation. The underlying dura is coagulated and opened at the entry point of the cannula providing adequate room to avoid hitting the dural edges. Piamater is coagulated and opened using no. 11 blade at the entry point of cannula. A cannula (length = 177 mm) is inserted through the pial opening to 15 mm above the target. The burr hole is then covered with surgicel and sealed using Tisseal glue to prevent CSF loss. The inner stylet of cannula is removed and a platinum-iridium or platinum/gold plated tungsten microelectrode with impedance range of 0.6–1.0-megaohm is introduced into the cannula for microelectrode recording. The microelectrode is then advanced through the brain matter using a motorized Microdrive system in submillimetric steps in an awake patient. The neuronal activities within the target are evaluated by passive manipulation and active movements of the extremities or orofacial structures every 1–2 mm along the length of the nucleus. The neuronal activity is amplified, filtered, displayed and recorded using a high-quality audio monitor, computer display and digital oscilloscopes [65]. Based on the microelectrode recordings and kinesthetic responses the borders and volume of the intended target is defined using either single or multiple parallel trajectories separated by 2–3 mm. Each neuronal structure has characteristic electrophysiological properties which assist in delineating the entry and exit points through that that structure such as STN neurons had a lower mean firing rate (37 Hz) and irregular pattern as compared to SNr (mean firing rate of 71 Hz and regular pattern) [66]. Following satisfactory electrophysiological recordings, the microelectrode is withdrawn into the guide tube ($\geq$3 mm) and macrostimulation is performed to delineate the thresholds of surrounding structures such as internal capsule, medial leminiscus, occulomotor nerve fibers and hypothalamus.

(c) Final electrode implantation: The data regarding location, characteristics of microelectrode recordings and the effects of macrostimulation are then evaluated and discussed by the whole team. Based on this evaluation, a "best-fit" to the Schaltenbrand and Bailey [67] atlas is created and final location of the DBS implantation is decided.

Stage 2: (Implantable pulse generator placement) is an outpatient procedure done under general anesthesia and involves connecting the distal end of electrode to the extension cable which is subsequently tunneled under the scalp and skin of neck into the subclavicular/abdominal area. Usually a linear incision in made below the clavicle and a subcutaneous pocket is dissected to accommodate the pulse generator. The extension cable is connected to the pulse generator.

We start deep brain stimulation 1 month after the second stage to allow adequate time for the surgical site to heal and for edema to subside. Chronic stimulation parameters are adjusted by a neurologist who is familiar with the patient condition. Usually the neurologist is part of the patient management team and participated in the evaluation, patient selection before surgery and intraoperative physiological mapping.

11.5 Conclusion

Unlike surgery for movement disorders, DBS surgery for OCD requires targeting multiple neural circuits to alleviate clinical symptoms in patients with medical refractory OCD. Technological advances and increased understanding of the OCD pathophysiology made it possible to delineate specific nodes for surgical intervention to maximize the clinical benefits associated with DBS. Furthermore, advances in imaging, neuronavigation and targeting techniques has improved the precision and safety profile of this minimally invasive surgery and made it a favored therapeutic option in patients with medical refractory OCD. DBS is now a FDA approved therapy under Human device exemption (HDE) status for patients with medical refractory OCD. DBS for OCD requires a close collaboration between expert group of multidisciplinary specialists such as psychiatrists, functional neurosurgeons, neurologist, neuropsychologist, neuroradiologist, biomedical engineers and bioethicist to manage these complex patients. The next generation DBS smart devices in the form of adaptive and responsive closed loop feedback devices based on chemical and electrical signals, add to the utility of this therapy for refractory OCD. Newer ablative techniques such as gamma knife, high intensity focused ultrasound or radiofrequency can be non-invasive alternative options in these complex patients. The rapidly advancing field of neuromodulation is likely to offer hope and benefit patients with medical refractory OCD. However, long-term randomized controlled studies are warranted to validate the efficacy of DBS therapy in patients with this clinical conundrum.

References

1. Ruscio AM, Stein DJ, Chiu WT, Kessler RC. The epidemiology of obsessive-compulsive disorder in the National Comorbidity Survey Replication. Mol Psychiatry. 2010;15:53–63.
2. Alonso P, Segalas C, Real E, Pertusa A, Labad J, Jimenez-Murcia S, Jaurrieta N, Bueno B, Vallejo J, Menchon JM. Suicide in patients treated for obsessive-compulsive disorder: a prospective follow-up study. J Affect Disord. 2010;124:300–8.
3. Kamath P, Reddy YC, Kandavel T. Suicidal behavior in obsessive-compulsive disorder. J Clin Psychiatry. 2007;68:1741–50.
4. Rasmussen SA, Eisen JL. The epidemiology and clinical features of obsessive compulsive disorder. Psychiatr Clin North Am. 1992;15:743–58.
5. Bjorgvinsson T, Hart J, Heffelfinger S. Obsessive-compulsive disorder: update on assessment and treatment. J Psychiatr Pract. 2007;13:362–72.
6. de Koning PP, Figee M, van den Munckhof P, Schuurman PR, Denys D. Current status of deep brain stimulation for obsessive-compulsive disorder: a clinical review of different targets. Current Psychiatry Rep. 2011;13:274–82.
7. Blomstedt P, Sjoberg RL, Hansson M, Bodlund O, Hariz MI. Deep brain stimulation in the treatment of obsessive-compulsive disorder. World Neurosurg. 2013;80:e245–53.
8. Robison RA, Taghva A, Liu CY, Apuzzo ML. Surgery of the mind, mood, and conscious state: an idea in evolution. World Neurosurg. 2013;80:S2–26.
9. Denys D. Pharmacotherapy of obsessive-compulsive disorder and obsessive-compulsive spectrum disorders. Psychiatr Clin North Am. 2006;29:553–84, xi.
10. Math SB, Janardhan Reddy YC. Issues in the pharmacological treatment of obsessive-compulsive disorder. Int J Clin Pract. 2007;61:1188–97.
11. Abudy A, Juven-Wetzler A, Zohar J. Pharmacological management of treatment-resistant obsessive-compulsive disorder. CNS Drugs. 2011;25:585–96.
12. Rasmussen SA, Eisen JL. Treatment strategies for chronic and refractory obsessive-compulsive disorder. J Clin Psychiatry. 1997;13:9–13.
13. Pallanti S, Quercioli L. Treatment-refractory obsessive-compulsive disorder: methodological issues, operational definitions and therapeutic lines. Prog Neuropsychopharmacol Biol Psychiatry. 2006;30:400–12.
14. Lapidus KA, Kopell BH, Ben-Haim S, Rezai AR, Goodman WK. History of psychosurgery: a psychiatrist's perspective. World Neurosurg. 2013;80:S27–e21–16.
15. Kopell BH, Greenberg B, Rezai AR. Deep brain stimulation for psychiatric disorders. J Clin Neurophysiol. 2004;21:51–67.
16. Lapidus KA, Kopell BH, Ben-Haim S, Rezai AR, Goodman WK. History of psychosurgery: a psychiatrist's perspective. World Neurosurg. 2013;80:e1–S27.
17. Goodman WK, Alterman RL. Deep brain stimulation for intractable psychiatric disorders. Annu Rev Med. 2012;63:511–24.
18. Heath RG, Monroe RR, Mickle WA. Stimulation of the amygdaloid nucleus in a schizophrenic patient. Am J Psychiatry. 1955;111:862–3.
19. Bickford RG, Petersen MC, Dodge HW Jr., Sem-Jacobsen CW. Observations on depth stimulation of the human brain through implanted electrographic leads. In: Proceedings of the staff meetings. Mayo Clinic. 1953;28:181–7.
20. Heath RG, Dempesy CW, Fontana CJ, Fitzjarrell AT. Feedback loop between cerebellum and septal-hippocampal sites: its role in emotion and epilepsy. Biol Psychiatry. 1980;15:541–56.
21. Johnson MD, Miocinovic S, McIntyre CC, Vitek JL. Mechanisms and targets of deep brain stimulation in movement disorders. Neurother: J Am Soc Exp Neurother. 2008;5:294–308.
22. McIntyre CC, Savasta M, Kerkerian-Le Goff L, Vitek JL. Uncovering the mechanism(s) of action of deep brain stimulation: activation, inhibition, or both. Clinical Neurophysiol: Official J Int Fed Clin Neurophysiol. 2004;115:1239–48.
23. McIntyre CC, Grill WM, Sherman DL, Thakor NV. Cellular effects of deep brain stimulation: model-based analysis of activation and inhibition. J Neurophysiol. 2004;91:1457–69.
24. Guo Y, Rubin JE, McIntyre CC, Vitek JL, Terman D. Thalamocortical relay fidelity varies across subthalamic nucleus deep brain stimulation protocols in a data-driven computational model. J Neurophysiol. 2008;99:1477–92.
25. Nuttin B, Cosyns P, Demeulemeester H, Gybels J, Meyerson B. Electrical stimulation in anterior limbs of internal capsules in patients with obsessive-compulsive disorder. Lancet. 1999;354(9189):1526.
26. Mindus P, Rasmussen SA, Lindquist C. Neurosurgical treatment for refractory obsessive-compulsive disorder: implications for understanding frontal lobe function. J Neuropsychiatry Clin Neurosci. 1994;6:467–77.
27. Nuttin BJ, Gabriels LA, Cosyns PR, Meyerson BA, Andreewitch S, Sunaert SG, Maes AF, Dupont PJ, Gybels JM, Gielen F, Demeulemeester HG. Long-term electrical capsular stimulation in patients with obsessive-compulsive disorder. Neurosurgery. 2003;52:1263–72.
28. Nuttin BJ, Gabriels LA, Cosyns PR, Meyerson BA, Andreewitch S, Sunaert SG, Maes AF, Dupont PJ, Gybels JM, Gielen F, Demeulemeester HG. Long-term

28. electrical capsular stimulation in patients with obsessive-compulsive disorder. Neurosurgery. 2008;62:966–77.

29. Abelson JL, Curtis GC, Sagher O, Albucher RC, Harrigan M, Taylor SF, Martis B, Giordani B. Deep brain stimulation for refractory obsessive-compulsive disorder. Biol Psychiatry. 2005;57:510–6.

30. Anderson D, Ahmed A. Treatment of patients with intractable obsessive-compulsive disorder with anterior capsular stimulation. Case report. J Neurosurg. 2003;98:1104–8.

31. Knutson B, Adams CM, Fong GW, Hommer D. Anticipation of increasing monetary reward selectively recruits nucleus accumbens. J Neurosci: Official J Soc Neurosci. 2001;21(16):Rc159.

32. Schultz W. Neural coding of basic reward terms of animal learning theory, game theory, microeconomics and behavioural ecology. Curr Opin Neurobiol. 2004;14:139–47.

33. Ruck C, Karlsson A, Steele JD, Edman G, Meyerson BA, Ericson K, Nyman H, Asberg M, Svanborg P. Capsulotomy for obsessive-compulsive disorder: long-term follow-up of 25 patients. Arch Gen Psychiatry. 2008;65:914–21.

34. Greenberg BD, Malone DA, Friehs GM, Rezai AR, Kubu CS, Malloy PF, Salloway SP, Okun MS, Goodman WK, Rasmussen SA. Three-year outcomes in deep brain stimulation for highly resistant obsessive-compulsive disorder. Neuropsychopharmacol: Official Publ Am Coll Neuropsychopharmacol. 2006;31: 2384–93.

35. Greenberg BD, Gabriels LA, Malone DA Jr, Rezai AR, Friehs GM, Okun MS, Shapira NA, Foote KD, Cosyns PR, Kubu CS, Malloy PF, Salloway SP, Giftakis JE, Rise MT, Machado AG, Baker KB, Stypulkowski PH, Goodman WK, Rasmussen SA, Nuttin BJ. Deep brain stimulation of the ventral internal capsule/ventral striatum for obsessive-compulsive disorder: worldwide experience. Mol Psychiatry. 2010;15:64–79.

36. Goodman WK, Foote KD, Greenberg BD, Ricciuti N, Bauer R, Ward H, Shapira NA, Wu SS, Hill CL, Rasmussen SA, Okun MS. Deep brain stimulation for intractable obsessive compulsive disorder: pilot study using a blinded, staggered-onset design. Biol Psychiatry. 2010;67:535–42.

37. Tsai HC, Chang CH, Pan JI, Hsieh HJ, Tsai ST, Hung HY, Chen SY. Acute stimulation effect of the ventral capsule/ventral striatum in patients with refractory obsessive-compulsive disorder—a double-blinded trial. Neuropsychiatric Dis Treat. 2014;10:63–9.

38. Knutson B, Wimmer GE, Kuhnen CM, Winkielman P. Nucleus accumbens activation mediates the influence of reward cues on financial risk taking. NeuroReport. 2008;19:509–13.

39. Liu X, Hairston J, Schrier M, Fan J. Common and distinct networks underlying reward valence and processing stages: a meta-analysis of functional neuroimaging studies. Neurosci Biobehav Rev. 2011;35:1219–36.

40. Sturm V, Lenartz D, Koulousakis A, Treuer H, Herholz K, Klein JC, Klosterkotter J. The nucleus accumbens: a target for deep brain stimulation in obsessive-compulsive-and anxiety-disorders. J Chem Neuroanat. 2003;26:293–9.

41. Aouizerate B, Cuny E, Martin-Guehl C, Guehl D, Amieva H, Benazzouz A, Fabrigoule C, Allard M, Rougier A, Bioulac B, Tignol J, Burbaud P. Deep brain stimulation of the ventral caudate nucleus in the treatment of obsessive-compulsive disorder and major depression. Case report. J Neurosurg. 2004;101:682–6.

42. Plewnia C, Schober F, Rilk A, Buchkremer G, Reimold M, Wachter T, Breit S, Weiss D, Kruger R, Freudenstein D. Sustained improvement of obsessive-compulsive disorder by deep brain stimulation in a woman with residual schizophrenia. IntJ Neuropsychopharmacol/Official Sci J Collegium Int Neuropsychopharmacol (CINP). 2008;11:1181–3.

43. Franzini A, Messina G, Gambini O, Muffatti R, Scarone S, Cordella R, Broggi G. Deep-brain stimulation of the nucleus accumbens in obsessive compulsive disorder: clinical, surgical and electrophysiological considerations in two consecutive patients. Neurol Sci: Official J Ital Neurol Soc Ital Soc Clin Neurophysiol. 2010;31:353–9.

44. Huff W, Lenartz D, Schormann M, Lee SH, Kuhn J, Koulousakis A, Mai J, Daumann J, Maarouf M, Klosterkotter J, Sturm V. Unilateral deep brain stimulation of the nucleus accumbens in patients with treatment-resistant obsessive-compulsive disorder: outcomes after one year. Clin Neurol Neurosurg. 2010;112:137–43.

45. Denys D, Mantione M, Figee M, van den Munckhof P, Koerselman F, Westenberg H, Bosch A, Schuurman R. Deep brain stimulation of the nucleus accumbens for treatment-refractory obsessive-compulsive disorder. Arch Gen Psychiatry. 2010;67: 1061–8.

46. Alexander GE, DeLong MR, Strick PL. Parallel organization of functionally segregated circuits linking basal ganglia and cortex. Annu Rev Neurosci. 1986;9:357–81.

47. Ardouin C, Pillon B, Peiffer E, Bejjani P, Limousin P, Damier P, Arnulf I, Benabid AL, Agid Y, Pollak P. Bilateral subthalamic or pallidal stimulation for Parkinson's disease affects neither memory nor executive functions: a consecutive series of 62 patients. Ann Neurol. 1999;46:217–23.

48. Woods SP, Fields JA, Troster AI. Neuropsychological sequelae of subthalamic nucleus deep brain stimulation in Parkinson's disease: a critical review. Neuropsychol Rev. 2002;12:111–26.

49. Mallet L, Mesnage V, Houeto JL, Pelissolo A, Yelnik J, Behar C, Gargiulo M, Welter ML, Bonnet AM, Pillon B, Cornu P, Dormont D, Pidoux B, Allilaire JF, Agid Y. Compulsions, Parkinson's disease, and stimulation. Lancet. 2002;360:1302–4.

50. Temel Y, Kessels A, Tan S, Topdag A, Boon P, Visser-Vandewalle V. Behavioural changes after

bilateral subthalamic stimulation in advanced Parkinson disease: a systematic review. Parkinson Relat Disord. 2006;12:265–72.

51. Witt K, Daniels C, Reiff J, Krack P, Volkmann J, Pinsker MO, Krause M, Tronnier V, Kloss M, Schnitzler A, Wojtecki L, Botzel K, Danek A, Hilker R, Sturm V, Kupsch A, Karner E, Deuschl G. Neuropsychological and psychiatric changes after deep brain stimulation for Parkinson's disease: a randomised, multicentre study. Lancet Neurol. 2008;7:605–14.

52. Krack P, Kumar R, Ardouin C, Dowsey PL, McVicker JM, Benabid AL, Pollak P. Mirthful laughter induced by subthalamic nucleus stimulation. Mov Disord. 2001;16:867–75.

53. Bejjani BP, Damier P, Arnulf I, Thivard L, Bonnet AM, Dormont D, Cornu P, Pidoux B, Samson Y, Agid Y. Transient acute depression induced by high-frequency deep-brain stimulation. N Engl J Med. 1999;340:1476–80.

54. Tommasi G, Lanotte M, Albert U, Zibetti M, Castelli L, Maina G, Lopiano L. Transient acute depressive state induced by subthalamic region stimulation. J Neurol Sci. 2008;273:135–8.

55. Fontaine D, Mattei V, Borg M, von Langsdorff D, Magnie MN, Chanalet S, Robert P, Paquis P. Effect of subthalamic nucleus stimulation on obsessive-compulsive disorder in a patient with Parkinson disease. Case report. J Neurosurg. 2004;100:1084–6.

56. Mallet L, Polosan M, Jaafari N, Baup N, Welter ML, Fontaine D, du Montcel ST, Yelnik J, Chereau I, Arbus C, Raoul S, Aouizerate B, Damier P, Chabardes S, Czernecki V, Ardouin C, Krebs MO, Bardinet E, Chaynes P, Burbaud P, Cornu P, Derost P, Bougerol T, Bataille B, Mattei V, Dormont D, Devaux B, Verin M, Houeto JL, Pollak P, Benabid AL, Agid Y, Krack P, Millet B, Pelissolo A. Subthalamic nucleus stimulation in severe obsessive-compulsive disorder. N Engl J Med. 2008;359:2121–34.

57. Chabardes S, Polosan M, Krack P, Bastin J, Krainik A, David O, Bougerol T, Benabid AL. Deep brain stimulation for obsessive-compulsive disorder: subthalamic nucleus target. World Neurosurg. 2013;80:S31–e31–38.

58. Greenberg BD, Rauch SL, Haber SN. Invasive circuitry-based neurotherapeutics: stereotactic ablation and deep brain stimulation for OCD. Neuropsychopharmacol: Official Publ Am Coll Neuropsychopharmacol. 2010;35:317–36.

59. Jimenez-Ponce F, Velasco-Campos F, Castro-Farfan G, Nicolini H, Velasco AL, Salin-Pascual R, Trejo D, Criales JL. Preliminary study in patients with obsessive-compulsive disorder treated with electrical stimulation in the inferior thalamic peduncle. Neurosurgery. 2009;65:203–9; discussion 209.

60. Nair G, Evans A, Bear RE, Velakoulis D, Bittar RG. The anteromedial GPi as a new target for deep brain stimulation in obsessive compulsive disorder. J Clin Neurosci: Official J Neurosurg Soc Australas. 2013;21(5):815–21.

61. Protection of Human Subjects. Use of psychosurgery in practice and research: report and recommendations of National Commission for the Protection of Human Subjects. Fed Reg. 1977;42:26318–32.

62. American Psychiatric Association. Diagnostic and statistical manual of mental disorders. Washington, DC: American Psychiatric Association; 2013.

63. Nuttin B, Gybels J, Cosyns P, Gabriels L, Meyerson B, Andreewitch S, Rasmussen SA, Greenberg B, Friehs G, Rezai AR, Montgomery E, Malone D, Fins JJ. Deep brain stimulation for psychiatric disorders. Neurosurg Clin N Am. 2003;14(2):xv–xvi.

64. Grant RA, Halpern CH, Baltuch GH, O'Reardon JP, Caplan A. Ethical considerations in deep brain stimulation for psychiatric illness. J Clin Neurosci: Official J Neurosurg Soc Australas. 2013;18:00251–8.

65. Baker KB, Lee JY, Mavinkurve G, Russo GS, Walter B, DeLong MR, Bakay RA, Vitek JL. Somatotopic organization in the internal segment of the globus pallidus in Parkinson's disease. Exp Neurol. 2010;222:219–25.

66. Hutchison WD, Allan RJ, Opitz H, Levy R, Dostrovsky JO, Lang AE, Lozano AM. Neurophysiological identification of the subthalamic nucleus in surgery for Parkinson's disease. Ann Neurol. 1998;44:622–8.

67. Schaltenbrand G, Bailey W. Introduction to stereotaxis with an atlas of the human brain. Stuttgart: Thieme; 1959.

Focused Ultrasound for the Treatment of Obsessive-Compulsive Disorder

12

Young Cheol Na, Hyun Ho Jung and Jin Woo Chang

Obsessive-compulsive disorder (OCD) is a disabling neuropsychiatric disorder characterized by recurrent and intrusive thoughts, desires, and/or images (obsessions) that lead to repetitive behavior aimed at reducing the associated anxiety (compulsions). Typical symptoms of OCD include fear of being contaminated by the environment, which patients try to ease by compulsively washing their hands until they become sore and chapped. Despite this effort, obsessive thoughts and the resulting behavior persist. Epidemiologic studies have revealed that about 1–2 % of the general population meet the diagnostic criteria for OCD at some time in their lives, with a lifetime prevalence of 2–3 % [4, 24, 27]. Despite the best available treatments including cognitive-behavioral therapy and medications, 10–20 % of patients with OCD remain refractory to conservative treatments [54].

Various neurosurgical approaches such as ablative procedures, deep brain stimulation (DBS), and gamma knife radiosurgery (GKRS) have been used for treating refractory OCD patients. Recently, transcranial magnetic resonance-guided focused ultrasound (MRgFUS) has been introduced as a novel thermal ablation method that is performed without opening the cranium [12, 26, 32, 36]. The appropriate targets, surgical procedures, technical considerations, advantages, potential risks, and clinical results of MRgFUS for OCD, will be discussed here.

12.1 Contemporary Neural Circuits in Obsessive-Compulsive Disorder

Although contemporary understanding of the neural circuits involved in psychiatric disorders is advancing rapidly, the exact neural circuits related to OCD are yet to be fully elucidated. Many earlier studies have revealed increased activity within the orbitofrontal cortex, anterior cingulate gyrus, and caudate nucleus [2, 45], whereas decreased activity has been observed in the dorsolateral prefrontal cortex [52]. A correlation has also been reported between decreased metabolism in the caudate nucleus and improvements in OCD symptoms after medical treatment [23]. Dysregulation of basal ganglia circuits has been demonstrated in the motor and OCD symptoms of Tourette syndrome. These circuits and some of the clinical features of OCD are also related to those of Parkinson's disease [30, 38]. These findings support the hypothesis that cortico-striato-thalamo-cortical (CSTC) loop functions are strongly implicated in the pathogenesis of OCD [3, 30]. Decreased frontal striatal control of limbic structures such as the amygdala results in an inadequate fear response in patients with OCD

Y.C. Na (✉) · H.H. Jung · J.W. Chang
Department of Neurosurgery, Brain Research Institute, Yonsei University College of Medicine, Seoul, Korea

B. Sun and A. De Salles (eds.), *Neurosurgical Treatments for Psychiatric Disorders*,
DOI 10.1007/978-94-017-9576-0_12
© Shanghai Jiao Tong University Press, Shanghai and Springer Science+Business Media Dordrecht 2015

and may also be responsible for the fear of contamination [52].

With this understanding of neural circuitry, three interconnected neural circuits have been proposed in the pathogenesis of OCD: the circuit of Papez, the basolateral circuit, and the CSTC loop [3]. The anterior nucleus of the thalamus projects to the cingulate gyrus through the anterior limb of the internal capsule (ALIC) in the circuit of Papez [25]. The dorsomedial nucleus of the thalamus projects to the orbitofrontal cortex via the ALIC in the basolateral circuit [3]. The thalamus also projects to the cerebral cortex via the ALIC in the CSTC loop, and these anatomical locations, together with the anterior cingulate gyrus and nucleus accumbens, are the most frequent targets in surgical treatments for OCD. Thus, knowledge of these interconnected neural circuits is critical for understanding the rationale behind the choice of certain targets for surgical intervention.

12.2 Surgical Strategies for Obsessive-Compulsive Disorder

Surgical strategies can be divided into two categories: ablation and neuromodulation. Various anatomical targets have been proposed for either approach. However, there are still controversies in the application of surgical procedures to anatomical targets in patients with OCD.

Ablative procedures offer benefits to about 45–65 % of patients with intractable OCD [21]. Anatomical targets include the anterior cingulate gyrus and anterior limb of the internal capsule. Considering the major role of the anterior cingulate gyrus in the neural circuits described above, neurosurgeons can target this structure for ablative therapy in patients with OCD. We have previously reported that bilateral anterior cingulotomy resulted in a mean improvement of 36 % in the Yale-Brown obsessive-compulsive scale (Y-BOCS). Among 14 cingulotomy patients, 6 met the criteria for responders, with a 35 % or higher improvement rating on Y-BOCS

12 months postoperatively. Most importantly, there was no significant cognitive dysfunction after cingulotomy [28]. Similar results have been reported after anterior capsulotomy, with a mean improvement in Y-BOCS of 33 % and no adverse cognitive effects [40, 42]. The invasive nature of ablative procedures means they can inevitably be associated with surgical complications such as intracerebral hemorrhage, epilepsy, and hydrocephalus. In addition, the operator cannot always estimate the exact size and location of the lesions until they are visualized in postoperative images. The development of GKRS has provided a noninvasive and accurate method for locating lesions without the need for invasive surgery. However, the use of a high dose of radiation is associated with an unpredictable risk of adverse effects [48, 49].

Several deep brain structures including the ALIC, nucleus accumbens (NAc), caudate nucleus, subthalamic nucleus (STN), and dorsomedial thalamus have been proposed as DBS targets. Nuttin et al. [39] reported a double-blinded study that achieved an improvement in Y-BOCS score of at least 35 % in 50 % of patients after bilateral anterior capsular DBS. The mean Y-BOCS score was 19.8 ± 8.0 during stimulation compared with 32.3 ± 3.9 with the stimulator turned off, and this stimulation-induced effect was maintained for at least 21 months after anterior capsular DBS. Along with the improvements seen after DBS of the anterior capsule, the ventral caudate nucleus [1] and NAc [50] have also been proposed as effective DBS targets in treatment-refractory patients with OCD and have yielded improvements in OCD symptoms. Unlike ablative procedures, DBS is reversible and adjustable based on symptoms or disease progression. However, DBS requires permanent implantation of at least one multi-contact electrode, lead extensions, and an implantable pulse generator (IPG). This means that the patient must be followed closely for device management, and undergo replacement of the IPG every 3–5 years. Furthermore, DBS devices are sensitive to high-energy electrical fields, which can switch them off or even cause a reset of the device. Despite the relatively effective outcomes described above, these limitations have urged investigators to find less-invasive and more precise methods.

12.3 Transcranial Magnetic Resonance Guided Focused Ultrasound

12.3.1 Brief History

The earliest applications of ultrasound in medicine were therapeutic. Initial reports on the biological effects of ultrasound appeared early in 1928 when Harvey and Loomis reported that high-intensity high-frequency ultrasound could bring about changes in living biological tissues [43, 51]. Although a few studies reported successful treatment outcomes using ultrasound [13, 47], therapeutic applications were hampered until the late 1990s, especially due to safety issues. With the development of improved ultrasound techniques and greater understanding of the effects of ultrasound on cells and tissues, such as the damage mechanisms, thresholds, and propagation properties through tissues, the therapeutic application of ultrasound has been realized [43].

Transcranial ultrasound has been used in pediatric neurosurgery to detect hydrocephalus and midline shifts in the brain. In adults, blood velocity in the carotid arteries may be monitored through the intact skull using the Doppler effect. Lynn et al. [34, 35] reported the earliest investigation of focused ultrasound for non-invasive ablation in 1942. Since the 1950s, the use of focused ultrasound to produce focal thermal lesions deep within the brain has been demonstrated in several studies [16–18]. Fry et al. [14] demonstrated that low-frequency (around 0.5 MHz) ultrasound could be focused through the skull. Later, this group also demonstrated the acoustic parameters and histological features of focal brain lesions produced in 10 craniectomized cats using intense focused ultrasonic beams [15]. Because the histological appearance of these lesions compared with previous thermal lesions was similar without the intervening skull,

they predicted the application of transcranial ultrasound in the clinical field.

Until the 1990s, the major obstacle to the use of transcranial focused ultrasound was the skull itself. Its deflecting effects and variable thickness affect wave propagation to such an extent that ultrasound could not produce a focal lesion. The generation of high temperatures within the skull was also a major concern due to energy absorption, which could damage the scalp, bone, and adjacent brain parenchyma. For this reason, previous focused ultrasound treatment of the brain required removal of the skull for energy delivery, resulting in an invasive procedure with additional risks and costs [14, 15, 17, 22]. As a result, many researchers agreed that therapeutic ultrasound energy could not be delivered through an intact skull. However, the development of phased array transducers compatible with magnetic resonance, which is the most progressive technological advancement, has rekindled interest in transcranial focused ultrasound. Combined with the utilization of temperature-dependent proton resonance frequency shift, which allows MR thermometry, these advances have yielded MRgFUS technology, which enables non-invasive, image-guided, and temperature-monitored MRgFUS interventions [29].

12.3.2 Biological Effects of Ultrasound

It was originally believed that diagnostic ultrasound would never produce biological damage. However, in the early 1990s, Child et al. [6] reported that diagnostic ultrasound could produce significant damage in mice. Two main biological effects are demonstrated when high intensity acoustic waves propagate through tissues: thermal, and non-thermal or mechanical effects [41, 43].

12.3.2.1 Thermal Effects
The principle of focused ultrasound is that a beam of ultrasound is brought to a focus on the target. As ultrasound waves propagate into attenuating materials such as tissue, the wave amplitude decreases with distance. This attenuation is

caused by wave absorption and scattering. Whereas absorption is thought of as a mechanism that converts some portion of the ultrasonic wave into heat, scattering can be thought of as changes to the direction of the wave. Wherever absorption takes place in tissues, the temperature will increase as long as the rate of heat production is greater than the rate of heat removal [41]. The thermal mechanism is relatively well understood because the increase in temperature produced by ultrasound can be calculated using the widely used bio-heat transfer equation [43]. With this equation, it is possible to estimate the thermal dose and evaluate whether the dose is high enough to destroy the tissue. Injurious effects in vitro generally occur at temperatures of 39–43 °C after a sufficient time period; at higher temperatures (≥44 °C) coagulation of proteins can occur [41]. Dickson and Calderwood [11] reported that exposures of long duration (5–100 h) were required for thermally induced cell death at 40 °C and no irreversible adverse effects were detected at temperatures below 40 °C.

The temperature of the focused volume may rise rapidly by more than 20 °C. Although the volume of destroyed tissue is small (typically 0.5 mL) for a single ultrasound beam, a more clinically relevant volume can be obtained from contiguous arrays of focused ultrasound lesions throughout the volume of interest [51].

12.3.2.2 Non-thermal or Mechanical Effects

Of the non-thermal effects, acoustically generated cavitation has received the most attention, and results principally from microbubbles in ultrasound contrast agents. Radiation forces can also be produced by the non-thermal effects of ultrasound.

Acoustic cavitation refers to ultrasonically induced activity occurring in a liquid or liquid-like material containing microbubbles that are either formed spontaneously or are present naturally. Under ultrasonic stimulation, these microbubbles oscillate and can collapse at sufficiently high ultrasonic pressure levels. This phenomenon is termed inertial cavitation because the bubble motion is dominated by the inertia of the liquid [41]. In general, inertial cavitation results when microbubbles expand during the acoustic cycle and then collapse rapidly due to oscillations and the rapid growth of the cavity [43]. This cavitation can generate a temperature increase, mechanical stress, and reactive free radicals [41]. Microbubble oscillation itself also produces mechanical stress due to the viscosity of the surrounding fluid, which opposes the oscillation, creating what are known as radiation forces [43]. The occurrence of cavitation and radiation forces depends precisely on the type of tissue being exposed, making it difficult to obtain a consistent response.

12.3.3 The MRgFUS System

For non-invasive, non-ionized thermal ablation with real time imaging and thermal feedback, MRgFUS is an attractive modality. This technique addresses the limitations described above by combining a large phased array, active water-cooling, an acoustic aberration correction algorithm, and computed tomography (CT) data for skull-thickness registration.

The large phased array transducer used in MRgFUS is composed of numerous transducer elements. It has been proven that large hemispherical phased arrays can deliver adequate energy through human skulls to ablate brain tissue in vivo without an excessive elevation of temperature on the skull surface [7, 8]. Current MRgFUS systems employ 1,024 hemispherical phased array transducers operating at a frequency of 650 kHz. The interface between the subject's head and the transducer is also filled with water to provide the acoustic path. The MRgFUS system includes a chiller (refrigeration unit) that keeps the water chilled to a constant temperature so that the skull-bone temperature remains within safe limits.

Acoustic aberration is created mostly by variations in the bony structure of the skull. The degree of compensation necessary for each transducer element is based on predicting the aberration along the acoustic path from each element to the target and calculating the relative phase and amplitude correction necessary for that element. The result of this compensation is that the acoustic energy contribution from each element will arrive at the focal point in phase. The phase/amplitude correction algorithm, based on ray acoustic methods, relies on an input that provides the bone density profile along a ray cast between each acoustic element and the target point. This information is extracted from a three-dimensional CT image of the skull.

The MRgFUS system combines a focused ultrasound delivery system with a conventional diagnostic 1.5 T or 3 T MRI scanner. This system provides a real-time therapy planning algorithm, thermal dosimetry, and closed-loop therapy control. The treatment process for MRgFUS is not very different conceptually from the system that is currently in clinical use for other soft tissue applications. The treatment begins with a series of standard diagnostic MR images to identify the location and shape of the area to be treated. The workstation uses the physician's designation of the target volume to plan the best way to cover the target volume with small spots called "sonications". These treatment spots are cylindrical in shape. Their size depends on the sonication power and duration. During the treatment, a specific MR scan, which can be processed to identify changes in tissue temperature, provides a thermal map of the treatment volume to confirm the therapeutic effect [53]. The thermal map is used to monitor the treatment in progress, and confirm that the ablation is proceeding according to plan, thus closing the therapy loop.

Before delivering a therapeutic dose of acoustic energy to the target site, confirmation of the alignment of the thermal spot within the target site is necessary. Therefore, several sub-threshold sonications (low power and short duration, usually 10–20 s) should be performed for which the peak tissue temperature (39–42 °C) is below the threshold for ablation but can still be visualized on MR thermography images. After this targeting confirmation procedure, sequential sonications of incremental acoustic energy levels can be applied to the site to induce tissue ablation, as indicated by peak temperatures of 53–60 °C.

12.3.3.1 Advantages of MRgFUS

As a non-invasive, non-ionized MR-guided procedure with real time imaging and thermal feedback, MRgFUS has several advantages. The treatment can be monitored in real-time using MRI and MR-thermography. This allows for immediate confirmation of the targeting process. Thermal lesioning can be performed discretely and accurately, and can be evaluated immediately. Unlike stereotactic radiosurgery, MRgFUS does not use ionizing radiation and does not carry the risk of radiation-induced tumorigenesis. Because the MRgFUS procedure is non-invasive, there is no scalp incision, no burr hole, and no electrode penetrating the brain, unlike radiofrequency lesioning. Thus, MRgFUS reduces the risk of hemorrhagic complications and this non-invasive procedure also eliminates the risk of infectious complications. Compared with DBS treatment, there is no implanted hardware, no concern about interference with external sources of electromagnetic noise, no need for extensive follow-up for programming, and no need for periodic battery replacement. This represents a much simpler treatment plan for all patients, and will save hours of clinic time for DBS device management and replacement. Additionally, health care costs will be greatly reduced. It will be possible to re-treat a patient who develops a recurrence after other surgical treatments.

12.3.3.2 Potential Risks of MRgFUS

Although ultrasound techniques have advanced enough to overcome many former issues, skull heating may still be sufficient to damage bone and/or adjacent soft tissues. The sonication times should be calculated to keep skull temperatures below dangerous levels, and a minimum of 10 min assigned for skull cooling will provide time for the skull to return to normal temperatures before any additional heating takes place. Tissues along the path to the target (scalp, dura, arachnoid) and brain tissues adjacent to the target, also can become heated to the point where tissue damage or a burn might occur. This heating can be caused directly by improper treatment targeting, irregularities on the skin surface, treatment volumes of tissue that are too close to the skin or bone, or the conduction of sufficient heat to cause a burn at the surface. The presence of microcalcification in the brain tissue may create additional heating effects along the beam path. By utilizing the CT data, the ultrasound beam can be prevented from passing through these calcified areas.

Secondary hot-spot formation at bone-tissue and air-tissue interfaces is also a major concern, especially at the base of the skull. Pulkkinen et al. reported [44] that therapeutic ultrasound devices can produce potentially dangerous heating of the base of the skull. They determined safety limits, which apply for the thermal treatments operating at a frequency of 230 kHz.

Blood brain barrier (BBB) disruption, edema, swelling, and hemorrhage outside and remote from the targeted area also can occur. Theoretically, these events may be due to heating effects and/or to the pressure wave of the ultrasound beam. An increased rate of cerebral hemorrhage has been reported in stroke patients concomitantly treated with intravenous tissue plasminogen activator (tPA) [10].

High-field MR-induced vertigo is often observed in users of high-field (≥ 2 T) MRI scanners who experience disorientation or the subtle perception of movement when working close to or within the bore tube of the magnet, and this can also torment patients during the procedure. The patients will manifest symptoms such as nausea, vomiting, and dizziness. Although these symptoms may be temporary in most cases and disappear when the subject moves out of the magnet, the sensation of vertigo may accompany longer exposure. In our experiences of treating essential tremor using MRgFUS, half of the patients (5 among 11 patients) suffered from MR-induced vertigo [5]. Three main hypotheses were proposed for this effect: induced currents, which modulate the firing rate of the vestibular hair cells, magneto-hydrodynamics, and tissue magnetic susceptibility differences [19].

There is a risk associated with subject motion during a sonication or between sonications. This could cause a movement of the tissue relative to the planned treatment volume on the system, and in extreme cases could result in the treatment of a point outside the planned treatment volume. Because the skull functions as a defocusing lens, the phase correction map computed for the target spot, will also become ineffective if the subject moves.

If the CT and MR volumes are not well aligned with each other, the tuning of the ultrasonic elements will be suboptimal and distortion will make it difficult to achieve an exact volume of heating. The protocols for image fusion are well-established and will be visually confirmed by clinicians experienced in stereotactic targeting. Observation of the location, size and pattern of areas heated by the low-power sonication trials will also provide direct confirmation of the accuracy of the MRgFUS focus. MR thermography allows for the confirmation of accuracy before the process of therapeutic sonications begins.

12.3.3.3 Treatment Procedure for MRgFUS

The patient's hair is carefully removed and the scalp examined for existing scars or any other lesions before the day of treatment. Just before applying head fixation, the patient's hair is shaved again to prevent thermal injury to the hair. Overall steps in the treatment procedure steps are performed as follows (Fig. 12.1).

1. The patient's head is placed in a MR-compatible stereotactic frame (similar to those used in stereotactic radiotherapy head fixation).
2. The patient is positioned supine and head-first on the MRgFUS therapy table.
3. A hemispherical helmet containing the transducer elements is positioned on the patient's head in the treatment position (this should be done according to measurements taken during the pre-operative imaging session).
4. A rubber diaphragm is attached to the patient's head and to the transducer to allow acoustic coupling between the ultrasound transducer and the scalp.
5. The immobilization system is secured over the patient's head to maintain a fixed position between the patient's head and the ultrasonic transducer.

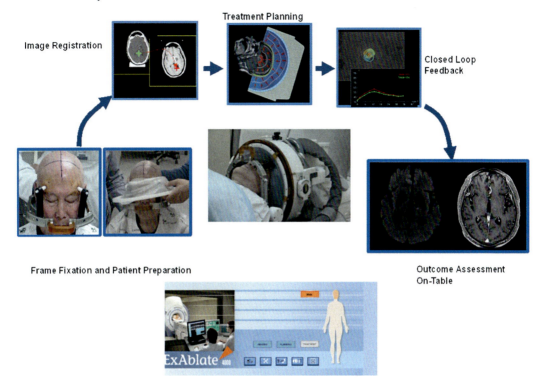

Fig. 12.1 Overall procedure of MRgFUS

6. A localizer scan (quick T1) and a T2 fast spin echo (T2-FSE) MR scan is obtained to allow further refinement of the transducer focal point with respect to the targeted zone.
7. Then, the interface within the rubber diaphragm is completely filled with degassed water to avoid air bubbles between the transducer and the scalp (active circulation, degassing, and cooling of this water is continuously maintained throughout the procedure to avoid undesired heating of the scalp and skull).
8. A series of MR images will be acquired to identify the target area, and plan the actual treatment:
   a. T2 Weighted imaging is examined along at least 2 axes: Axial and Sagittal.
   b. Other MR imaging series may also be acquired.
9. The pre-treatment MRI and CT image datasets are registered to the T2 weighted MR images acquired in the previous steps. This image fusion of pre-operative MR assists in the accurate delineation of the target area and determination of a safe sonication pathway:
   a. The fusion of the CT data is required for the computation of phase correction values to correct for skull aberration, and identification of intracranial calcifications.
   b. Scars on the scalp are designated to ensure the ultrasound beam avoids these specific areas.
10. The treating physician defines the treatment volume and plan. A commercial workstation automatically computes the number of sonications, and the phase and amplitude corrections (per sonication spot) necessary

for the system to produce a focal spot at each of the desired locations.

11. A central point in the targeted area is targeted by a low-dose sonication with a sublethal energy level to confirm the targeting accuracy on the MR images. Focal point position and/or transducer location are adjusted as necessary.

12. To enhance the procedure safety and to reduce some of the inherent risks of thermal lesioning of brain tissue:

    a. MRgFUS treatment is performed as a series of sonications with small increments in power within the designated target volume in the conscious patient.

    b. The patient is examined by the clinical team during and after each sonication for neurologic signs and symptoms.

    c. Sonication starts with low energy prior to permanent thermal ablation. Low-energy sonication non-destructively warms the target. The warming is captured by the MR thermometry and the MR thermal images are displayed to the treating physician in real time. The physician then verifies that the warming is centered on the anatomical target. This allows the centering of the permanent thermal lesion in the correct location.

    d. The titration of escalating focal sonications continues up to 60 °C within a 5 mm diameter centered on the target point, or until side effects are reported by the subject or observed by the clinical team.

13. After MRgFUS treatment, a series of MR images is acquired to assess the treatment effects.

12.4 Capsulotomy Using MRgFUS for Obsessive-Compulsive Disorder

There are no previous clinical reports on MRg-FUS for OCD, and the world's first clinical trial was conducted in our institute. This will be discussed below.

12.4.1 Patient Selection

Details about inclusion and exclusion criteria are listed in Table 12.1. Using these criteria, 4 patients with OCD were selected and treated with MRgFUS. OCD was diagnosed by a psychiatrist according to the criteria of the Diagnostic and Statistical Manual of Mental Disorders, 4th edition (DSM-IV). All patients were refractory to medications and cognitive behavioral therapy (CBT), had suffered from OCD for at least 3 years, and their Y-BOCS scores were more than 28, as listed in Table 12.1. Refractoriness to medication was defined as a lack of improvement after taking more than two different types of serotonin reuptake inhibitors at the maximum tolerable dose for more than 12 weeks. Refractoriness to CBT was defined as a lack of response after one year of therapy, or after 20 sessions. Before MRgFUS, all patients took medication stably, and medication doses were not changed during the entire follow-up period. The patient demographics and clinical characteristics are presented in Table 12.2.

12.4.2 Procedures

The fundamental procedures are described above and have also been described in detail in our previous papers. The MRgFUS was performed using a 3 T MRI system (GE Medical System, Milwaukee, WI), and the ExAblate 4000 (InSightec, Haifa, Israel), which features a 30-cm diameter, hemispherical 1,024 element phased-array transducer operating at 650 kHz and held by a mechanical positioner. The patient's scalp was closely shaved and the head was fixed with a Cosma-Roberts-Wells stereotactic frame (Radionics, USA) after injection of local anesthetic. A circular flexible silicone membrane with a central hole was stretched around the patient's head and sealed to the outer face of the transducer to contain the degassed and chilled (15–20 °C) water that was circulated between the head and the transducer. After the patient entered the MRI room, the stereotactic frame was fixed to the table, which was part of the ExAblate 4000

Table 12.1 Inclusion and exclusion criteria

Inclusion criteria
1. Men and women, between 18 and 80 years
2. Subjects who are able and willing to give consent and able to attend all study visits
3. OCD refractory to adequate trials of medication and behavioral therapy by psychiatrist (more than 12 weeks at the maximum tolerated dose)
4. Bilateral anterior limb of internal capsule can be target by the MRgFUS device. (The anterior limb of internal capsule must be apparent on MRI such that targeting can be performed with direct visualization)
5. Able to communicate sensations during the MRgFUS treatment
6. Definitive diagnosis of OCD, according to the criteria of the Diagnostic and Statistical Manual of Mental Disorder fourth edition (DSM-IV), with disease duration of more than 3 years, with diagnosed psychosocial dysfunction
7. A score on the Y-BOCS of more than 28
8. OCD medication regimen is stable for at least 30 days before enrolment
9. Subjects with diagnosed psychosocial dysfunction influenced by OCD
Exclusion criteria
1. Subjects with unstable cardiac status including:
a. Unstable angina pectoris on medication
b. Patients with documented myocardial infarction within last 40 days to protocol entry
c. Congestive heart failure NYHA Class IV
2. Subjects exhibiting any behavior(s) consistent with ethanol or substance abuse as defined by the criteria outlined in the DSM-IV as manifested by one (or more) of the following occurring within a 12 month period:
a. Recurrent substance use resulting in a failure to fulfill major role obligations at work, school, or home (such as repeated absences or poor work performance related to substance use; substance-related absences, suspensions, or expulsions from school; or neglect of children or household)
b. Recurrent substance use in situations in which it is physically hazardous (such as driving an automobile or operating a machine when impaired by substance use)
c. Recurrent substance-related legal problems (such as arrests for substance related disorderly conduct)
d. Continued substance use despite having persistent or recurrent social or interpersonal problems caused or exacerbated by the effects of the substance (for example, arguments with spouse about consequences of intoxication and physical fights)
3. Severe hypertension (diastolic BP > 100 mm Hg on medication)
4. Subjects with standard contraindications for MR imaging such as non-MRI compatible implanted metallic devices including cardiac pacemakers, size limitations, etc.
5. Known intolerance or allergies to the MRI contrast agent (e.g. Gadolinium or Magnevist) including advanced kidney disease
6. Subjects receiving dialysis
7. History of abnormal bleeding and/or coagulopathy
8. Receiving anticoagulant (e.g. warfarin) or antiplatelet (e.g. aspirin) therapy within 1 week of focused ultrasound procedure or drugs known to increase risk or hemorrhage (e.g. Avastin) within 1 month of scheduled focused ultrasound procedure
9. Active or suspected, acute or chronic uncontrolled infection or known life-threatening systemic disease
10. History of intracranial hemorrhage
11. Cerebrovascular disease (multiple CVA or CVA within 6 months)

(continued)

Table 12.1 (continued)

12. Individuals who are not able or willing to tolerate the required prolonged stationary supine position during treatment (can be up to 4 h of total table time)

13. Symptoms and signs of increased intracranial pressure (e.g. headache, nausea, vomiting, lethargy, and papilledema)

14. Subjects unable to communicate with the investigator and staff

15. Presence of any other neurodegenerative disease like Parkinson-plus syndromes suspected on neurological examination. These include:

    a. Multisystem atrophy

    b. Progressive supranuclear palsy

    c. Dementia with Lewy bodies

    d. Alzheimer's disease

16. Subjects diagnosed with idiopathic Parkinson's disease

17. Presence of significant cognitive impairment as determined with a score ≤ 24 on the Mini Mental Status Examination (MMSE)

18. History of immunocompromise, including patient who are HIV positive

19. Subjects with a history of seizures within the past year

20. Subjects with risk factors for intraoperative or postoperative bleeding:

    a. Platelet count less than 100,000 mm^{-3}

    b. PT > 14 s

    c. PTT > 36 s

    d. INR > 1.3

    e. Documented coagulopathy

    f. Patients receiving medications that are known to induce or contribute to Hemorrhages

21. Subjects with any types of brain tumors, including metastases

22. Any illness that in the investigator's opinion preclude participation in this study

23. Pregnancy or lactation

24. Subjects with history of aneurysms, including newly diagnosed condition

25. Subjects who have had deep brain stimulation or a prior stereotactic ablation of anterior cingulated gyrus

26. OCD medication regimen is not stable for at least 30 days before enrolment

27. Legal incapacity or limited legal capacity

28. Subjects with remarkable atrophy and poor healing capacity of the scalp (>30 % of the skull area traversed by the sonication pathway)

29. Are participating or have participated in another clinical trial in the last 30 days

device. Presonication MRI was performed, and images were fused with computed tomography (CT) and other MR sequences to determine the target coordinates. We targeted the bilateral ALIC (7 mm anterior to the anterior margin of the anterior commissure in the same anterior commissure-posterior commissure (AC-PC) plane, extending 2–3 mm along the capsule in a coronal view). Several sub-threshold heatings with low-power sonications of 10 s duration were applied to induce peak temperatures of 40–42 °C. This allowed us to visualize the exact position and size of the thermal spot and the overall safety profile of the applied sonication parameters. Then, high-power sonications were applied with stepwise increases in acoustic power and energy to achieve a peak temperature in the target region of 51–56 °C for more than 3 s duration. All these sonication processes were guided by MRI and MR thermometry. The goal was to make 10-mm

12 Focused Ultrasound for the Treatment of Obsessive-Compulsive Disorder

Table 12.2 Demographics and clinical characteristics of the patients at baseline

Case no.	Sex/age	Symptoms (obsession/compulsion)	Duration (years)	Medicaiton	CBT	Y-BOCS	HAM-A	HAM-D
1	M/24	Contamination fear/hand washing Counting	11	Escitalopram Valproic acid	Ineffective	38	34	27
2	M/29	Contamination fear/hand washing	17	Fluoxetine Escitalopram Buspirone	Ineffective	34	17	18
3	M/22	Aggressive obsession Compulsive washing Counting	13	Sertaline Clomipramine Aripiprazole Risperidone	Ineffective	35	31	25
4	F/44	Pathologic doubt/checking	24	Fluoxetine Olanzapine	Ineffective	34	26	20
Mean (±S.D.)			16.3(±5.7)			35.3(±1.9)	27(±7.4)	22.5(±4.2)

No. number; *CBT* cognitive behavioral therapy; *Y-BOCS* Yale-Brown obsessive-compulsive disorder scale; *HAM-A* Hamilton anxiety scale; *HAM-D* Hamilton depression scale; *S.D.* standard deviation

sized elliptical lesions by adjusting the sonication center. After every sonication, the patient was evaluated physically and neurologically in the MR room by a neurosurgeon and a psychiatrist to check for any adverse effects. The number of sonications for full lesioning ranged from 23 to 36, each of 10–31 s. The total procedure time was 5–7 h. All patients were fully awake and responsive during the entire procedure. After MRgFUS, they were monitored for about 24 h in the intensive care unit.

T1-weighted imaging with and without contrast enhancement, T2-weighted imaging, diffusion-weighted imaging (DWI), and fluid-attenuated inversion recovery (FLAIR) sequences were performed to detect the lesion after sonication. Axial, sagittal, and coronal T1- and T2-weighted fast spin echo images were obtained before and after MRgFUS and compared with changes in MRI immediately, 1 week, 1 month, and 6 months after MRgFUS.

Y-BOCS, Hamilton Rating Scale for Depression (HAM-D), and Hamilton Rating Scale for Anxiety (HAM-A) were assessed by psychiatrists at baseline, 1 week, 1 month, 3 months and 6 months after MRgFUS.

Potential adverse effects and any changes in a patient's neurological and physical states were evaluated at every visit by a neurosurgeon and a

psychiatrist. The study protocol for OCD001 is presented on the web site for Clinical Trials (http://www.clinicaltrials.gov/ct2/show/NCT019 86296?term=OCD001&rank=2).

12.4.3 Clinical Outcomes

The mean Y-BOCS score of 35.3 ± 1.9 at baseline improved to 23.5 ± 4.9 at 6 months after MRgFUS. The mean improvement rate was 33 ± 11 %. Although only two of the four patients achieved the criteria for a full response (more than 35 % improvement in Y-BOCS) during the 6 months of follow-up, all four patients experienced a sequential improvement in the Y-BOCS score. Considering the habitual behavior of patients with OCD, it may take a longer time to detect a definitive treatment effect. The mean HAM-A score at baseline was 27 ± 7.4 and also improved to 8.3 ± 6 after 6 months. The sequential mean improvement rates were 62 % at 1 week, 66.7 % at 1 month, 66.7 % at 3 months, and 69.4 % at 6 months after MRgFUS. All four patients experienced significant improvement 1 week after MRgFUS and this improvement was maintained throughout the 6 months. The mean HAM-D score at baseline was 22.5 ± 4.2 and also improved to 8.8 ± 3.3 after 6 months with a

61.1 % improvement rate. The sequential improvement rates were 52.2 % at 1 week, 64.4 % at 1 month, 55.6 % at 3 months, and 61.1 % at 6 months after MRgFUS. The HAM-D score also improved soon after MRgFUS, similar to the HAM-A score (Fig. 12.2).

There were no significant and/or permanent complications including physical, neurological, and psychological changes in any patients.

12.4.4 Image Outcomes After MRgFUS

All MRgFUS was initially performed in the right hemisphere, and the operator could not find any signal changes in the right ALIC in MR images during right hemisphere sonications. However, hyperintense signal changes in the right ALIC appeared in T2-weighted images during sonications of the contralateral left hemisphere. There

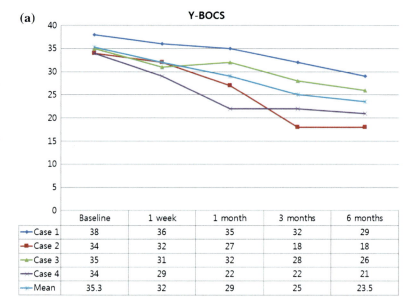
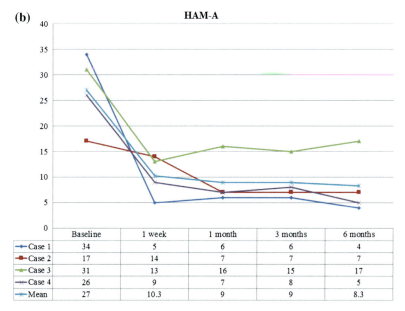

Fig. 12.2 The clinical course of obsessive-compulsive, depression, and anxiety symptoms. **a** The Y-BOCS score at baseline, 1 week, 1 month, 3 months, and 6 months after MRgFUS. **b** The HAM-A score at baseline, 1 week, 1 month, 3 months, and 6 months after MRgFUS. **c** The HAM-C score at baseline, 1 week, 1 month, 3 months, and 6 months after MRgFUS

Fig. 12.2 (continued)

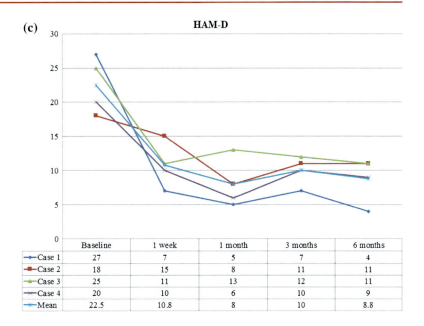

was also a subtle enhancement of the ALIC immediately after the procedure and we hypothesized that this enhancement was due to the partial breakdown of the BBB. One week after MRgFUS, thermal lesions became more prominent on MR images with a prominent improvement in the HAM-A scores and the HAM-D scores. However, the subtle enhancement disappeared on MR images. As we hypothesized earlier, restoration of the BBB would play a role in the disappearance of enhancement. Perilesional edema was also noted 1 week after MRgFUS, but faded away after 1 month. After 6 months, although hyperintense signals were was still noted in T2-weighted images, the total size of the lesions decreased slightly, and appeared smaller compared with the images taken 1 week and 1 month after MRgFUS (Fig. 12.3).

12.4.5 Future Perspectives of MRgFUS for Treating OCD

In earlier neurosurgical approaches for the management of OCD, Mindus et al. [37] demonstrated the potential advantages of radiofrequency thermal capsulotomy in patients with severe OCD. Thereafter, radiofrequency thermal capsulotomy has been accepted as an effective treatment option. However, this procedure has serious surgical risks such as intracranial hemorrhage. Moreover, the exact size and location of the lesion in ALIC could not be guaranteed for each patient, which creates uncertainty regarding the therapeutic effect [48]. GKRS is a noninvasive procedure that can be used to make a lesion in the ALIC. However, GKRS can also have unpredictable and permanent adverse effects due to high doses of radiation, although the exact dose has not been defined yet [48, 49]. Despite many advantages, none of these ablative techniques could monitor the lesion during procedures. Thus, the operator could not adjust the size and/or location of the lesion during the procedures [31, 33, 48, 49]. Although DBS has advantages such as adjustability and reversibility, it also has drawbacks such as hardware-related complications, infection, hemorrhage, expense, and maintenance demands.

By contrast, MRgFUS enables neurosurgeons to perform a safe and accurate lesion in the ALIC by real-time, closed-loop monitoring of MR

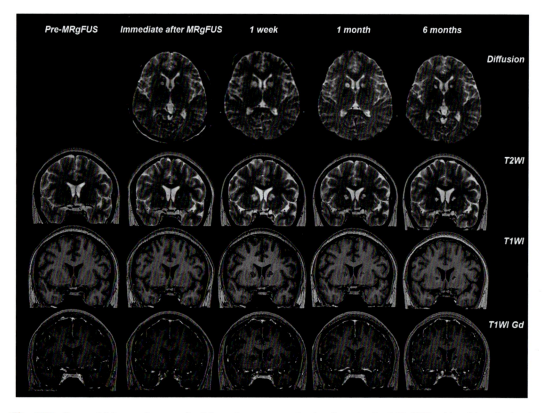

Fig. 12.3 Sequential image changes after bilateral anterior capsulotomy using MRgFUS. The size of the bilateral lesion in the anterior limb of the internal capsule was maximal at 1 week after MRgFUS with mild perilesional edema. One month after MRgFUS, the lesion stabilized and the edema disappeared

thermometry, without injuries in adjacent deep brain structures. Y-BOCS scores improved after 6 months, with a mean 33 ± 11 % improvement. The sequential improvement pattern after MRgFUS resembled other conventional neurosurgical treatments [9, 20, 46], although full response of Y-BOCS (more than 35 % improvement) was achieved in half of the total number of patients. Interestingly, significant improvements in both the HAM-D and HAM-A scores were detected after only 1 week, and were maintained for the whole follow-up period. Based on these results, neurosurgeons can realistically expand the scope of MRgFUS to treat other psychological disorders, especially depression. After inclusion of more patients and longer follow-up periods, we can expect MRgFUS to be adopted as a safe and effective neurosurgical option for refractory OCD patients.

12.5 Conclusion

There have always been attempts to finds safer and more effective methods for treating disease. In the era of neurosurgery and with the advent of focused ultrasound and MR thermography, MRgFUS enables neurosurgeons to make accurate, safe, and effective thermal lesions in deep brain structures. Even with our limited experience, we can predict the success of MRgFUS for treating refractory OCD patients.

References

1. Aouizerate B, Cuny E, Martin-Guehl C, Guehl D, Amieva H, Benazzouz A, Fabrigoule C, Allard M, Rougier A, Bioulac B, Tignol J, Burbaud P. Deep brain stimulation of the ventral caudate nucleus in the treatment of obsessive-compulsive disorder and major depression. Case report. J Neurosurg. 2004;101:682–6.
2. Baxter LR. Brain imaging as a tool in establishing a theory of brain pathology in obsessive compulsive disorder. J Clin Psychiatry. 1990;51 Suppl 22–25; discussion 26.
3. Bear RE, Fitzgerald P, Rosenfeld JV, Bittar RG. Neurosurgery for obsessive-compulsive disorder: contemporary approaches. J Clin Neurosci: Official J Neurosurg Soc Australas. 2010;17:1–5.
4. Bjorgvinsson T, Hart J, Heffelfinger S. Obsessive-compulsive disorder: update on assessment and treatment. J Psychiatr Pract. 2007;13:362–72.
5. Chang WS, Jung HH, Kweon EJ, Zadicario E, Rachmilevitch I, Chang JW. Unilateral magnetic resonance guided focused ultrasound thalamotomy for essential tremor: practices and clinicoradiological outcomes. J Neurol Neurosurg Psychiatry. 2014.
6. Child SZ, Hartman CL, Schery LA, Carstensen EL. Lung damage from exposure to pulsed ultrasound. Ultrasound Med Biol. 1990;16:817–25.
7. Clement GT, Sun J, Giesecke T, Hynynen K. A hemisphere array for non-invasive ultrasound brain therapy and surgery. Phys Med Biol. 2000;45:3707–19.
8. Clement GT, White J, Hynynen K. Investigation of a large-area phased array for focused ultrasound surgery through the skull. Phys Med Biol. 2000;45:1071–83.
9. D'Astous M, Cottin S, Roy M, Picard C, Cantin L. Bilateral stereotactic anterior capsulotomy for obsessive-compulsive disorder: long-term follow-up. J Neurol Neurosurg Psychiatry. 2013;84:1208–13.
10. Daffertshofer M, Gass A, Ringleb P, Sitzer M, Sliwka U, Els T, Sedlaczek O, Koroshetz WJ, Hennerici MG. Transcranial low-frequency ultrasound-mediated thrombolysis in brain ischemia: increased risk of hemorrhage with combined ultrasound and tissue plasminogen activator: results of a phase II clinical trial. Stroke; J Cereb Circ. 2005;36:1441–6.
11. Dickson JA, Calderwood SK. Temperature range and selective sensitivity of tumors to hyperthermia: a critical review. Ann N Y Acad Sci. 1980;335:180–205.
12. Elias WJ, Huss D, Voss T, Loomba J, Khaled M, Zadicario E, Frysinger RC, Sperling SA, Wylie S, Monteith SJ, Druzgal J, Shah BB, Harrison M, Wintermark M. A pilot study of focused ultrasound thalamotomy for essential tremor. N Engl J Med. 2013;369:640–8.
13. Field SB, Bleehen NM. Hyperthermia in the treatment of cancer. Cancer Treat Rev. 1979;6:63–94.
14. Fry FJ, Barger JE. Acoustical properties of the human skull. J Acoust Soc Am. 1978;63:1576–90.
15. Fry FJ, Goss SA, Patrick JT. Transkull focal lesions in cat brain produced by ultrasound. J Neurosurg. 1981;54:659–63.
16. Fry WJ. Intense ultrasound in investigations of the central nervous system. Adv Biol Med Phys. 1958;6:281–348.
17. Fry WJ, Barnard JW, Fry EJ, Krumins RF, Brennan JF. Ultrasonic lesions in the mammalian central nervous system. Science (N Y, NY). 1955;122:517–8.
18. Fry WJ, Barnard JW, Fry FJ, Brennan JF. Ultrasonically produced localized selective lesions in the central nervous system. Am J Phys Med. 1955;34:413–23.
19. Glover PM, Cavin I, Qian W, Bowtell R, Gowland PA. Magnetic-field-induced vertigo: a theoretical and experimental investigation. Bioelectromagnetics. 2007;28:349–61.
20. Greenberg BD, Gabriels LA, Malone DA Jr, Rezai AR, Friehs GM, Okun MS, Shapira NA, Foote KD, Cosyns PR, Kubu CS, Malloy PF, Salloway SP, Giftakis JE, Rise MT, Machado AG, Baker KB, Stypulkowski PH, Goodman WK, Rasmussen SA, Nuttin BJ. Deep brain stimulation of the ventral internal capsule/ventral striatum for obsessive-compulsive disorder: worldwide experience. Mol Psychiatry. 2010;15:64–79.
21. Greenberg BD, Price LH, Rauch SL, Friehs G, Noren G, Malone D, Carpenter LL, Rezai AR, Rasmussen SA. Neurosurgery for intractable obsessive-compulsive disorder and depression: critical issues. Neurosurg Clin N Am. 2003;14:199–212.
22. Guthkelch AN, Carter LP, Cassady JR, Hynynen KH, Iacono RP, Johnson PC, Obbens EA, Roemer RB, Seeger JF, Shimm DS, et al. Treatment of malignant brain tumors with focused ultrasound hyperthermia and radiation: results of a phase I trial. J Neurooncol. 1991;10:271–84.
23. Hansen ES, Hasselbalch S, Law I, Bolwig TG. The caudate nucleus in obsessive-compulsive disorder. Reduced metabolism following treatment with paroxetine: a PET study. Int J Neuropsychopharmacol Official Sci J Collegium Int Neuropsychopharmacologicum (CINP). 2002;5:1–10.
24. Hollander E. Obsessive-compulsive disorder: the hidden epidemic. J Clin Psychiatry. 1997;58(Suppl 12):3–6.
25. Jang SH, Yeo SS. Thalamocortical tract between anterior thalamic nuclei and cingulate gyrus in the human brain: diffusion tensor tractography study. Brain Imaging Behav. 2013;7:236–41.
26. Jolesz FA. MRI-guided focused ultrasound surgery. Annu Rev Med. 2009;60:417–30.
27. Karno M, Golding JM, Sorenson SB, Burnam MA. The epidemiology of obsessive-compulsive disorder in five US communities. Arch Gen Psychiatry. 1988;45:1094–9.
28. Kim CH, Chang JW, Koo MS, Kim JW, Suh HS, Park IH, Lee HS. Anterior cingulotomy for refractory obsessive-compulsive disorder. Acta Psychiatr Scand. 2003;107:283–90.

29. Kyriakou A, Neufeld E, Werner B, Paulides MM, Szekely G, Kuster N. A review of numerical and experimental compensation techniques for skull-induced phase aberrations in transcranial focused ultrasound. Int J Hyperth: Official J Eur Soc Hyperth Oncol, N Am Hyperth Group. 2014;30:36–46.

30. Lapidus KA, Kopell BH, Ben-Haim S, Rezai AR, Goodman WK. History of psychosurgery: a psychiatrist's perspective. World Neurosurg. 2013;80:S27–e21-16.

31. Lippitz BE, Mindus P, Meyerson BA, Kihlstrom L, Lindquist C. Lesion topography and outcome after thermocapsulotomy or gamma knife capsulotomy for obsessive-compulsive disorder: relevance of the right hemisphere. Neurosurgery. 1999;44:452–58; discussion 458–60.

32. Lipsman N, Schwartz ML, Huang Y, Lee L, Sankar T, Chapman M, Hynynen K, Lozano AM. MR-guided focused ultrasound thalamotomy for essential tremor: a proof-of-concept study. Lancet Neurol. 2013;12:462–8.

33. Lopes AC, Greenberg BD, Noren G, Canteras MM, Busatto GF, de Mathis ME, Taub A, D'Alcante CC, Hoexter MQ, Gouvea FS, Cecconi JP, Gentil AF, Ferrao YA, Fuentes D, de Castro CC, Leite CC, Salvajoli JV, Duran FL, Rasmussen S, Miguel EC. Treatment of resistant obsessive-compulsive disorder with ventral capsular/ventral striatal gamma capsulotomy: a pilot prospective study. J Neuropsychiatry Clin Neurosci. 2009;21:381–92.

34. Lynn JG, Zwemer RL, Chick AJ. The biological application of focused ultrasonic waves. Science (N Y, NY). 1942;96:119–20.

35. Lynn JG, Zwemer RL, Chick AJ, Miller AE. A new method for the generation and use of focused ultrasound in experimental biology. J Gen Physiol. 1942;26:179–93.

36. Martin E, Jeanmonod D, Morel A, Zadicario E, Werner B. High-intensity focused ultrasound for noninvasive functional neurosurgery. Ann Neurol. 2009;66:858–61.

37. Mindus P, Nyman H. Normalization of personality characteristics in patients with incapacitating anxiety disorders after capsulotomy. Acta Psychiatr Scand. 1991;83:283–91.

38. Muller N, Putz A, Kathmann N, Lehle R, Gunther W, Straube A. Characteristics of obsessive-compulsive symptoms in Tourette's syndrome, obsessive-compulsive disorder, and Parkinson's disease. Psychiatry Res. 1997;70:105–14.

39. Nuttin BJ, Gabriels LA, Cosyns PR, Meyerson BA, Andreewitch S, Sunaert SG, Maes AF, Dupont PJ, Gybels JM, Gielen F, Demeulemeester HG. Long-term electrical capsular stimulation in patients with obsessive-compulsive disorder. Neurosurgery 2003;52:1263–72; discussion 1272–64.

40. Nyman H, Andreewitch S, Lundback E, Mindus P. Executive and cognitive functions in patients with extreme obsessive-compulsive disorder treated by capsulotomy. Appl Neuropsychol. 2001;8:91–8.

41. O'Brien WD Jr. Ultrasound-biophysics mechanisms. Prog Biophys Mol Biol. 2007;93:212–55.

42. Oliver B, Gascon J, Aparicio A, Ayats E, Rodriguez R, Maestro De Leon JL, Garcia-Bach M, Soler PA. Bilateral anterior capsulotomy for refractory obsessive-compulsive disorders. Stereotact Funct Neurosurg 2003;81:90–5.

43. Phenix CP, Togtema M, Pichardo S, Zehbe I, Curiel L. High intensity focused ultrasound technology, its scope and applications in therapy and drug delivery. J Pharm Pharm Sci: Publ Can Soc Pharm Sci, Soc Can Sci Pharm. 2014;17:136–53.

44. Pulkkinen A, Huang Y, Song J, Hynynen K. Simulations and measurements of transcranial low-frequency ultrasound therapy: skull-base heating and effective area of treatment. Phys Med Biol. 2011;56:4661–83.

45. Rauch SL, Jenike MA, Alpert NM, Baer L, Breiter HC, Savage CR, Fischman AJ. Regional cerebral blood flow measured during symptom provocation in obsessive-compulsive disorder using oxygen 15-labeled carbon dioxide and positron emission tomography. Arch Gen Psychiatry. 1994;51:62–70.

46. Roh D, Chang WS, Chang JW, Kim CH. Long-term follow-up of deep brain stimulation for refractory obsessive-compulsive disorder. Psychiatry Res. 2012;200:1067–70.

47. Rubin D, Kuitert JH. Use of ultrasonic vibration in the treatment of pain arising from phantom limbs, scars and neuromas; a preliminary report. Arch Phys Med Rehabil. 1955;36:445–52.

48. Ruck C, Karlsson A, Steele JD, Edman G, Meyerson BA, Ericson K, Nyman H, Asberg M, Svanborg P. Capsulotomy for obsessive-compulsive disorder: long-term follow-up of 25 patients. Arch Gen Psychiatry. 2008;65:914–21.

49. Sheehan JP, Patterson G, Schlesinger D, Xu Z. Gamma knife surgery anterior capsulotomy for severe and refractory obsessive-compulsive disorder. J Neurosurg. 2013;119:1112–8.

50. Sturm V, Lenartz D, Koulousakis A, Treuer H, Herholz K, Klein JC, Klosterkotter J. The nucleus accumbens: a target for deep brain stimulation in obsessive-compulsive- and anxiety-disorders. J Chem Neuroanat. 2003;26:293–9.

51. ter Haar G. Intervention and therapy. Ultrasound Med Biol. 2000;26(Suppl 1):S51–4.

52. van den Heuvel OA, Veltman DJ, Groenewegen HJ, Dolan RJ, Cath DC, Boellaard R, Mesina CT, van Balkom AJ, van Oppen P, Witter MP, Lammertsma AA, van Dyck R. Amygdala activity in obsessive-

compulsive disorder with contamination fear: a study with oxygen-15 water positron emission tomography. Psychiatry Res. 2004;132:225–37.

53. Vykhodtseva N, Sorrentino V, Jolesz FA, Bronson RT, Hynynen K. MRI detection of the thermal effects of focused ultrasound on the brain. Ultrasound Med Biol. 2000;26:871–80.

54. Zhang QJ, Wang WH, Wei XP. Long-term efficacy of stereotactic bilateral anterior cingulotomy and bilateral anterior capsulotomy as a treatment for refractory obsessive-compulsive disorder. Stereotact Funct Neurosurg. 2013;91:258–61.

Deep Brain Stimulation for Tourette Syndrome

13

Jianuo Zhang, Yan Ge and Fangang Meng

13.1 Instruction

Tourette syndrome (TS) is a chronic neurobehavioral disorder characterized by waxing and waning motor and phonic tics that persist for at least 12 months [1]. It is also a multifactorial neurodevelopmental disorder that affects up to 1 % of children as well as many adults worldwide. The first clear description of this condition, published by Georges Albert Édouard Brutus Gilles de la Tourette in 1885 [2], noted childhood onset of stereotyped, abnormal movements and vocalizations (called tics), heritability, coprolalia (the utterance of obscene or socially offensive words), echolalia (repeating other people's words), and waxing and waning of symptoms; this description remains accurate and relevant today.

Tics generally occur in episodes and are preceded by premonitory sensations in the majority of patients. As many as 90 % of patients with TS have comorbid psychiatric conditions, such as obsessive compulsive behavior (OCB), attention deficit hyperactivity disorder (ADHD), or exhibit self-injurious behavior (SIB), depression and anxiety [3]; of these, OCB and ADHD are the most common, each occurring in up to 50 % of patients [4].

Once thought to be relatively rare, the prevalence of TS may in fact be as high as 50/10,000 in the general population [5]. The condition is approximately 10-fold more common in children than in adults, with a prevalence of up to 299/10,000 in 13- to 14-year-old children. In addition, TS is approximately 3 times more common in males than females. The onset of tics occurs at a mean age of 5–7 years, and severity appears to peak around age 10 years [5]. Symptoms may improve or even remit over time without treatment, and this tends to occur in the 3rd decade. However, no patient or clinical characteristics predictive of spontaneous resolution have been found [4].

13.2 Diagnosis

Instruments used to diagnose TS include the Diagnostic and Statistical Manual, 4th edition (DSM-IV) [6], the World Health Organization International Classification of Disease and Related Health Problems, 10th edition (ICD-10) [7] and the Tourette's Syndrome Classification Study Group (TSCSG) criteria [8]. According to the TSCSG, a diagnosis of *definite Tourette's syndrome* requires motor and/or phonic tics to be witnessed by a reliable examiner or to be captured in a video recording [8]. A patient may be considered to have *Tourette's syndrome by history* if a family member or close friend witnesses the tics and is able to provide a description to a reliable examiner that is accepted as indicative of TS. A diagnosis of TS is made when multiple motor tics and at least one vocal tic are present

J. Zhang (✉) · Y. Ge · F. Meng
Department of Neurosurgery, Beijing Tiantan Hospital, Capital Medical University, Beijing, China

B. Sun and A. De Salles (eds.), *Neurosurgical Treatments for Psychiatric Disorders*,
DOI 10.1007/978-94-017-9576-0_13
© Shanghai Jiao Tong University Press, Shanghai and Springer Science+Business Media Dordrecht 2015

(not necessarily concurrently), develop before the age of 18 years, and last for more than 1 year from their onset, although the intensity and frequency of tics may wax and wane during this period. Other potential causes of tics, including direct physiological effects of drugs (such as cocaine), or medical conditions (such as stroke, Huntington disease, or postviral encephalitis), should also be excluded. Moreover, tics can sometimes resemble choreic, myoclonic movements and stereotypies, but the presence of premonitory urges and the ability to temporarily suppress tics can help to distinguish TS from other movement disorders, where ADHD, OCB, SIB, or non-obscene socially inappropriate behaviors are also present.

13.3 Course of the Syndrome

The natural history of TS is fairly well understood. Tics usually emerge in childhood between the ages of 4 and 6 years and then increase in severity, peaking between the ages of 10 and 12 years. Motor tics generally precede the development of vocal tics, and onset of simple tics often predates that of complex tics. Tics tend to decline in severity during adolescence and, by early adulthood, most individuals experience markedly reduced numbers of tics or are free of tics. Tics that appear during adulthood are often attributable either to reemergence of childhood tics or to other factors, such as drugs, trauma, and stroke or brain infection. Onset of psychiatric conditions, especially ADHD, can precede the development of tics, present concurrently, or emerge after the appearance of tics. These comorbidities sometimes follow a similar clinical course to the tics, but in other cases they differ greatly. Some features of psychiatric conditions, such as mood disorders and SIB, often persist or worsen during adulthood, irrespective of tic severity. Certain factors and events, such as stress, anxiety, and fatigue, can increase the occurrence of tics, whereas others, such as tasks requiring concentration and motor skills, including musical and athletic performances and/

or physical exercise, can reduce or even temporarily halt tics. In addition, some individuals can voluntarily delay or suppress their tics for a short time; however, tics often reemerge with increased intensity and/or frequency.

The severity of tics and psychiatric disorders in patients with TS ranges from mild to severe. In some individuals, severe tics (for example, of the neck) can lead to self-inflicted pain, injury, and disability. However, for many patients with TS, the psychiatric comorbid disorders are more problematic than the tics, and can have a profoundly negative effect on quality of life. These individuals often live with various degrees of impairment in their academic and professional development, as well as reduced psychosocial wellbeing. Nonetheless, many individuals with TS lead successful lives, and can be unusually gifted and highly creative.

13.4 Pathophysiology

Anatomical and neurochemical changes that underlie the clinical manifestations of TS are unclear [9]. However, several studies provide evidence that both functional and structural alterations in the basal ganglia and other neuronal systems have a role in the complex symptomatology of the disorder. These changes could lead to alterations in filtering or sensorimotor gating mechanisms, resulting in urges to perform motor and vocal activities that are inappropriate, poorly timed, excessive, and/or very frequent [9].

Neuropathological studies in patients with TS demonstrate a reduction of up to 60 % in the number of fast-spiking γ-aminobutyric acid-releasing (GABAergic) and cholinergic interneurons in the caudate nucleus and putamen. Such individuals also demonstrate a decreased number of parvalbumin-positive GABAergic neurons in the globus pallidus externa (GPe), whereas the number of these neurons is markedly increased in the globus pallidus interna (GPi). These findings need to be confirmed in future studies, but they raise the possibility that defects in neuronal migration occurring during CNS development lead to altered basal ganglia circuitry and function [10, 11].

Brain imaging studies in patients with TS have produced inconsistent and sometimes conflicting results. Magnetic resonance imaging (MRI), for example, reveals considerable alterations in the volumes of certain neuroanatomical structures, including a notable reduction in the volume of the caudate nucleus and an increase in the volume of the hippocampus, amygdala, and thalamus. Similar studies have also reported thinning of sensory and motor cortical areas in individuals with this disorder. Functional MRI studies of patients with TS who were performing tasks to control their tics demonstrated alterations in the activity of various cortical, limbic, and basal ganglia areas. These observations might reflect either how the brain is affected by TS or how it seeks to compensate for the illness.

Overall, patients with TS seem to exhibit hypoactivity in the basal ganglia and hyperactivity in motor and/or premotor areas, consistent with the structural neuroimaging findings. Exactly how the above-mentioned neuroanatomical changes are related to TS is not clear, although an increasing body of evidence suggests that alterations in basal ganglia function, specifically within the corticostriatal–thalamocortical circuitry and perhaps also the dopaminergic nigrostriatal pathway, play a role in the pathophysiology of this disorder. Ablation or electrical stimulation of the globus pallidus internal segment or thalamic nuclei has been reported to reduce the severity of tics. Similarly, dopamine D_2 receptor antagonists, such as haloperidol and pimozide, and dopamine-depleting agents, such as tetrabenazine, are effective in alleviating the motor symptoms of TS. By contrast, drugs that increase dopamine levels and/or activity in the brain, such as levodopa, also increase the frequency of tics. Notably, other neuronal pathways, including noradrenergic, serotoninergic, histaminergic, glutaminergic, GABAergic, and cholinergic systems, have been implicated in TS, perhaps because drugs that target these systems can improve some symptoms of the disorder.

13.5 Therapy

The early attempts to treat individuals with TS are considered, by today's standards, bizarre, inventive, and largely ineffective. These approaches included application of leeches to the skin, cooling of the body, static electricity, hydrotherapy, spinal elongation, and the use of various chemical agents, such as herbs. To date, no cure exists for TS, but several rational approaches are now available for management of the disorder, although they are not universally effective. Importantly, the complex presentation of motor dysfunction, psychiatric features, and psychosocial impairments in individuals with TS clearly require a multifactorial approach to management of the disorder.

After a diagnosis is obtained, educating the patient, their parents, and other interested parties (for example, a child's teachers) about TS can help to define appropriate expectations for these individuals, as well as to optimize the patient's treatment strategy. Indeed, for most children with TS, addressing the many popular misconceptions about the disorder among their peers often leads to informed and improved relationships and can substantially reduce the burdens associated with this condition. Medication is not necessary for many individuals with TS, especially those with only mild tics. However, for those with moderate to severe tics or psychiatric comorbidities, which are often more problematic than the tics, several pharmacological agents are available, although such treatments frequently produce ineffective results, whereby the risks associated with treatments outweigh the benefits. Some patients with TS find that professional counseling, guidance, and psychotherapy sessions are invaluable, whereas others, such as children with learning impairments, might benefit from access to specialist educational and disability services. Behavioral and surgical approaches to TS are also currently being investigated and are expected to become accessible treatment options in the future for some people with this disorder. Treatment for TS is, therefore, highly personalized, and optimization requires effort from both the care provider and the patient.

13.6 Pharmacological Therapy

During the 1960s and 1970s, researchers showed that the dopamine D_2 receptor blocker haloperidol could reduce tic severity in patients with TS. These findings led to the investigation of many other potential drug treatments for the disorder. Notably, none had been specifically developed to treat TS; instead, these agents were all in use for other indications, both neurological (such as schizophrenia) and non-neurological (such as hypertension), before they were found to be effective in the treatment of TS. Haloperidol and pimozide are currently the only FDA-approved medications for this syndrome. These two drugs and other medications can be used to reduce tic severity, as well as some of the psychiatric comorbidities associated with TS.

Physicians typically follow a sequential approach to treating tics in people with TS. α-Adrenergic agonists, such as guanfacine and clonidine, are the usual first-line treatment. These two drugs are recommended for individuals with mild tics, since these medications are associated with fewer adverse effects than are other classes of drugs. Second-line treatment (used owing to lack of efficacy of α-adrenergic agonists) consists of antipsychotic agents, which are the most effective drugs for treating TS. However, these agents are associated with serious adverse effects. Antipsychotic drugs are classified as either typical or atypical; the typical agents are dopamine D_2 receptor antagonists (such as haloperidol, pimozide and fluphenazine), whereas the atypical antipsychotic drugs are dopaminergic and serotonergic receptor antagonists (such as risperidone and aripiprazole). Atypical antipsychotic drugs are preferred over typical ones as the atypical agents carry a lower risk of extrapyramidal and other adverse effects (such as tardive dyskinesias). In addition, atypical antipsychotic drugs improve behavioral comorbidities, as well as tics, in patients with TS.

Other medications beneficial for treating TS include benzodiazepines, such as clonazepam, topiramate, and injections of botulinum toxin into the muscle groups associated with bothersome or disabling tics (for example, those of the eyelids, neck, or larynx). Some case reports suggest that tetrabenazine, a dopamine-depleting agent, can reduce tic severity in patients with TS, but double-blind studies are required to define its efficacy [3, 5, 12].

As previously mentioned, psychiatric comorbidities often pose a greater problem than tics for people with TS. The stimulant drug methylphenidate, the α-adrenergic agonists guanfacine and clonidine, and the selective norepinephrine reuptake blocker atomoxetine, can improve ADHD in patients with TS. Initial concerns that stimulant drugs could worsen tics and other features of TS have been refuted by the results of further studies. Cognitive behavioral therapy, selective serotonin reuptake inhibitors such as fluoxetine, and both typical and atypical antipsychotic drugs have all been used to treat OCB in patients with TS.

13.7 Behavioral Therapy

Behavioral therapies for patients with TS aim to teach the individual how to modify the environmental factors that influence their tic severity, as well as offer skills that can be used by the individual to optimize their management of the symptoms of the disorder. The therapeutic potential of these approaches, such as habit reversal training and exposure with response prevention, has long been known, but these approaches have not been investigated as extensively as pharmacological interventions for TS. In recent years, however, major advances have been made in behavioral therapies for TS. A randomized controlled trial in children and adolescents with TS or chronic tic disorders showed that comprehensive behavioral intervention for tics (CBIT), an enhancement of the widely used habit reversal training method for treating behavioral disorders, significantly reduced tic severity in almost 50 % of patients. CBIT is a promising therapy that should be further developed and tested in future studies, and will probably become accessible to many people with TS.

13.8 Surgical Therapy

Although it is frequently self-limited, some patients remain symptomatic and require chronic treatment. The standard treatment is pharmacologic involving mainly neuroleptics, 2-adrenergic agonists, and sometimes benzodiazepines. In some cases, behavioral treatment may provide temporary control of symptoms but certain patients prove medically untreatable or experience unbearable side effects from the medication. It is these patients who are potential candidates for neurosurgical interventions. During the past few decades, many ablative procedures have been performed in an attempt to treat intractable TS. In total, 65 patients underwent ablative surgery varying from "tailored" stereotactic operations to more rigorous prefrontal lobotomies, which were lobotomy, limbic leucotomy, leucotomy, cingulotomy, campotomy, thalamotomy, dentatotomy, coagulation, ablative surgery, and stereotactic surgery.

In 1962, Baker [13] described TS as an "involuntary paroxysmal hyperkinesis involving the entire skeletal musculature" and reported the first leucotomy for TS. The procedure was complicated by a frontal lobe abscess, which was aspirated. In the same year, Cooper [14] published the case of a 16-year-old girl, and a right chemothalamectomy was performed, followed by a left chemothalamectomy 1 year later. Cooper reported that after the surgery, the patient experienced substantial tic reduction and was fully functional. Two years later, Stevens [15] published long-term follow-up results of a 37-year-old man who had undergone the first prefrontal lobotomy, carried out by James Watts in 1955. In 1970, Hassler and Dieckmann [16] reported the results of bilateral thalamotomies in 3 patients with intractable TS. They performed more than 10 coagulations of the intralaminar and medial thalamic nuclei, and, in case of facial tics, in the ventro-oralis internus (Voi). Only the effects with respect to tics were reported, which improved after surgery by 100 % in Patient 1, 90 % in Patient 2, and 70 % in Patient 3. No details regarding the tic-rating method were provided. Nadvornik and associates [17]

described a case of stereotactic dentatotomy and bilateral frontal leucotomy. Beckers [18] published the outcome of neurosurgical treatment in 3 TS patients. Two stereotactic operations (target unclear) were performed on Patient 1 (female) with a interval of 1 year between surgeries. Patient 2 (male) underwent a bilateral campotomy and prefrontal leucotomy in two surgical sessions. A bilateral leucotomy was performed on the third patient (female). The author observed that these stereotactic interventions resulted in partial tic reduction. Nevertheless, surgery was not advocated as a good treatment option for intractable TS because of the side effects, which were not specified. In 1978, Wassmann and associates [19] briefly mentioned a female patient who had undergone a prefrontal lobotomy but they did not provide any information regarding the outcome. Asam and colleagues [20] provided a brief (and incomplete) review of the literature on surgical interventions for TS and reported their experience with two TS patients. The patients were male, 14 and 15 years old, with a disease duration of 5 and 11 years, respectively. Their first patient underwent stereotactic surgery (target unclear) with temporary relief of tics. Postoperatively, this patient developed a spastic hemiplegia. Coagulation of the left zona incerta (ZI) was performed in the second patient, who also experienced a postoperative hemiplegia. The same patient was operated on 15 months later, for unclear reasons, in the contralateral ZI. Postoperatively, this patient developed hemiplegia of the left side and became quadriplegic. According to the authors, temporary relief of symptoms was achieved in this patient. Later, tics reoccurred in combination with complex dystonic movements. They concluded that surgical intervention in TS may produce temporary improvement of tics but that surgery can be accompanied by severe side effects. In 1982, Hassler [21] updated the material on stereotaxic surgery for psychiatric disturbances in Schaltenbrand's textbook and briefly mentioned his experience with thalamic surgery in 15 patients suffering from intractable TS. No details were provided about the outcome.

In 1987, Cappabianca and coworkers [22] published the long-term results of 3 patients described initially by de Divitiis and associates [23], and of 1 new patient. In addition, they provided a review of (all) operated patients. Their operation was based on stereotactic coordinates proposed by Hassler and Dieckmann. The intralaminar and dorsomedian nuclei of the thalamus were coagulated bilaterally in 1 patient and unilaterally in 3 patients. The authors reported temporary tic improvement in 2 patients lasting a few months, a slight reduction in compulsive symptoms in 1 patient, and almost complete tic regression in the fourth. Follow-up examinations of these patients were several years earlier than one would expect when considering the publication year. Robertson and associates [24] reported on a 19-year-old man with disease onset at the age of 5.5 years, presenting with a variety of verbal and motor tics. The tics were treated successfully with the D_2 receptor antagonist, sulpiride; however, compulsions could not be treated. Stereotactic limbic leucotomy was performed involving bilateral lesions in the lower medial quadrants of the frontal lobes and separate lesions in the anterior cingulum (limbic leucotomy). Postoperatively, compulsions disappeared within 6 weeks. Side effects consisted of apathy, general intellectual impairment, organizational problems, and difficulties in concentration. After 2 years, the patient was socially independent and free from SIB. Robertson and colleagues concluded that limbic leucotomy should be considered an effective treatment in TS patients with severe self-injurious behavior, but emphasized that long-term effects on tics required further assessment. Again, the authors did not mention the method of tic evaluation, the impact or the time course of side effects, or criteria for the diagnosis of TS. In 1993, Sawle and colleagues reported on the results of bilateral limbic leucotomy in a 45-year-old man suffering from TS. The symptoms consisted of severe SIB, obsessions and compulsions [25], and vocal and motor tics. Long-term trials of pharmacologic and behavioral therapy had failed. During limbic leucotomy, bilateral coagulations were performed on the anterior hypothalamus and cingulate gyrus. In a personal communication to Rauch and coworkers [26], Sawle remarked that the actual targets were those of conventional limbic leucotomy (cingulotomy plus thermocoagulation of the frontothalamic fibers). According to the authors, the surgery had no direct effect on tics whereas the compulsions were reduced. Nineteen months after surgery, however, there were no longer any signs of tics and the patient reported excellent improvement with regard to his obsessions. Leckman and associates [27] in 1993 reported on a 40-year-old man suffering from TS and OCB who underwent surgery. Disease onset was at the age of 3 years with motor tics. Vocal tics appeared later, and checking and cleaning compulsions were present, as was SIB. Symptoms failed to respond to medication trials. The patient underwent bilateral stereotactic infrathalamic lesioning and anterior cingulotomy. Postoperatively, the obsessions and compulsions improved, but the patient continued to experience severe motor and vocal tics. Three weeks later, the left infrathalamic and cingulated lesions were repeated. During this second surgical session, the infrathalamic lesion was extended more inferiorly within the borders of the red nucleus and a subsequent coagulation was performed in the H fields of Forel. The patient experienced severe neurological deficits postoperatively including dysarthria, dysphagia, handwriting and gait problems, mild hemiparesis, abnormal extraocular movements, axial rigidity, and bradykinesia. The authors suggested that these side effects were due to extension of the infrathalamic lesion. Long-term, tics and OCB returned. The authors concluded that brain lesioning not only influences pathological symptoms, but also damages physiological functioning.

One year later, Baer and coworkers [28] reported on the effects of cingulotomy in a patient with TS and OCB. The patient was a 35-year-old man with OCB and associated TS with onset at age 5 years. He failed to respond to either behavioral therapy or medication. The patient underwent two cingulotomies with an interval of 18 months between procedures. After the first and second operation, there was no clear effect on his tics. This procedure, however, resulted in an improvement in OCB. The authors concluded that cingulotomy alone was not an effective treatment for TS. In 1995, Rauch and colleagues [28] published a comprehensive review of neurosurgical treatments for TS. They provided detailed information regarding the different neurosurgical approaches by summarizing the available literature. In their report, emphasis was placed on the rationale for the different targets. Mention was made, however, regarding 3 patients who underwent bilateral anterior cingulotomies and infrathalamic lesioning, which had not been published previously. The first patient was a 34-year-old woman with severe TS, OCB, and bipolar disorder. The patient underwent an anterior cingulotomy plus infrathalamic lesioning. Tic counting using videotapes, performed by Rauch and co-workers, revealed a decrease in the number of tics from 18 to 2 tics/min. The second patient was a 40-year-old man suffering from self-injurious motor tics, coprolalia, and OCB. The third patient was not described in detail. The latter 2 patients underwent the same procedure as the first, with a poor outcome. Furthermore, the second patient experienced dysarthria and swallowing, handwriting, and gait problems, postoperatively. Only a moderate improvement in tics and OCB was observed. The third patient experienced no improvement in symptoms at all. In addition, Rauch and associates noted a case published in the Russian literature by Korzenin in 1991. This involved a 19-year-old man with TS and associated OCB who underwent bilateral cryothalamotomy (ventrolateral nuclei) with good results observed at a 1-year follow-up. Several years later, Korzenev and colleagues [29] published results of their surgical treatment of 4 intractable TS patients. They concluded that stereotactic surgery was an effective method of treatment for severe incurable TS. However, in their article no description of the TS patients was provided with respect to patient characteristics, tics, surgical target, or method of evaluation.

Many different lesioning procedures have been performed in TS throughout the history of surgical treatment of this disorder. Frontal lobe operations included prefrontal lobotomies and bimedial frontal leucotomies. The limbic system was targeted during limbic leucotomy and anterior cingulotomy. Thalamic operations included lesioning of the medial, intralaminar, and ventrolateral thalamic nuclei. Infrathalamic lesions were performed at the level of Forel's fields (campotomies) and the zona incerta, and cerebellar surgeries included dentatotomies. In an attempt to achieve total control of symptoms, more complex operations have been performed, such as combined anterior cingulotomies and infrathalamic lesioning.

13.9 Deep Brain Stimulation

Deep brain stimulation (DBS) is a reversible and adjustable neurosurgical technique involving the implantation of stimulating electrodes that send continuous electrical impulses to specific target areas in the brain. Following implantation of the electrodes, the stimulator settings are adjusted at follow-up endpoints to achieve optimal results with minimal adverse effects.

In 1999, the first DBS was performed for intractable TS, with the target for thalamic stimulation based on the thalamotomies described by Hassler [30]. Since then, different targets have been used. While DBS is a well-established treatment option for different neurological disorders, including Parkinson's disease, dystonia, and tremor, its use in TS is still experimental.

13.10 Deep Brain Stimulation in Tourette Syndrome

Although DBS has shown potential in the treatment of refractory TS, there are numerous issues still to be resolved: (1) The proper indications for DBS and the definition of 'refractoriness' to conventional treatments, (2) the choice of target area on the basis of the clinical picture, (3) the suitability of general anesthesia during DBS, (4) postoperative issues, such as follow-up evaluation techniques, and (5) optimization of pulse generator settings.

13.10.1 Patient Selection

Useful recommendations for patient selection have been provided by the Tourette Syndrome Association (TSA) [4]. However, on the basis of the waxing and waning nature of the clinical picture of TS and considering the rather frequent behavioral comorbidities that limit patient compliance, indication for DBS can be difficult. Moreover, the widespread view that DBS should be considered an adjunctive therapy for conservative or noninvasive/nonsurgical treatments (such as botulinum toxin infiltration) is the most uncertain issue as criteria for the definition of 'refractoriness' are still not clearly defined.

DBS is used on the basis of a documented lack of response or presence of unbearable adverse effects over a minimum of 6 months' treatment with conventional (typical and atypical neuroleptics) or innovative treatments (including dopamine depletors such as tetrabenazine), while selective serotonin reuptake inhibitors (fluvoxamine 25–100 mg) are also administered for obsessive-compulsive comorbidity, alone or in association with clorimipramine 25–100 mg/day. ADHD is treated with clonidine 75–150 mg/day or guanfacine 5 mg or higher/day, while nonresponsive isolated tic manifestations can be treated with botulinum toxin infiltration at the involved districts (including the cricoarythenoid muscles for phonic tics) [31, 32].

Patients were selected from our specialty clinic of thousands of TS patients and all potential subjects were screened by a multidisciplinary team including a neurologist, neurosurgeon, neuropsychologist, psychiatrist, and ethicist, and were also required to have followed a psychobehavioral approach for at least 6 months without clinical success. Surgery should be considered if a patient continues to demonstrate clinical signs incompatible with normal social functioning, or if the symptoms are life threatening. A study by Servello et al. reported that 2 of 18 patients underwent DBS because their refractory neck twisting tics caused cervical myelopathy requiring spinal surgery. Following DBS, the neck torsion bouts decreased significantly, motor impairment was stabilized and a motor rehabilitation program was established [33].

Moreover, in order to be eligible for DBS, patients should demonstrate compliance with previous treatments. Compliance should be assessed in terms of (1) adherence to pharmacological protocols, (2) completion of follow-up visits, and (3) adherence to psychobehavioral training programs. The rational to use different targets is that all targets belong to the ventral striatal-thalamo-cortical circuitries which are thought to be dysfunctional in TS.

13.10.2 Target Choice

In TS patients, the most often used targets of stimulation are the thalamus (centromedian-parafascicular complex; CM–Pf) and the globus pallidus internus (GPi). In the literature, however, seven different targets have been described so far in patients with chronic tics: thalamus (CM–Pf) and CM–Spv [substantia periventricularis/nucleus ventralis oralis intermedius (Voi)], GPi (posteroventrolateral and anteromedial part), nucleus accumbens (NA), anterior limb of the internal capsule (AIC), and subthalamicus nucleus (STN).

One of the most commonly used targets for DBS in the treatment of TS, the CM-Pf, part of the intralaminar nucleus of the thalamus, is involved in sensorimotor basal ganglia circuitry [34, 35]. The anterior CM-Pf is able to influence cells involved in tremor generation located in a wide area including the ventral oral anterior and posterior (VoA and VoP) nuclei [36]. The intralaminar nuclei and CM-Pf convey multimodal stimulatory signals to the striatum, and are thus involved in attention and arousal in response to stimulation. Stimulation of the CM-Pf and VoA complex has proved to be effective in the treatment of behavioral aspects of TS as well as alleviation of tics [33]. In a study of 18 patients reported by one center treated with DBS of the CM-Pf and VoA, all patients responded well with significant, although varied, reductions in severity and frequency of tics and in behavioral comorbidities after DBS. The mean total Yale

Global Tic Severity Scale (YGTSS) scores were reduced from 41.1 (SD 8.3) prior to DBS to 28.6 (SD 17.5) post-DBS ($p < 0.001$) and similar reductions were seen in YGTSS motor, phonic, and social impairment scores (all $p < 0.001$ vs. baseline) [33]. In a recent case report, a woman with severe refractory TS despite DBS of the anterior internal capsule achieved significant improvement in tic control at 3 months following bilateral centromedian thalamic stimulation (reduction in total tic score: 42 % compared with pre-DBS baseline and 27 % compared with DBS of the postinternal capsule) and a reduction in psychiatric side effects such as altered mood and impulse control compared with internal capsule stimulation [38].

Although the CM-Pf is often thought to be the preferred target for DBS [33, 35], alternative locations such as the nucleus accumbens and the GPi are not to be excluded; favorable outcomes in patients with TS have been reported with DBS of both the nucleus accumbens and the GPi.

The anteromedial part of the GPi acts as a limbic relay for output pathways of the basal ganglia, and continuous high frequency stimulation of this region has been shown to ameliorate dystonia. Stimulation of the GPi is able to modify the neuronal activity of the VoA nucleus. The VoA nucleus is involved in initiating planned movement and suppressing unwanted movement, whereas the VoP nucleus plays a role in the sensations of touch, itching, temperature, taste and arousal, in addition to body position. Recently, in a double blind, randomized study in 3 patients with severe, refractory TS, bilateral stimulation of the GPi produced a significant and greater reduction in tic severity (assessed using the Yale Global Tic Severity Scale; YGTSS) than stimulation of the CM-Pf [38].

The nucleus accumbens is presumed to have a modulatory activity on amygdaloid basal ganglia-prefrontal cortex circuitry and, as the activity of its neurons is modulated by dopamine and a high proportion of cells have high concentrations of dopamine D_1 and D_3 receptors, the nucleus accumbens is believed to also be involved in addiction and OCB [39]. The effectiveness of DBS of the nucleus accumbens has been demonstrated in patients with severe OCB and anxiety disorder. In a 37-year-old woman with severe refractory TS, DBS administered to the anterior limb of the internal capsule (electrode terminating in the nucleus accumbens) provided significant reduction in tic frequency and severity at 18 months after surgery [12]. Tic reduction was also shown following DBS of the nucleus accumbens in a 26-year-old male patient with severe tics and SIB; coprolalia and tics involving self-harm were almost completely resolved [40].

The optimal area for the final DBS electrode implantation within the chosen target nucleus was studied with intraoperative microrecordings in at least two monopolar electrode tracks, acquired at steps of 1–0.5 mm from 8–10 mm above to 1 mm below the neuroradiologically estimated position of the target nucleus. Undergoing studies are evaluating firing patterns in order to characterize a neurophysiological target thus increasing DBS precision.

We retrospectively assessed long-term clinical outcomes of 13 TS patients, who were refractory to pharmacological and psychotherapeutic treatment, and underwent DBS targeting the GPi, using data from Beijing Tiantan Hospital database from January 1 2006 to May 31 2013. The primary outcome was a change in tic severity as measured by the YGTSS and the secondary outcome was a change in associated behavioral disorders and mood as measured by the Tourette Syndrome–Quality of Life Scale (TSQOL) assessment. The results showed that the average reduction in the total YGTSS scores at last follow-up (mean 43 months, range 13–80 months) compared with those at baseline were reduced by 52 % (range 4–84 %), and mean improvement rates at 1, 6, 12, 18, 24, 30, and 36 months relative to baseline were 13, 22, 29, 34, 42, 47, and 55 %, respectively. We noticed significant improvements in tic symptoms after 6 months of DBS programming ($p < 0.05$), as assessed by paired t-test. TSQOL scores improved by an average of 46 % (range 11–77 %). Our study provides the largest reported GPi DBS case series of 13 treatment-refractory TS patients with the longest follow-up. Our results support the potential beneficial effect of GPi DBS for reducing disabling tics and improvement in quality of life. The details are as follows.

Totally, thirteen patients (12 males and 1 female) with TS were selected to undergo GPi DBS (Tables 13.1 and 13.2) due to the severe disability arising from their tics. All patients failed treatment with α-adrenergic agonists, ≥2 dopamine receptor antagonists, benzodiazepine, and behavioral therapy. Preoperatively, each of these patients was evaluated by a specialist and identified to fulfill Diagnostic and Statistical Manual of Mental Disorders (Fourth Edition) [6] criteria for TS. The DBS procedure was approved by the Neuromodulation Committee at Beijing Tiantan Hospital. Preoperatively, and again after optimization of DBS parameters, each patient was tested with the YGTSS, as detailed in supplementary materials. A YGTSS score of 35/ 50 (motor and vocal tic severity on a 0–50 scale) or higher for 1 year is a marker of disease severity sufficient to warrant consideration for DBS. All patients had severe tic disorders with functional impairment and YGTSS > 35/50 (motor and vocal tic severity on a 0–50 scale). In addition, tics were the major symptom causing disability in all patients and their comorbid conditions were stably treated.

In brief, patients were fixed with a Leksell G stereotactic head frame (ElektaAB, Stockholm, Sweden) on the morning of surgery and transferred to an MRI suite to obtain MRI (3.0 T) scans. Image data were then transferred to a Surgiplan Workstation (Elekta, Sweden) in the operation room to visualize the individual pallidal target [41–43]. The target was the GPi located on fused MRI images with the following coordinates: GPi was 3 mm anterior to the midcommissural point, 18–21 mm lateral to the midplane of the third ventricle, and 4–6 mm below the intercommissural line. Target coordinates were adapted according to the width of the third ventricle and anterior commissure-posterior commissure (AC-PC) length. During planning, visible vessels were avoided in the planned trajectory. A Leksell stereotactic frame was used,

with microelectrode recording to document electrode location in relation to the patient's individual anatomy. Full details of the neurosurgical procedure were published previously. After placement of a burr hole, in line with the planned trajectory, extracellular single-unit microelectrode recordings were performed. Recording started 15 mm above target and continued until 4 mm beneath target (LeadPoint, Medtronic, Minneapolis, MN, USA) in 0.5–1 mm steps. In all 13 patients, microelectrode recordings clearly showed GPi electrical signals. The signals demonstrated a high frequency and high amplitude firing pattern with high background noise. Electrical activity was rhythmic and in some cases "tremor cells" could be detected. Tentative stimulation usually mildly relieved the hypertension of muscles, while the involuntary movement seldom improved. Subsequently, the quadripolar electrode (model 3387; Medtronic) with the deepest contact (contact 0) at the level of the GPi target was implanted, and a temporary test stimulation was performed below the best electrical signal (0–3+, frequency 185 Hz, pulse width 90 μs) to assess stimulation-induced side effects. Stimulus intensity was gradually increased in steps of 0.1 mA, until unwanted side effects occurred or until a maximum stimulus intensity of 5.0 mA. Finally, this definite electrode was fixed in the burr hole with acrylic cement, and connected to an externalized extension cable. DBS was always performed bilaterally. CT scans were performed on the operative day to evaluate electrode position and detect asymptomatic hemorrhage. MRI was also performed on the next day of the operation to evaluate the electrode position. Once agreement between the neurologist, the neurosurgeon, and the psychiatrist was obtained regarding potential beneficial effects, an implantable pulse generator (IPG) was implanted as a separate procedure, under general anesthesia, within 1 week (Kinetra model 7428, Medtronic).

After the second procedure, stimulation parameters were adjusted during a 4-week unblinded period to determine the most effective parameters on tics with the lowest amplitude.

13 Deep Brain Stimulation for Tourette Syndrome

Table 13.1 Clinical characteristics of ten patients with Tourette syndrome

Patient	Tic symptoms	Associated behavioral disorders	Socioprofessional status	Medication before surgery	Medication 1 year after surgery
1[a]	Eye blinking, head banging, shoulder shrugs, jerks of legs facial grimaces	None	Employed	Haloperidol 4 mg bid	Haloperidol 4 mg bid
2[b]	Facial grimaces, shoulder shrugs flexion arm, shouting, coprolalia	None	Employed	None	None
3	Shoulder shrugs, grunting, echolalia	None	Employed	None	None
4	Echolalia	OCB	Employed	None	None
5	Head banging, shoulder shrugs, shouting	None	Employed	Haloperidol 4 mg bid	Haloperidol 4 mg bid
6[b]	Head banging, shoulder shrugs, shouting	None	Employed	Haloperidol 4 mg bid, pimozide 4 mg/day	None
7[b]	Head banging, neck extension	None	Employed	Haloperidol 4 mg bid	None
8	Facial grimaces, shoulder shrugs flexion arm, shouting, coprolalia	OCB ADHD	Unemployed	Haloperidol 4 mg bid, pimozide 4 mg/day	Haloperidol 4 mg bid
9	Shoulder shrugs, shouting	ADHD	Unemployed	None	None
10	Eye blinking, coughing, head banging, shouting, bird noises	None	Employed	None	None
11	Eye blinking, coughing, head banging, shouting	None	Employed	None	None
12[a]	Head banging, shoulder shrugs neck extension, coprolalia, elevation shoulder	OCB ADHD	Unemployed	Risperidone 2 mg bid, mirtazapine, 45 mg bid, citalopram 40 mg/day	Risperidone 2 mg bid, mirtazapine, 45 mg bid, citalopram 40 mg/day
13	Eye blinking, head banging	None	Unemployed	None	None

All patients failed treatment with α-adrenergic agonists, ≥2 dopamine receptor antagonists, benzodiazepine, and behavioral therapy before the surgery

OCB obsessive-compulsive behavior; *ADHD* attention-deficit hyperactivity disorder anxiety

[a] There was no charge in the implantable pulse generator *IPG* of patient 1, but it was changed or removed for unknown reasons. Patient 12 reported anxiety, agitation, depression, and constant tiredness that did not vary with stimulation adjustment. Eventually this patient had his electrodes removed, and the IPG was not implanted

[b] Symptoms of patient 2 almost completely resolved, but patients 6 and 7 thought there was almost no change in their disorders. Thus the implanted systems of the 3 patients were removed 4–5 years after the operation

Table 13.2 Patients operated on for GPi DBS for TS

Patient	Sex	Age at tic onset	Age at DBS	Motor tics	Phonic tics	Target	DBS surgery complications	Side effects	Follow-up time (m)
1	M	8	16	C	None	GPi	None	None	80
2	M	9	19	C	S	GPi	Pyosis of the head	None	60
3	M	13	20	S	S	GPi	Subcutaneous hydrops of the chest	Anxiety	53
4	M	3	18	S	S	GPi	None	None	54
5	M	11	20	C	S	GPi	None	None	57
6	M	10	28	C	S	GPi	None	None	54
7	F	20	21	C	None	GPi	None	None	47
8	M	12	18	C	S	GPi	None	Agitation	38
9	M	10	17	C	S	GPi	None	Agitation	36
10	M	6	34	C	S	GPi	None	None	14
11	M	13	28	C	S	GPi	None	Anxiety	22
12	M	7	23	C	C	GPi	None	Anxiety, agitation depression, tiredness	17
13	M	7	20	C	None	GPi	None	None	13

M male; *F* female; *DBS* deep brain stimulation; *S* simple; *C* complex; *m* month; *Gpi* globus pallidus internus

Sequential monopolar stimulation through each contact was delivered on four consecutive days with a pulse width of 60 μs and a frequency of 130 Hz. During this period the voltage was progressively increased until unwanted side effects occurred. Once the final electrode active contacts were chosen (monopolar or bipolar), the frequency, pulse width and voltage were adapted to obtain the best clinical effect on tic reduction and side effects.

Tables 13.1 and 13.2 present an overview of the 13 patients. Mean age at DBS was 21.7 years (SD, 5.0 years). All patients failed treatment with α-adrenergic agonists, ≥2 dopamine receptor antagonists, benzodiazepine, and behavioral therapy. YGTSS scores at the last visit compared to those at baseline were reduced in all 13 patients. Table 13.3 presents quantitative results of YGTSS assessments for each patient at sequential follow-up visits. Table 13.4 presents quantitative results of TSQOL assessments at the last follow-up. Figure 13.1 presents the mean YGTSS scores and the SD of the 13 patients at sequential follow-up examinations.

13.10.3 Electrode Localization and Stimulation Settings

Each Medtronic 3387 electrode has 4 contacts at the distal tip, conventionally named 0–3 for the left hemisphere and 4–7 for the right hemisphere; site, voltage, pulse width, and frequency of stimulation can be controlled by external programming through an implanted battery. Usually, it took as long as 6 months before optimal stimulation settings were identified (Table 13.5). The majority of our TS patients had a configuration of double monopolar with 0–2-/C+ and 4–6-/C+, while several other patients had configurations of monopolar (1-/C+ and 5-/C+), and bipolar (1–3+ and 5–7+), all with bilateral amplitude ≤3.6 V, pulse width ≤120 μs, and rate ≤185 Hz.

13 Deep Brain Stimulation for Tourette Syndrome

Table 13.3 Yale Global Tic Severity Scale (YGTSS) assessments at sequential follow-up

Patient	YGTSS baseline	1 month	6 months	12 months	18 months	24 months	30 months	36 + months	Final follow-up improvement rate (%)
1	58	43	35	27	30	30	26	24	19 (67.2)
2	61	53	48	37	33	27	24	15	10 (83.6)
3	74	53	47	43	36	33	26	19	17 (77.0)
4	74	65	46	53	38	27	28	26	21 (71.6)
5	47	43	40	35	31	24	21	10	8 (83.0)
6	45	42	43	39	36	32	27	25	18 (60.0)
7	48	45	41	37	33	29	25	23	22 (54.2)
8	93	87	78	67	63	55	67	59	48 (48.4)
9	73	65	67	64	59	55	48	46	46 (37.0)
10	58	53	45	38	–	–	–	–	35 (39.7)
11	58	51	48	45	43	39	–	–	36 (37.9)
12[a]	94	94	92	90	–	–	–	–	90 (4.3)
13	42	34	31	29	–	–	–	–	25 (40.5)
Mean[b]	60.9	52.8	47.4	42.8	40.2	35.1	32.4	27.4	25.4 (58.3)
SD[b]	15.1	14.1	13.0	12.6	11.6	11.3	15.1	15.5	13.1 (–)
Improvement rates[b] (%)	–	13.3	22.2	29.7	34.0	42.4	46.8	55.0	58.3 (–)
Mean[c]	63.5	56	50.8	46.5	40.2	35.1	32.4	27.4	30.4 (52.1)
SD[c]	17.1	17.7	17.6	17.8	11.6	11.2	15.1	15.5	21.8 (–)
Improvement rates[c] (%)	–	11.8	20	26.8	36.7	44.7	49.0	56.9	52.1 (–)

Motor and phonic tic number, frequency, intensity, complexity, and interference are scored 0–5 each, and the overall impact of tics on activities scored out of 50. The total is thus in the 0–100 range

If case 12 was not included, the Mean, SD and the improvement rates were different

DBS deep brain stimulation; *SD* standard deviation

[a] The DBS electrodes of case 12 was pulled out and the IPG was not implanted

[b] Patient 12 was not included in the value of mean and SD because the electrodes of patient 12 were pulled out and the IPG was not implanted

[c] The mean and SD scores of all the 13 patients

13.10.4 Effects

The mean YGTSS score was 63.5 (range 42–94, SD, 17.1) at baseline and 30.4 (range 8–90, SD, 21.8) at the last follow-up (average 43 months, range 13–80 months) with a mean percentage reduction of 52 % (range 4–84 %). The mean improvement rates at 1, 6, 12, 18, 24, 30, and 36 months relative to baseline were 13, 22, 29, 34, 42, 47, and 55 %, respectively (Table 13.3; Fig. 13.1). Additionally, motor and vocal tic severity on a 0–50 scale are shown in Table 13.6. Notably, five (patients 1, 2, 4, 8, 9) of 13 patients, who were younger than 20 years of age at the time of DBS implantation, yielded excellent post DBS outcomes (the mean YGTSS improvement rate was 62 % with range of 37–84 %). The mean TSQOL score of all studied patients was 53.2 (range 43–73) preoperatively and 28.9 (range 13–65) postoperatively with a mean percentage reduction in TSQOL score of 46 % (range 11–77 %, Table 13.4). Almost all patients showed an improvement in well-being as assessed by the TSQOL scale ($p < 0.05$, by paired t-test). Taken together, our study demonstrated that almost all patients experienced a reduction in YGTSS scores and significant improved tic symptoms. YGTSS improvement rate was noticed at 6 months after DBS surgery ($p < 0.05$, by paired t-test) (Table 13.3).

Table 13.4 Tourette Syndrome–Quality of Life Scale (TSQOL) assessments at the final follow-up

Patient	TSQOL baseline (overall)	Final follow-up	Improvement rates (%)
1	48	21	56.3
2	53	15	71.7
3	58	27	53.4
4	55	33	40.0
5	57	13	77.2
6	48	18	62.5
7	43	21	51.2
8	68	42	38.2
9	49	35	28.6
10	43	27	37.2
11	54	31	42.6
12	73	65	11.0
13	43	28	34.9
Mean[a]	51.6	25.9	49.8
Mean[b]	53.2	28.9	45.7

DBS deep brain stimulation. TSQOL was transformed to a 0–100 range (lower scores reflecting better quality of life)
[a] If case 12 was not included, the mean TSQOL score was 51.6 preoperatively and 25.9 postoperatively with a percentage reduction of 49.8 %
[b] The mean TSQOL score was 53.2 preoperatively and 28.9 postoperatively with a mean percentage reduction of 45.7 % at the last follow-up

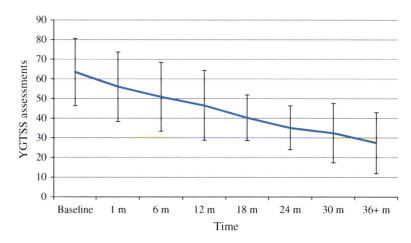

Fig. 13.1 Yale Global Tic Severity Scale (YGTSS) assessments of the studied patients at different time points before and after DBS

Furthermore, 9 of 13 patients found jobs and were able to financially support their families. We also identified that comorbid psychiatric symptoms remained stable or slightly improved in almost all patients according to the consulting psychiatrists, and most patients attained a self-reported higher level of social functioning.

13.10.5 Surgical Accuracy, Complications, and Side Effects of Stimulation

No immediate complications were reported in our cases. Patient 2 complained of pyosis of the head 2 years after the operation. Notably, his

13 Deep Brain Stimulation for Tourette Syndrome

Table 13.5 Program parameters

Patient	Active contacts (left)	Amplitude (V)	Pulse width (μs)	Frequency (Hz)	Active contacts (Right)	Amplitude (V)	Pulse width (μs)	Frequency (Hz)
1	C+ 0- 2-	3.1	90	185	C+ 4- 6-	3	120	185
2	C+ 0-	3.2	90	185	C+ 4-	3.3	90	185
3	C+ 1- 3-	3	90	185	C+ 4- 7-	3.1	90	185
4	1- 3+	3.2	120	185	5- 7+	3.3	90	185
5	C+ 2- 3-	3	90	185	C+ 5- 6-	3.2	90	185
6	C+ 2-	3.5	90	185	C+ 6-	3.3	90	185
7	C+ 0- 2-	2.8	120	160	C+ 4- 6-	2.9	120	160
8	C+ 1-	3.4	90	185	C+ 6-	3.5	90	185
9	C+ 0- 2-	3.3	90	185	C+ 4- 6-	3.4	90	185
10	C+ 0- 2-	2.7	90	160	C+ 4- 6-	2.5	120	160
11	C+ 1-	2.8	90	185	C+ 5-	2.8	90	185
12	0- 3+	3	90	185	5- 7+	3.3	90	185
13	C+ 1- 3-	3.4	90	185	C+ 5- 7-	3.3	90	185

Table 13.6 Yale Global Tic Severity Scale Scores (YGTSS) in 13 TS patients with DBS

Case	Pre-DBS				Post-DBS			
	Motor-subscore	Vocal-subscore	Impairment subscore	Total score	Motor-subscore	Vocal-subscore	Impairment subscore	Total score
1	23	0	35	58	12	0	18	30
2	18	11	32	61	7	0	20	27
3	19	15	40	74	6	7	20	33
4	19	13	42	74	6	3	18	27
5	10	9	28	47	8	1	15	24
6	10	8	27	45	8	4	20	32
7	18	0	30	48	9	0	20	29
8	25	22	46	93	17	13	25	55
9	17	13	43	73	14	11	30	55
10	17	11	31	58	10	8	20	38
11	16	14	28	58	13	9	23	45
12	25	23	46	94	23	22	45	90
13	17	0	25	42	9	0	20	29
Average	18.0	10.7	34.8	63.1	11.0	6.0	22.6	39.5

symptoms were almost completely resolved, and he attained a self-reported higher level of social functioning (demonstrated by engagement and subsequent marriage). Subsequently, with the patient's request, we removed the battery, electrode, and extension cables 5 years after the operation. The patient has not reported any further symptoms. The DBS electrodes of case 12 were removed 1 week after implantation due to the absence of clinical benefit during programming and persistent requests from the patient and his family members. In addition, the electrodes of patients 6 and 7 were removed 4 years after the operation, and both patients obtained substantial benefit from the DBS and returned to normal life. Patient 3 experienced subcutaneous hydrops of the chest and signs of infection 3 years after surgery. Unsurprisingly, some patients complained of mood disorders, for instance, patients 3 and 11 reported anxiety; patients 8 and 9 experienced agitation. However, these symptoms were resolved by careful programming. Patient 12 complained of anxiety, agitation, depression, and constant tiredness that was not amenable to stimulation adjustment, and eventually, his electrodes were removed.

Our recommendations are given against the background that up to now there are no randomized controlled studies available including a sufficiently large number of patients. Hence, it cannot entirely be excluded that at least in some of the patients beneficial effects following DBS were related to placebo effects or to the waxing and waning course of the symptomatology. Therefore, the aim in the near future must be conduct blinded controlled trials including a sufficient number of patients and/or to share databases to combine samples to obtain a sufficiently large sample size. This is best established by collaborating among centers and sharing databases.

13.11 Complementary and Alternative Therapies

Some individuals with TS assert that acupuncture, hypnosis, dietary supplements, and/or homeopathic remedies reduce both the frequency and severity of tics to various degrees. Although these approaches could be beneficial for some individuals, their effectiveness has not yet been confirmed in well-designed, large clinical trials.

References

1. Bloch MH, Leckman JF. Clinical course of Tourette syndrome. J Psychosom Res. 2009;67(6):497–501.
2. de la Tourette GG. Étude sur une affection nerveuse caractérisée par de l'incoordination motrice accompagnée d'écholalie et de coprolalie (French). Arch Neurol. 1885;9:158–200.
3. Robertson MM. Tourette syndrome, associated conditions and the complexities of treatment. Brain. Mar 2000;123(3):425–62.
4. Mink JW, Walkup J, Frey KA, et al. Patient selection and assessment recommendations for deep brain stimulation in Tourette syndrome. Mov Disord. 2006;21(11):1831–8.
5. Leckman JF. Tourette's syndrome. Lancet. 2002;360 (9345):1577–86.
6. DSM-IV-TR. Diagnostic and Statistical Manual of Mental Disorders. 4th ed. Washington: American Psychiatric Association; 2000. p. 111–4.
7. ICD-10. International Classification of Disease and Related Health Problems. Classification of mental and behavioural disorders: clinical descriptions and diagnostic guidelines. 10th ed. Geneva: World Health Organization; 1992, p. 284–6.
8. TSCS Group. Definitions and classification of tic disorders. The Tourette Syndrome Classification Study Group. Arch Neurol. 1993;50:1013–16.
9. Jankovic J. Tourette's syndrome. N Engl J Med. 2001;345:1184–92.
10. Peterson BS, Skudlarski P, et al. A functional magnetic resonance imaging study of tic suppression in Tourette syndrome. Arch Gen Psychiatry. 1998; 55:326–33.
11. Singer HS, Minzer K. Neurobiology of Tourette's syndrome: concepts of neuroanatomic localization and neurochemical abnormalities. Brain Dev. 2003;25 (Suppl 1):S70–84.
12. Flaherty AW, Williams ZM, et al. Deep brain stimulation of the anterior internal capsule for the treatment of Tourette syndrome: technical case report Neurosurgery. 2005;57(suppl 4):E403.
13. Baker EFW. Gilles de la Tourette syndrome treated by bimedial leucotomy. Can Med Assoc J. 1962;86:746–7.
14. Cooper IS. Dystonia reversal by operation in the basal ganglia. Arch Neurol. 1962;7:64–74.
15. Stevens H. The syndrome of Gilles de la Tourette and its treatment. Med Ann District Columbia. 1964; 36:277–9.
16. Hassler R, Dieckmann G. Stereotaxic treatment of tics and inarticulate cries or coprolalia considered as motor obsessional phenomena in Gilles de la Tourette's disease. Rev Neurol (Paris). 1970; 123:89–100.
17. Nadvornik P, Sramka M, Lisy L, Svicka I. Experiences with dentatotomy. Confin Neurol. 1972; 34:320–4.

18. Beckers W. Gilles de la Tourette's disease based on five own observations. Arch Psychiatr Nervenkr. 1973;217:169–86.
19. Wassman ER, Eldridge R, Abuzzahab S Sr, Nee L. Gilles de la Tourette syndrome: clinical and genetic studies in a midwesterncity. Neurology. 1978;28: 304–7.
20. Asam U, Karrass W. Gilles de la Tourette syndrome and psychosurgery. Acta Paedopsychiatr. 1981;47: 39–48.
21. Hassler R. Stereotaxic surgery for psychiatric disturbances. In: Schaltenbrand G, Walker AE, editors. Stereotaxy of the human brain. New York: Thieme-Stratton Inc.; 1982. p. 570–90.
22. Cappabianca P, Spaziante R, Carrabs G, de Divitiis E. Surgical stereotactic treatment for Gilles de la Tourette's syndrome. Acta Neurol (Napoli). 1987;9:273–80.
23. de Divitiis E, D'Errico A, Cerillo A. Stereotactic surgery in Gilles de la Tourette syndrome. Acta Neurochir (Wien) 1977; (Suppl. 24):73.
24. Robertson M, Doran M, Trimble M, Lees AJ. The treatment of Gilles de la Tourette syndrome by limbic leucotomy. J Neurol Neurosurg Psychiatry. 1990;53:691–4.
25. Sawle GV, Lees AJ, Hymas NF, Brooks DJ, Frackowiak RS. The metabolic effects of limbic leucotomy in Gilles de la Tourette syndrome. J Neurol Neurosurg Psychiatry. 1993;56:1016–9.
26. Rauch SL, Baer L, Cosgrove GR, Jenike MA. Neurosurgical treatment of Tourette's syndrome: a critical review. Compr Psychiatry. 1995;36:141–56.
27. Leckman JF, de Lotbiniere AJ, Marek K, Gracco C, Scahill L, Cohen DJ. Severe disturbances in speech, swallowing, and gait following stereotactic infrathalamic lesions in Gilles de la Tourette's syndrome. Neurology. 1993;43:890–4.
28. Baer L, Rauch SL, Ballantine HT Jr, et al. Cingulotomy for intractable obsessive compulsive disorder. Prospective long-term follow-up of 18 patients. Arch Gen Psychiatry. 1995;52:384–92.
29. Korzenev AV, Shoustin VA, Anichkov AD, Polonskiy JZ. Nizkovo- los VB, Oblyapin AV. Differential approach to psychosurgery of obsessive disorders. Stereotact Funct Neurosurg. 1997;68: 226–30.
30. Vandewalle V, van der Linden C, Groenewegen HJ, Caemaert J. Stereotactic treatment of Gilles de la Tourette syndrome by high frequency stimulation of thalamus. Lancet. 1999;353:724.
31. Porta M, Maggioni GR, Ottaviani F, Schindler A: Treatment of phonic tics in patients with Tourette's syndrome using botulinum toxin type A. Neurol Sci. 2003;24:420–3.
32. Porta M, Sassi M, et al. Tourette's syndrome and role of tetrabenazine: review and personal experience. Clin Drug Investig. 2008;28:443–59.
33. Servello D, Porta M, et al. Deep brain stimulation in 18 patients with severe Gilles de la Tourette syndrome refractory to treatment: the surgery and stimulation. J Neurol Neurosurg Psychiatry. 2008;79: 136–42.
34. Priori A, Giannicola G, Krauss JK, Simpson RK Jr, et al. Concepts and methods in chronic thalamic stimulation for treatment of tremor: technique and application. Neurosurgery. 2001;48:535–43.
35. Houeto JL, Karachi C, et al. Tourette's syndrome and deep brain stimulation. J Neurol Neuro surg Psychiatry. 2005;76:992–5.
36. Katayama Y, Kano T, et al.: Difference in surgical strategies between thalamotomy and thalamic deep brain stimulation for tremor control. J Neurol 2005;252 (suppl 4):IV17–IV22.
37. Welter ML, Mallet L, et al. Internal pallidal and thalamic stimulation in patients with Tourette syndrome. Arch Neurol. 2008;65:952–7.
38. Sturm V, Lenartz D, et al. The nucleus accumbens: a target for deep brain stimulation in obsessive compulsive and anxiety-disorders. J Chem Neuroanat. 2003;26:293–9.
39. Kuhn J, Lenartz D, et al. Deep brain stimulation of the nucleus accumbens and the internal capsule in therapeutically refractory Tourette syndrome. J Neurol. 2007;254:963–5.
40. Hirabayashi H, Tengvar M, Hariz MI. Stereotactic imaging of the pallidal target. Mov Disord. 2002;17 (Suppl 3):S130–4.
41. Hu W, Klassen BT, Stead M. Surgery for movement disorders. J Neurosurg Sci. 2011;55:305–17.
42. Schiefer TK, Matsumoto JY, Lee KH. Moving forward: advances in the treatment of movement disorders with deep brain stimulation. Front Integr Neurosci. 2011;5:69.

Stereotactic Neurosurgery for Drug Addiction

14

Guodong Gao and Xuelian Wang

Drug addiction is also known as drug dependence. A committee of experts from WHO defined drug addiction as a mental, and sometimes a physical, state caused by the interaction of the drug with the organism. Individuals addicted to a drug exhibit a compulsive and continuous drug-taking behavior along with other reactions. The aim of these reactions is either to experience euphoria or to avoid the discomfort caused by drug withdrawal. The core feature of addiction is that the addicts know that the behavior is pernicious but they cannot control their intake. Drug addiction includes two parts, physiological dependence (physical dependence) and psychological dependence (psychic dependence). Physiological dependence is a physiological adaptation state caused by repeated drug consumption and displays drug tolerance and withdrawal syndrome. Psychological dependence is the euphoria caused by drug consumption and underlies the need for continuous consumption to experience the euphoria repeatedly. It is the main cause for relapse into drug addiction.

The survey results announced by the United Nations Office of Drug-inspection and Crime-defense (UNODC) on June 25, 2007 indicate that around 200 million people (equivalent to 5 % of the world population at that time) showed drug-taking behavior in 2006. Each year, among drug addicts, about 100 thousand people die and 10 million people become incapacitated worldwide. The investigation of Substance Abuse and Mental Health Services Administration indicated that about 22.3 million above-12-year-old people (equivalent to 8.9 % of the whole population at that time) had used drugs at least once in 2010. The data announced by National Ban Drug Commission and Ministry of Public Security of China showed that by the end of 2010, there were 15.45 million registered drug addicts and among them, there were 10.65 million (69 %) were heroin addicts. By November of 2011, there were 17.8 million registered drug addicts under 35 years, which amount to 87 % of all addicts, and the actual total may be far higher.

At present, the methods for treating drug addiction in China mainly include replacement therapy, non-replacement therapy, Chinese herbs therapy, acupuncture, and electro-acupuncture therapy. *Replacement therapy* uses drugs with pharmacologic actions similar to opioids to replace the addiction drugs. In this method, consumption of the replacement drugs are gradually reduced over time until addiction ceases to exist. Methadone and buprenorphine are representatives of replacement drugs. *Non-replacement therapy* employs central-acting α_2 receptor agonist to decrease withdrawal symptoms. Clonidine and lofexidine are representative non-replacement drugs. Withdrawal symptoms for these drugs are weaker than those for replacement drugs. *Chinese herbs, acupuncture, and electro-acupuncture*

G. Gao (✉) · X. Wang
4th Military Medical University, Tang Du Hospital,
Xi an 710038, Shan Xi, China
e-mail: gguodong@fmmu.edu.cn

therapy can cause withdrawal within a short time but cannot efface the psychological dependence caused by addiction drugs, and therefore, cannot prevent relapse effectively. This problem exists for all noninvasive treatment methods available at present. Addicts fall into the vicious circle of drug taking, withdrawal, and relapse. The relapse rate of withdrawal within a half year is 97–100 %. Therefore, relapse prevention is a problem that defies a solution by these methods and poses a challenge, to both the medical community and human society.

Following the development of experimental studies and stereotactic and functional surgery, it is possible to reduce the psychological dependence on drugs effectively by intervening in key cerebral nuclei for drug addiction used minimal invasive surgery and adjust the function of addictive cycle in the brain. Stereotactic and functional surgery is an important branch of modern neurosurgery that can be regarded as a frontier discipline. During several decades of development, stereotactic surgery has been widely applied to non-organic brain diseases whose main symptoms are characterized by movement disorders, psychiatric diseases, and several types of pain and seizure disorders. This surgical procedure has gradually become a component of integrated treatment strategies that may include pharmacotherapy and other conservative therapies. Over the years, some neurosurgeons with expertise in functional brain disease have attempted to treat drug addiction by targeting brain lesions with stereotactic technology. From 2000 to 2004, such operations were performed in several hospitals in China, but this caused widespread public concern and extensive debate. In November of 2004, China's Ministry of Public Health subsequently banned these operations as a clinical service, but continues to support this technology as part of clinical research projects. This chapter will describe the history of stereotactic surgery for the treatment of drug addiction, the neurological basis of this method, the surgical techniques involved, the assessment of outcomes, and the prospects for the use of this technique in the future.

14.1 History of Stereotactic Surgery for Drug Addiction

Stereotactic technology had been applied to psychosurgery since the late 1950s. It enables accurate localization of target sites and reduces the operation wound size and subsequent complication rate. Since the 1960s, published papers have reported that the cingulate gyrus, hypothalamus, and frontal white matter could be treatment targets for opioid and alcohol addiction [1–3]. An Indian scholar, Kanaka, reported in 1978 [3] that 73 drug addicts had undergone stereotactic ablation of anterior cingulate gyrus lesions, with an efficacy rate of 60–80 %. Medvedev et al., from the Human Brain Research Institute of the Russian Academy of Sciences, has completed 348 cases of bilateral stereotactic cingulotomy to treat drug addiction since 1998. He followed-up 187 of these cases over 2 years and determined that 62 % of the patients did not relapse, while 13 % of patients had dramatically reduced the levels of drug-taking; some had been able to resume work, and only minor operative complications were recorded in this series [4]. However, due to lack of long-term follow-up results, this study's focus can be applied to only psychosurgery rather than drug addiction. For example, Medvedev considered that bilateral stereotactic cingulotomy can help addicts choose the right selection when faced to the drugs by the treatment results of reduced the compulsive drug-taking behavior in addicts. Therefore, this report did not raise much interest.

Guodong Gao from the Neurosurgery Department of Tangdu Hospital, the Fourth Military Medical University, Xi'an, China, used stereotactic surgery to create bilateral lesions in the nucleus accumbens (NAc) to treat patients with opioid addiction in 2000 [5, 6]. He reported that 45 % of the 42 patients had not relapsed 1 year postoperatively with only rare adverse reactions [5, 6]. Subsequently, more than 10 hospitals performed this operation in China until 2004, which sharply increased the number of patients who received this therapy to over 1,000. However, due to varying equipment quality, technologies, and practice experience in these hospitals, it has been difficult to objectively evaluate this huge case series. In addition, increasing numbers of scholars realized that the rapid spread of this surgical method was not suitable as it was still in the clinical research phase. Their major concerns were that the neural mechanisms of drug addiction remain unknown, and unforeseen long-term complications may occur since the areas targeted in such operations are involved in many advanced brain functions, such as reward, cognition, behavioral decision-making, and learning-memory. It is true that the potential for such risks are unknown, and the operation could carry high risks. In addition, this surgical technique has other potential negative factors, including its intrinsic aggressive nature, controversial efficacy rates, and unknown long-term outcomes and complications. Based on these factors, China's Ministry of Public Health banned such operations from clinical services in November 2004, and has only permitted this technology to be applied as part of clinical research projects. For similar reasons, Russian officials had previously banned this therapeutic method in 2002.

14.2 Pathophysiology of Drug Addiction

The pathophysiology mechanism is extremely complex. Although different addiction drugs are quite different in their chemical structure, acute target sites, and pharmacological effect, the major common features resulting in drug abuse, and finally drug addiction, are the effects of reward and reinforcement. There is sufficient evidence to show that the NAc and cerebral cortex are the final neural substrates producing the reinforcement effect of opioid. Olds and Milner discovered a mesencephalon-limbic dopamine (DA) system, which is composed of a mesencephalon-protocerebrum-extrapyramidal circle with the NAc as the center of this circle. The cerebral nucleus related to rewarding system involves the ventral tegmental area (VTA), NAc,

arcuate nucleus, amygdaloid nucleus, locus coeruleus, and periaqueductal gray, and so on.

Although there are other independent reinforcement pathways of opiates addiction, the main mechanism is that opioids act on dopaminergic neuron via opiate receptor to induce reinforcement. The other independent reinforcement ways may include the following: (i) Opioids directly spur increased DA release and prevent DA reabsorption; (ii) Opioids restrain the action of gamma-aminobutyric acid (GABA) by acting on the μ receptors on GABAergic interneurons thereby removing the inhibitory effect of GABA on DA neurons in the VTA and increase DA release in its target region; (iii) Opioids directly spur increased DA release, which then excites related neurons, inducing euphoria. The opioids-opiates receptor-dopaminergic neuron pathway is the specific cycle responsible for DA involvement in the rewarding process. The drug consumption/stimulation, DA release, rewarding effect, and drug-seeking behavior show a mutually promoting relationship. Blocked DA receptors can weaken this reinforcement. In opiate addiction, DA level increases in the brain and is adaptively balanced at a high level. Once the drug intake ceases, DA content decreases gradually and then withdrawal symptoms and drug-seeking behavior emerge. Among the DA receptors, D_2 particularly functions in the rewarding effect. In opiate-addiction rats without the D_2 receptor gene, the drug-seeking behavior and conditioned place preference still exist, but are restrained. These results reinforce that the DA system has an important role in the psychological dependence in opiates addiction.

Acute administration of most of the addiction drugs can activate the DA neurological circuits within the NAc and cerebral cortex, which are part of the rewarding system, and can induce reward and reinforcement effects. Cocaine and DA transporter act together to prevent DA reabsorption. As a result, DA concentration in the synaptic spaces of NAc neurons increases. Benzedrine specifically increases monoamine neurotransmitter release and simultaneously accelerates DA release in NAc neurons. Therefore, benzedrine and cocaine have similar reinforcement and mental stimulation effect. Animal studies have shown that ablation of either the cell mass in the VTA or the nerve pathway between the VTA and medial forebrain bundle, or termination of the nerve pathway in the ending of nerve fiber in the NAc and forebrain cortex or in the related ventral pallidum dramatically decrease the rewarding effect of addiction drugs (especially cocaine and benzedrine). Brain circuits involved in the chronic effect of long-term administration of addiction drugs include not only circuits regulating the acute rewarding effect but also circuits involved in learning and memory, which participate in processing and storage of the pleasant rewarding stimuli induced by the drugs. These brain circuits are important for drug addiction. Using positron emission tomography (PET), it has been shown that addiction drug-induced changes in the hippocampus, amygdaloid nucleus, and other related brain areas are accompanied by a desire for the drug. Further, metabolic changes related to the desire for drugs have been reported to occur in some brain regions, including the limbic system and related cerebral cortex.

14.3 Rationale of Surgery for Drug Addiction

Using a Cartesian coordinate system and taking the midpoint between the anterior commissure and posterior commissure as the origin, stereotactic surgery can obtain the spatial value of any position in the brain. The core technology enables accurate location of a lesion, so that biopsies and device implantation can be performed through minimal invasion [7]. Only a small keyhole needs to be drilled through the skull during stereotactic surgery; therefore, only a small volume of tissue is damaged around the target lesion. At present, stereotactic surgery is mainly used for treating movement disorders (e.g., Parkinson's disease, myodystony, and essential tremor) and psychosurgery (e.g., obsessive compulsive disorder

[OCD]). The common difficulties encountered include determining appropriate targets and locating them accurately.

Target selection is of vital importance for the effectiveness of stereotactic operations for drug addiction. Unfortunately, existing experimental and clinical research data does not provide definitive conclusions. A literature review found that the current targets for the treatment of drug addiction were either the cingulate gyrus or the NAc [4–6, 8, 9]. Some hospitals have targeted multiple brain areas for combined lesioning. However, this may cause more neural damage and potential complications. Furthermore, if multiple sites are targeted, then assessing the relationship between a region and curative effects becomes more difficult.

The cingulate gyrus is part of the limbic system. Cingulotomy has been used to relieve cancer-related pain since the 1960s. This technique is safer than other neurosurgical methods, such as amygdalohippocampotomy or leucotomy, and remains an effective treatment for intractable depression, OCD, and anxiety disorders. Many studies have selected the cingulate gyrus as the target for stereotactic surgery for drug addiction, principally because many researchers believe that compulsive drug-seeking behavior is similar to the compulsive behavior observed in OCD [10].

Addiction is an acquired behavior, and its regular pattern is characterized as both habitual and compulsive. Underlying this pattern are pathological changes in several neurological circuits caused by the long-term intake of drugs. A pathological reward effect in the neurological circuits of the mesolimbic-dopamine system can trigger compulsive drug taking. The NAc, which is an intersection point of this system, participates widely in pathological reward mechanisms. Functional research regarding the NAc has shown that its shell is involved in the direct effect of drugs and increases the reinforcement mechanism of drug taking. The shell and core of NAc participate in unconditioned and conditioned stimulus-aroused drug-seeking motivations, respectively. They can also maintain formed drug-seeking behavior patterns, which lead to drug seeking and relapse. The NAc forms the main dopaminergic connection between the ventral and dorsal striatum. In addition, glutamatergic projections between the anterior cingulate gyrus and NAc core comprise the common path of drug addiction relapse due to numerous factors [11–13].

Drug addiction involves several types of brain functions, including reward, emotion, learning-memory, motivation, and behavioral decision-making. Several neural nuclei and neurological circuits are involved in addiction. As the NAc is the intermediary between the limbic system and motor cortex, it integrates information regarding reward-based emotions and participates in the transition from motivation to behavior, thus playing a significant role in the mechanism of addiction. Therefore, targeting the NAc during surgery could theoretically reduce drug-seeking behavior and effectively prevent relapse.

14.4 Clinical Studies

Stereotactic surgery for drug addiction is in the exploratory phase at present. The irreversible damage caused by the ablation of target areas in the human brain has triggered controversy. Due to technological developments in the novel stereotactic neurosurgery technique of deep brain stimulation (DBS), this technique is gradually replacing the ablation procedures. DBS involves location of targets by stereotactic technology and subsequent placement of an electrode, which improves symptoms by stimulating the target site. Although similar to stereotactic surgery, DBS has the advantages of causing lesser brain damage and being adjustable. DBS had been successfully applied for the treatment of movement disorders such as Parkinson's disease. In addition, research on the use of DBS for intractable psychiatric disorders, including OCD, major depression, anxiety disorder, and anorexia nervosa, as well as for pain

and persistent vegetative states, has reached the clinical research stage [14–16]. Using DBS and more specific target areas, researchers can explore new disease types within ethically approved limits. The possibility of using of DBS for drug addiction may be a worthy to discuss. Some Chinese centers have conducted research on DBS for drug addiction and received good preliminary results [17].

In a prospective study conducted by our center, we compared the clinical effects and complications for DBS in four different NAc subregions, and found the medial-posterior shell of the NAc to be the best target area, with the highest response rate and lowest complication rate [18] (Figs. 14.1 and 14.2).

Using stereotactic technology, we precisely planted an electrode in the target region, and then stimulated it to affect functioning of the related cerebral nuclei, improve the symptom, and control the condition. DBS has the following advantages: *non-destructive* (DBS does not cause much damage to the brain tissue, is very safe, and electrodes can be planted bilaterally at the same time), *adjustability* (the disease can be best controlled by adjusting the parameters for DBS), and *reversibility* (the adverse reaction related to DBS can be relieved by adjusting the parameters).

The distinguishing feature of our center's DBS for drug addiction is that we can simultaneously stimulate the NAc and anterior limb of internal capsule (ALIC) using a single electrode. We applied the path analysis function of the image analysis software in the stereotactic system to place the far-end contacts of an electrode in the NAc and the proximal contact of electrode in the ALIC. Therefore, we can stimulate both the regions simultaneously. We have included the ALIC in our research considering the compulsivity of drug addiction [10] and the effectiveness of ALIC therapy for OCD [19, 20] (Figs. 14.3 and 14.4).

The centers of the small and big circles indicate the NAc and ALIC, respectively.

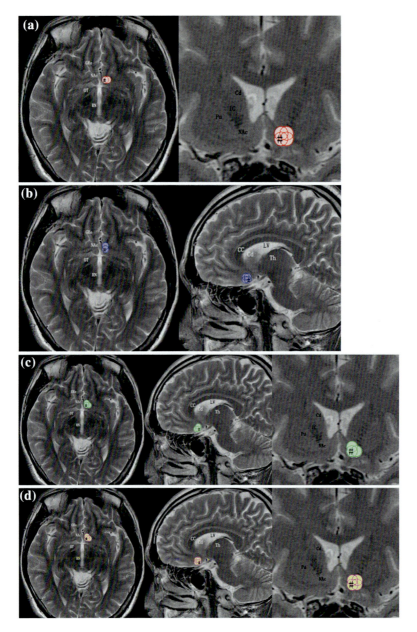

Fig. 14.1 The schematic diagram of lesion loci. **a** Group A (axial and coronal views). *CC* corpus callosum; *Cd* caudate nucleus; *GRe* gyrus rectus; *Ic* internal capsule; *LV* lateral ventricle; *NAc* nucleus accumbens; *OT* optical tract; *Pu* putamen; *RN* red nucleus; *Th* thalamus; *hash* (#) indicates initial lesion. **b** Group B (axial and sagittal views). *CC* corpus callosum; *Cd* caudate nucleus; *GRe* gyrus rectus; *Ic* internal capsule; *LV* lateral ventricle; *NAc* nucleus accumbens; *OT* optical tract; *Pu* putamen; *RN* red nucleus; *Th* thalamus; *hash* (#) indicates initial lesion. **c** Group C (axial, sagittal, and coronal views). *CC* corpus callosum; *Cd* caudate nucleus; *GRe* gyrus rectus; *Ic* internal capsule; *LV* lateral ventricle; *NAc* Nucleus accumbens; *OT* optical tract; *Pu* putamen; *RN* red nucleus; *Th* thalamus; *hash* (#) indicates initial lesion. **d** D group (axial, sagittal, and coronal views). *CC* corpus callosum; *Cd* caudate nucleus; *GRe* gyrus rectus; *Ic* internal capsule; *LV* lateral ventricle; *NAc* Nucleus Accumbens; *OT* optical tract; *Pu* putamen; *RN* red nucleus; *Th* thalamus; *hash* (#) indicates initial lesion

14 Stereotactic Neurosurgery for Drug Addiction

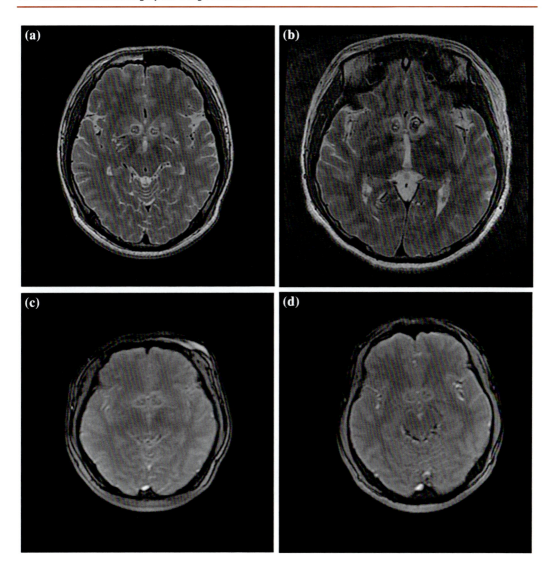

Fig. 14.2 Post-operative MRI images of patients. Post-operative MRI scans showing the condition of the lesion foci in four patients belonging to four different surgical groups. **a** MRI of a patient from group A (axial views, T2-weighted image). **b** MRI of a patient from group B (axial views, T2-weighted image). **c** MRI of a patient from group C (axial views, T1-weighted image). **d** MRI of a patient from group D (axial views, T1-weighted image)

14.5 How to Perform the Surgery

14.5.1 Aim

The aim of stereotactic surgery for drug addiction is to directly affect the key cerebral nuclei involved in drug addiction in order to control functioning of the addiction circuit, thereby weakening the psychological dependence on drugs and finally avoiding relapse to ensure complete recovery from addiction.

14.5.2 Indications

1. Patients diagnosed with drug addiction in accordance with the Chinese Classification

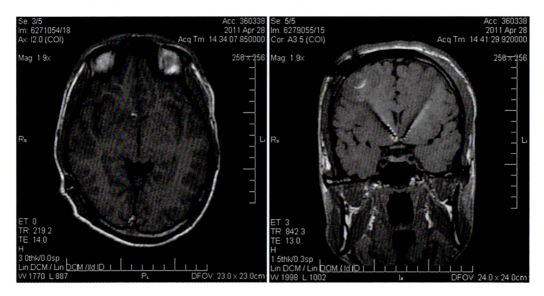

Fig. 14.3 Post-operative MRI of a patient subjected to NAc-ALIC DBS for drug addiction

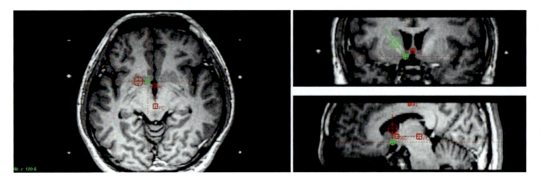

Fig. 14.4 Schematic diagram of NAc-ALIC DBS

and Diagnostic Criteria of Mental Disorders (Revision of Second Edition; CCMD-II-R).
2. Patients with a history of drug abuse >3 years with at least three relapses despite systematic conservative treatments.
3. Patients aged between 18 and 70 years.
4. Patients and their families volunteer to undergo surgery, and agree to comply with the treatment.
5. Patients have completed the physiological detoxification treatment (discontinued all drugs for at least 7–10 days and acute withdraw symptoms have disappeared, with negative results for the morphine urine and naloxone tests).

14.5.3 Contraindications

1. Patients who are reluctant to give up drugs and are forced to stay in hospital by their family.
2. Patients who have contraindications for stereotactic neurosurgery.
3. Patients who have obvious mental disorders, personality disorders, and social disability in accordance with the diagnostic standard of CCMD-II-R.
4. Patients who have severe communicable diseases, such as AIDS, syphilis, and viral hepatitis.
5. Patients who have obvious learning difficulties or concomitant degenerative brain diseases.

14.5.4 Preoperative Assessment

Collection for basic information
The collection includes patients' history of drug abuse, kind of drug, drug dosage, history of treatment, height, weight, and other indexes of health condition.

Assessment for mental condition
Note: Considering the actual situation, at least choose one to two scales in each of following aspect:

1. Assessment for addiction severity
   Opiate Addiction Severity Inventory (OASI)
   Opiate Withdrawal Scale (OWS)
2. Assessment for general mental condition
   Symptom Checklist 90 (SCL-90)
3. Assessment for neuropsychological function

Personality

Minnesota Multiphasic Personality Inventory (MMPI)
Eysenck Personality Questionnaire (EPQ)
16 Personality Factor Questionnaire (16PF)

Mood

Beck Depression Inventory (BDI)
Beck Anxiety Inventory (BAI)
Hamilton Anxiety Scale (HAMA)
Hamilton Depression Scale (HAMD)

Cognition

Wechsler Adult Intelligence Scale-Revised by China (WAIS-RC)
Raven Standard Progressive Matrices Test-Revised by China (RSPM-RC)
Wechsler Memory Scale-Revised by China (WMS-RC)
Clinical Memory Scale (CMS)
4. Assessment for life quality and social function
Short Form 36 Health Survey Questionnaire (SF-36)
Quality of life Scale for Drug Addicts (QOL-DA)

14.5.5 Preoperative Preparation

1. Patients have completed the physiological detoxification treatment.
2. Morphine urine test and naloxone test are negative.
3. MRI or CT of the brain to screen intracranial organic lesions.
4. Preoperative assessment (see Sect. 14.5.4)
5. Neurosurgery preoperative normal examination.
6. Fasting for solids and liquids.
7. Mental preparation for operation.

14.5.6 Operative Procedure

1. Type of anesthesia: Total intravenous anesthesia + endotracheal intubation
2. Operation methods:
   Operation methods include traditional ablation surgery and DBS surgery.

Stereotactic Ablation Surgery

Targets Bilateral NAc is the prime target. More targets can be added if there are any concomitant mental symptoms. However, there is no necessity for multiple targets in a single operation.

Surgery Procedure After the pedestal of the stereotactic apparatus is installed, patients undergo thin-slice MRI or CT (depth of stratum 2 mm, distance of stratum 0 mm). The obtained images are processed using a computer workstation to determine coordinate values in accordance with the Schaltenbrand–Wahren Stereotaxic Atlas [21]. The range of NAc coordinate values are 5–6 mm under the line joining the anterior and posterior commissure; 16–17 mm anterior to the brain midpoint; and 5–7 mm lateral to the brain midline. With the patients in a supine position, the surgeons make an approximate 3-cm incision 11 cm dorsal to the ophryon and 2.5 cm from the midline. Next, two bone holes are drilled on the skull and the dura mater is incised. After arresting the bleeding and fulguratively incising the cortex, using the stereotactic device, the surgeons guide the electrode to the target site and ablate it. After ablation is completed and the bleeding has stopped, the incision on the scalp is sutured.

Parameters of Ablation Temperature: 80 °F; Time: 60 s; Specification of radio frequency stylus: 1.6×4.0 mm or 1.6×5.0 mm; Volume of lesion: $2 \times 2 \times 8$ mm^3.

Stereotactic DBS Surgery

Targets The prime targets are bilateral NAc or bilateral NAc + ALIC.

Surgery Procedure Up until the step of location, DBS surgery and stereotactic ablation surgery are the same. After affirming NAc's coordinate values, the surgeon can set and confirm the "skull approach" using the path analysis function of the image analysis software in the stereotactic system in order to place the far-end contacts of the electrode in the NAc and the proximal contact of the electrode in the ALIC. In this skull approach, a bilateral, small-disc-shaped incision is made on the scalp, two bone holes are drilled in the skull, and the dura mater incised. Used the guide bow of the stereotactic apparatus, the electrodes are guided to the targets and fixed. The guide bow of stereotactic apparatus are removed, the bleeding is stopped, and the incision in the scalp is sutured. After recovery from general anesthesia, the temporary stimulator can be turned on. The instant effect and side reaction can then be observed. If there are no obvious side reactions within 1 week postoperatively and the review MRI shows no deviation in the location of electrodes, the subskin impulsator can be planted in the pre-thoracic skin under local anesthesia.

Stimulating electrode and stimulation's related parameters *Stimulating Electrode* Medtronic model 3387 (Medtronics, Inc., Minneapolis, Minnesota), four-contact electrode, contact length 1.5 mm, and the space between contacts length is 1.0 mm. *Stimulation mode*: monopolar or bipolar stimulation mode, single or multiple contact stimulation mode, continuous stimulation mode, high frequency and fixed pulse width, gradually increased voltage. Stimulation parameter 130 Hz, 90 µW, 4.0–7.0 V.

14.5.7 Operative Response Evaluation

The standard for successful rehabilitation from drug addiction is that the patients can refrain from consuming any kind of drug for 1 year, and that within the first year, the morphine urine and naloxone tests are negative at any given time. The evaluative criteria for the curative effect are based on the occurrence of relapse and withdrawal duration as follows: (1) *Good*: Refrained from all kinds of drugs over 12 months postoperatively; (2) *Improvement*: Refrained from all kinds of drugs 6–12 months postoperatively; (3) *Ineffective*: Consumed any kind of drug within 6 months postoperatively.

14.5.8 Postoperative Follow-Up

Face-to-face follow-up is conducted at postoperative months 1, 3, 6, 12, 18, and 24, respectively. The scope of examination is as follows:

1. Effectiveness: Relapse, retention rate and time of drug addiction, dose and frequency of drug relapse, and changes in the levels of craving and euphoria.
2. Safety: Changes in e general physiological parameters (e.g., blood pressure, temperature, weight), appetite and sexual desire; comparison of the preoperative and postoperative values of multiple indexes for psychological assessment (memory, intelligence, personality, etc.); incidence of nonspecific complications (e.g., bleeding and infection); and incidence of specific neurological complications (e.g., central high fever, aconuresis, anterograde amnesia, and dysfunction in motivation-forming).
3. Verification of lesion targeting: A repeated thin-slice MRI conducted within 6 months postoperatively in order to verify the location of the targeted lesion.

14.5.9 Complications

1. Non-specific complications: Include complications not related to functions of the target area and related closely to the wound itself. These mainly include fever, infection, headache, incontinence of urine, and epilepsy. The occurrence rate of non-specific complications is 10 %, and these complications are usually transient and mild and can disappear after appropriate handling.
2. Specific complications: Refers to complications related closely to the function of the lesion target. These mainly include personality changes, aprosexia, memory complaints, interest changes, mild affective disorder, hyposphraesia, and parasexuality. The occurrence rate of specific complications is 10 %, and these complications usually disappear gradually after appropriate handling.

14.5.10 Unresolved Questions

1. Stereotactic surgery is more than a surgical method to treat drug addiction; it also concerns about psychotherapy and social support. It is a holistic treatment model and can overcome psychological dependence, reduce the relapse rate post-operatively. However, this surgery treatment is not the only approach to drug addiction. It is only adopted when other conservative treatment methods failed repeatedly.
2. For success of this surgical treatment, patients' cooperation is the most important factor. Patients and their family realizing the harmful effects of drug addiction and volunteering to receive the treatment are the prime premise and guarantee the success of this surgical treatment.
3. At our institute, this method yielded good results, in that the patients received detoxification for 7–10 days and waited until all withdrawal symptoms disappeared (The morphine urine and naloxone tests were negative.), before the stereotactic operation was performed. The reasons for this stringent condition is that the interaction between physiological and psychological dependence can easily lead to relapse.
4. Some patients still report chronic protracted withdrawal symptoms, which include refractory insomnia, anxiety, and pain in the limb joints and muscles, after completion of the detoxification treatment and attainment of negative results for morphine urine and naloxone tests. For such cases, some medication can be used. However, Chinese medicines free of risk of addiction are preferred over "easy-to-cause addiction" Western medicines like adanon, tramagetic, dilantin, and triazolam. If a Western medicine has to be selected, the medications daily decreasing principle is more helpful.
5. Postoperative specific and non-specific complications are mainly related to brain edema around the target. The complications can be prevented by precise stereotactic technology and apparatus, abundant clinical experience, and timely symptomatic treatment.

14.6 Follow-up Results: A Multicenter Study in China

Most clinical reports have indicated that stereotactic surgery can effectively prevent relapse in drug addiction [4–6, 8, 9]. After this treatment, over half of patients show no relapses and, among those who relapse, intake dose and drug-taking frequency is markedly dropped [4–6, 8, 9]. The incidence of nonspecific complications, such as bleeding and infection, is low [4–6, 8, 9]. Among specific complications, central high fever and aconuresis are common shortly after the operation, but these resolve after symptomatic treatment is applied. These complications may arise due to edema around the targeted lesion [6]. Some patients have been reported to shown anterograde amnesia and dysfunction in motivation forming, which is characterized by silence, apathy, lack of interest, lack of proactive behaviors, idleness, and social withdrawal [22]. These patients usually recover after some months of rehabilitation.

Most researchers who have applied stereotactic surgery for treating drug addiction consider it to be safe and effective. Although evidence-based medical evidence to support this opinion is lacking, pilot studies have indicated that this surgery is effective in terms of short-term outcomes. However, regrettably, most pilot studies did not verify the location and volume of the targeted lesion and did not analyze the relationship between the lesion location, targeted volume, and treatment effectiveness. Most pilot studies only reported follow-up results within 1 postoperative year, and gave no indication about the long-term effects of this treatment.

In contrast to these positive reports, many experts have raised questions about the safety and efficacy of this surgery. Furthermore, the ethical issues concerning this surgery have become a matter of contention [23, 24]. The Chinese "11th Five Years" scientific support plan project, entitled the *"Clinical reevaluation of current prevention of relapse"* (No. 2007BAI0703), was completed in 2010. An independent third-party committee of experts evaluated the safety and efficacy of stereotactic surgery comprehensively and scientifically, with the aim of reaching an impartial and compelling conclusion.

The follow-up results showed that 17 centers in China had adopted stereotactic surgery for drug addiction, and 1,167 patients had undergone this surgery until November of 2004. From them, 8 centers participated in the follow-up study, and 769 patients were included in the study. The study selected 150 patients by applying a completely random digital method. After completion of follow-up, of the 150 patients, 122 patients agreed for a face-to-face interview, and 28 patients were either lost during follow-up or refused for a face-to-face interview. Non-relapse was judged by the conformity of patients and their families' denial of drug-taking behavior, negative results for both morphine urine and naloxone tests, and negative results for hair drug-content detection. The conservative non-relapse rate of this follow-up study was 50 % (75/150),

and the longest non-relapse time was 8 years. And among the 47 cases of patients who relapsed, 34 relapsed within 1 year postoperatively. The study identified that the following as main reasons for relapse in this sequence: negative events in life, lack of social and family care, drug traffickers' lure, psychological dependence for drugs, and body discomfort caused by chronic protracted withdrawal symptoms. The occurrence rate of non-specific complications was 9.0 % (11/122), and all of them were resolved within 6 months post-operatively. The occurrence rate of specific complications was 7.4 % (9/122), and most of them improved gradually with time. Among the 122 patients, 75.4 % had different kinds of regular work, and 84.6 % patients were financially independent. Compared with patients who did not undergo the surgery, patients who did lived a better life postoperatively. Moreover, quality of life for patients who did relapse for 5 or more years postoperatively was similar to that of normal people.

In conclusion, drug treatment should constitute a system that includes the following three continuous processes: detoxification, relapse prevention, and societal return. In this chapter, we have summarized our successful clinical experience at achieving a curative effect through preoperative physiological detoxification, accurate and appropriate ablation of the NAc, and positive cognitive behavior modification. In addition to other treatment methods, a standardized stereotactic technique can help humans overpower the demon of drug addiction in the future.

References

1. Dieckmann G, Schneider H. Influence of stereotactic hypothalamotomy on alcohol and drug addiction. Appl Neurophysiol. 1978;41(1–4):93–8.
2. Jansson B, Nystrom S. Lobotomy as a therapeutic alternative in drug addiction. Lakartidningen. 1968;65 (24):2444–5.
3. Kanaka TS, Balasubramaniam V. Stereotactic cingulumotomy for drug addiction. Appl Neurophysiol. 1978;41(1–4):86–92.
4. Medvedev SV, Anichkov AD, Polyakov YI. Physiological mechanisms of the effectiveness of

bilateral stereotactic cingulotomy against strong psychological dependence in drug addicts. Hum Physiol. 2003;29(4):492–7.

5. Gao G, Wang X, He S, et al. Clinical study for alleviating opiate drug psychological dependence by a method of ablating the nucleus accumbens with stereotactic surgery. Stereotact Funct Neurosurg. 2003;81(1–4):96–104.

6. Wang X, He S, Heng L et al. Follow-up of nucleus accumbens lesion for treatment of drug dependence. Chinese Journal of Neurosurgery. 2005;10.28;21(10).

7. Fu X, Niu C. Stereotactic and Functional Neurosurgery Anhui Science and Technology Publishing House. 2004

8. Xu M, Wang C, Jiang C. Bilateral cingulotomy for the treatment of heroin dependence. Chinese Journal of Minimally Invasive Neurosurgery. 2005;10 (4):162–3.

9. Yang K, Xi S, Wang K et al. Stereotactic bilateral nucleus accumbens lesion for the treatment of opioid dependence. Chinese Journal of Stereotactic and Functional Neurosurgery. 2005;18(3):135–9.

10. Orellana C. Controversy over brain surgery for heroin addiction in Russia. Lancet Neurol. 2002;1(6):333.

11. Everitt BJ, Robbins TW. Neural systems of reinforcement for drug addiction: from actions to habits to compulsion. Nat Neurosci. 2005;8 (11):1481–9.

12. Belin D, Everitt BJ. Cocaine seeking habits depend upon dopamine-dependent serial connectivity linking the ventral with the dorsal striatum. Neuron. 2008;57 (3):432–41.

13. Kalivas PW, McFarland K. Brain circuitry and the reinstatement of cocaine-seeking behavior. Psychopharmacology. 2003;168(1–2):44–56.

14. Bittar RG, Kar-Purkayastha I, Owen SL, et al. Deep brain stimulation for pain relief: a meta-analysis.

J Clin Neurosci: Official J Neurosurg Soc Australas. 2005;12(5):515–9.

15. Wichmann T, Delong MR. Deep brain stimulation for neurologic and neuropsychiatric disorders. Neuron. 2006;52(1):197–204.

16. Yamamoto T, Katayama Y. Deep brain stimulation therapy for the vegetative state. Neuropsychological Rehabil. 2005;15(3–4):406–13.

17. Zhou H, Xu J, Jiang J. Deep brain stimulation of nucleus accumbens on heroin-seeking behaviors: a case report. Biol Psychiatry. 2011;69:e41–2.

18. Li N, Wang J, Wang XL, Chang CW, Ge SN, Gao L, et al. Nucleus accumbens surgery for addiction. World Neurosurg. 2012. pii:S1878–8750(12) 01106–0, doi:10.1016/j.wneu.2012.10.007.

19. Greenberg BD, Gabriels LA, Malone DA Jr, Rezai AR, Friehs GM, Okun MS, et al. Deep brain stimulation of the ventral internal capsule/ventral striatum for obsessive-compulsive disorder: worldwide experience. Mol Psychiatry. 2010;15 (1):64–79.

20. Anderson D, Ahmed A. Treatment of patients with intractable obsessive-compulsive disorder with anterior capsular stimulation: case report. J Neurosurg. 2003;98:1104–8.

21. Schaltenbrand G, Wahren W. Atlas for stereotaxy of the human brain. Stuttgard: Thieme; 1977.

22. Heng L, Wang X, He S, et al. Complications of nucleus accumbens leasions for the treatment of drug dependence. Chinese Journal of Stereotactic and Functional Neurosurgery. 2006;19(1):5–8.

23. Hang J. Reflections on neurosurgery detoxification. Chinese Journal of Pain Medicine. 2005;11(1):45–6.

24. Qu X, Qiu Z. Our views for the treatment of drug addiction by neurosurgery. Medicine and Philosophy. 2004;25(12):32.

Surgical Treatments for Anorexia Nervosa

15

Bomin Sun, Dianyou Li, Wei Liu, Shikun Zhan, Yixin Pan and Xiaoxiao Zhang

Abstract

Anorexia nervosa (AN) is a severe psychiatric disorder with high rates of morbidity and mortality. An estimated 21 % of patients experience a chronic course despite treatment with the best available medications and behavioral therapies. Existing data suggest that lesioning and deep brain stimulation can benefit a large proportion (ranging from 60 to 80 %) of patients with medically intractable AN. Long-term serious adverse events are very infrequent. Functional neuroimaging studies have increased our understanding of the mechanisms of disease development and therapeutic action. At our institution, we grade AN on a four-point scale based on patient clinical characteristics and our surgical experience over the past 8 years. This scale is particularly useful for guiding the selection of surgical procedures. Such treatment options include deep brain stimulation or lesioning of the nucleus accumbens, anterior capsulotomy, and anterior cingulotomy. Data suggest that surgical treatment is a viable option for intractable AN, and can alleviate suffering and improve the quality of life of patients with these disabling disorders.

Keywords

Anorexia nervosa · Surgery · Deep brain stimulation · Capsulotomy · Cingulotomy

15.1 Introduction

Anorexia nervosa (AN) is one of the most challenging psychiatric disorders which usually begins in adolescence and is characterized by a refusal to maintain body weight at or above a minimally normal weight for age and height, an intense fear of gaining weight, a relentless drive for thinness, and a disturbance in the way one's bodyweight and shape experienced. Amenorrhea

B. Sun (✉) · D. Li · W. Liu · S. Zhan · Y. Pan · X. Zhang
Department of Stereotactic and Functional Neurosurgery, Ruijin Hospital, Shanghai Jiaotong University School of Medicine, 197 Ruijin Er Road, Shanghai 200025, China
e-mail: Bominsun@sh163.net.cn

B. Sun and A. De Salles (eds.), *Neurosurgical Treatments for Psychiatric Disorders*,
DOI 10.1007/978 94-017-9576-0_15
© Shanghai Jiao Tong University Press, Shanghai and Springer Science+Business Media Dordrecht 2015

is also often present in female patients. Other features include disturbed body image, heightened desire to lose more weight, and pervasive fear of fatness [1, 2]. The average point prevalence rate of AN is 0.3–1 % in young females and approximately one tenth of that rate in males. Lifetime prevalence is 2.2 % among females [3, 4].

Anorexia nervosa, which has one of the highest excessive mortality rates of all psychiatric disorders, causes remarkable agony for the patients and their families. Suicide or medical complications are the major causes of mortality for those with AN [5, 6]. Long-lasting malnutrition can lead to numerous severe physical complications, including osteoporosis, gastrointestinal and cardiac complications, liver damage, electrolyte disturbances, and eventually multiple organ failure [7]. AN psychiatric comorbidities include major depressive disorder (MDD; 50–70 % of AN patients), anxiety disorder (>60 %), obsessive-compulsive disorder (OCD; >40 %) [8, 9]. Personality disorders and alcohol or substance abuse may also be present (12–27 %) among those with the binging-purging subtype of AN, in whom the rate of impulsive behavior is also higher than in the restricting subtype of AN [10].

In an extensive literature review, it reported that less than half (46.9 %) of surviving patients recover from AN, one-third (33.5 %) improve partially, and in 20.8 % (0–79 %) the disease takes on a chronic course [11, 12]. AN patients with a duration of illness longer than 10 years are very unlikely to recover [11, 13, 14]. Besides, linkage studies further confirmed that AN, major depressive disorder(MDD), anxiety, OCDs and addictive disorders shared about a third of genetic risk factors [15]. And there is evidence indicates that the presence of depressed mood may be a risk factor for AN, which could lead to worse outcomes and greater rates of relapse in AN patients [5, 16]. These psychotic disorders may have significant overlap in the anatomic structures.

15.2 Neurocircuitry of Anorexia Nervosa

The neurocircuitry underlying food intake is complex and the precise mechanism of AN is still unclear. Since no single factor has been shown to be either necessary or sufficient for development of AN, a multifactorial threshold model is likely the most appropriate explanatory model of illness [14]. The biology and neural circuitry of AN are research "hotspots", with most disease models focusing on factors that underlie pathological mood, anxiety, reward, body perception, inhibition, alexithymia, and appetite [17]. Much of this work on AN is driven by neuroimaging, which has been used extensively to show both structural and functional differences between patients with AN, those recovered from AN, and healthy controls.

Individuals with AN typically exhibit distinctive temperament and personality traits, which often first occur in childhood before the onset of AN, may even contribute to the development of AN, and often persist after recovery [18]. Many of these traits are likely encoded in neural circuits, for example, characteristic harm avoidance is positively associated with dopamine (DA) D2/D3 receptor binding in the dorsal caudate [19], and perfectionism and obsessive personality traits are associated with exaggerated cognitive control by the dorsolateral prefrontal cortex (DLPFC). The DLPFC may become excessively involved in inhibitory processes to dampen information processing through reward pathways [20]. The anxious temperament of patients with AN leads to a variety of dysfunctional behaviors thought to serve as a means of coping with adverse mood. Functional brain imaging demonstrates that decreased activation of fronto-striatal circuits, including the ventral striatum, anterior cingulate cortex (ACC), and supplementary motor area (SMA), may underlie the impaired cognitive flexibility in patients with AN, which results in the stereotypical and ritualistic behaviors to control eating and weight [21].

Considerable data indicate that individuals with AN exhibit disturbances in DA and serotonin (5-HT) systems. 5-HT might play a role in altered satiety, impulse control, and mood, whereas DA is implicated in motivation, executive functions (i.e. inhibitory control, salience attribution, and decision-making), and the aberrant reward effects of food. Recent studies of AN, using positron emission tomography (PET) and single photon emission computed tomography (SPECT) with 5-HT-specific radio ligands, consistently show alterations in 5-HT1A and 5-HT2A receptor and 5-HT transporter activity in cortical and limbic structures, which may be related to anxiety, behavioral inhibition, and body image distortions [17]. Depletion of 5-HT levels reduces anxiety in acutely ill patients and those recovered from AN [22]. Starvation may reduce pathologically increased DA levels that are associated with anxious temperament [20].

The processing of food reward is complex and modulated by cognitive, emotional, and biological factors involving learned behaviors and genetic predispositions. The motivation to eat and approach food is a critical part of the reward pathway and is particularly disturbed in AN. It is possible that food has little reward value in AN, and thus may be associated with corresponding responses in the orbitofrontal cortex (OFC) or the striatum [19]. Recent imaging studies provide evidence for disturbed gustatory processing in patients with AN, which involves the anterior insula as well as striatal regions [18]. Genetic, pharmacological, and physiological data show that individuals with AN and those recovered from AN exhibit altered striatal DA function [23, 24]. DA disturbances could contribute to altered modulation of appetitive behaviors as well as symptoms of anhedonia, dysphoric mood, asceticism, and increased motor activity [25]. These results raise the possibility that individuals with AN have altered appetitive mechanisms that may involve either sensory, interoceptive, or reward processes. These disturbances in the modulation of reward and emotion may increase vulnerability to dysregulated appetitive behaviors. Individuals with AN may be able to inhibit appetite and have extraordinary self-control due to exaggerated dorsal cognitive circuit function [17].

In addition to the reward pathway, several other neural circuits contribute to AN. The insular cortex serves to integrate processing from many of the structures relevant to AN, and thus may be critical for AN. It has therefore been hypothesized that a rate limiting dysfunction of neural circuitry integrated by the insula may account for the clinical phenomena of AN [26]. However, the exact neural circuitry of anorexia remains unclear. Neuroimaging, neurophysiological, and lesion studies implicate the ventral (limbic) and dorsal (cognitive) neural circuits, which may be of particular relevance for understanding behavior in AN. The ventral neurocircuitry consists of the amygdala, insula, ventral striatum, ventral regions of the ACC and OFC, and mediates identification of and responses to stimuli. By contrast, the dorsal circuitry consists of the hippocampus, dorsal regions of the ACC, DLPFC, and parietal cortex, and may be involved in the modulation of selective attention, planning, and effortful regulation of affective states [27, 28].

Key regions involved in fear perception include the amygdala, hippocampus, insular cortex, ACC, striatum, and prefrontal cortex (PFC) [29]. In response to visual food cues, patients with AN display stronger activation of the bilateral amygdala, medial PFC, ACC, and striatum than healthy controls. Thus, food cues trigger arousal, fear, and avoidance in patients with AN [30]. Fear circuitry is also involved in the extinction of fearful memories. Furthermore, inhibitory projections from the medial PFC/OFC to the amygdala are important for this extinction. In this regard, individuals suffering from eating disorders exhibit faster fear learning and heightened resistance to the extinction of conditioned responses [21].

In a recent 18F-FDG PET/CT study of patients with AN, we observed that hypermetabolism in the frontal lobe, hippocampus, and lentiform nucleus decreases after deep brain stimulation of the nucleus accumbens (NAcc-DBS) [31]. Lipsman et al. [32] also reported decreased hypermetabolism of the anterior cingulate, insular, and parietal lobes after sub-callosal cingulate-DBS, together with substantial improvements in body mass index (BMI) and mood. These results demonstrate the importance of these brain regions for AN.

It remains unknown whether disturbances in neural circuits occur prior to or secondary to malnutrition. It has been proposed that structural and functional alterations in the insula and frontal cortex, including areas that contribute to reward and anxiety processing, such as orbito-frontal and cingulate regions, could predispose individuals to developing EDs and that the adaptive changes in these circuits may occur in response to malnutrition [33]. Thus, structural and functional alterations in specific brain regions, together with neurotransmitter-mediated changes, are implicated in the etiopathology of AN. Additional studies are required to further elucidate the etiopathology and neurocircuitry of AN.

15.3 Non-invasive Treatments

Anorexia nervosa is usually a chronic illness which could annoyed one's whole lifetime. Current psychotherapeutic interventions and pharmacological therapies for AN are far from universally effective. Surprisingly, there is no high-level evidence [category A, according to National Institute for Health and Clinical Excellence (NICE) guidelines] regarding the efficacy of pharmacological or psychotherapeutic interventions. Furthermore, only family interventions meet category B criteria (well-conducted studies but no randomized controlled trials) [34, 35]. Variants of family therapy are effective in adolescents but there is little evidence regarding their efficacy in adults [36].

Selective serotonin reuptake inhibitors (SSRIs) are the main stay of pharmacological treatment for AN symptoms or weight restoration; however, the American Psychiatric Association does not support the use of SSRIs in the management of underweight patients with AN [37]. There are only limited data available for atypical antipsychotics; olanzapine may help increase weight and decrease obsessive symptoms in chronic severe AN outpatients, but practice guidelines do not recommend routine use [38–40].

Although there are many available treatments for AN, almost 20 % of the patients are refractory to all current medical treatments and at risk for premature death. The standardized mortality ratio over the first 10 years is about 10 % [11, 12, 41]. For treatment-refractory AN, surgical management may be an alternative therapy.

15.4 Neurosurgical Management of Anorexia Nervosa

15.4.1 History of Neurosurgery in Anorexia Nervosa

Experimental neurosurgical approaches for AN have been proposed for over half a century. The first case report of a prefrontal leucotomy for the treatment of AN was published in 1950 [42]. The patient was a 21-year-old female and received a transorbital leucotomy, followed by a full prefrontal leucotomy as a result of disease relapse. Two months after the second surgery, the patient experienced significant weight gain and increased appetite. In the next 20 years, 16 patients with AN who underwent prefrontal leucotomies were evaluated and reported [43–49]. In a similar manner to the first publication, most patients experienced significant weight gain and greater interest in food; however, a number developed complications. For example, 3 patients experienced continued psychiatric symptoms including depression, anxiety, and panic disorder. In addition, 1 patient committed suicide approximately 4 months after the operation [43, 44, 46]. A study in 1976 reviewed the management of AN patients who underwent stereotactic limbic leucotomies [50–53]. All patients reported significant weight gains and improvements in other psychiatric disorders.

Modern stereotactic psychosurgery for AN has experienced a naissance over the past 10 years. The approaches of modern procedures have focused on the creation of smaller, more targeted stereotactic lesions with an eye toward enhancing the safety and efficacy of the procedure and diminishing the complications. Different from the interventions used in the past, most procedures are performed today with the help of CT or MRI guiding. The high resolution of MRI provides the exact location of the target which declined the severe adverse effects obviously. These procedures are relatively safe, minimally invasion, effective, with less side effects and complications comparing to prefrontal lobotomy. In 2007, Dr. Bomin et al. [54] presented the results of surgical treatment for 20 AN patients in whom previous psychiatric and pharmaceutical therapies were ineffective. Fifteen of these patients underwent bilateral NAcc DBS. Two months after stimulation, anorexic patients gained between 17 and 44 pounds, and many experienced significant improvements in obsessive-compulsive behaviors and symptoms of anxiety. Twelve patients with the binging-purging subtype of AN did not experience significant weight gain by 6 months after stimulation. These patients then received bilateral anterior capsulotomies, and showed significant improvements in both in eating behavior and psychiatric symptoms. Follow-up results at 38 months were also reported for four AN patients who received bilateral NAcc DBS [55]. Following these studies, several different centers have reported successful DBS and lesioning procedures for treatment of AN [50–53].

Two stereotactic procedures are commonly used for AN: DBS and ablative procedures. DBS targets the NAcc or pre-and sub-callosal components (SCC) of the ACC, whereas ablative procedures include capsulotomy, NAcc lesioning, and cingulotomy (Fig. 15.1).

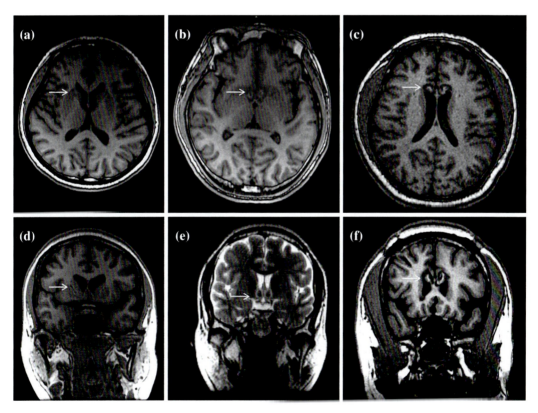

Fig. 15.1 MRI slices showing the typical lesions of capsulotomy, NAcc lesion, and cingulotomy. **a** Axial view of capsulotomy. **b** Coronal view of capsulotomy. **c** Axial view of NAcc lesion. **d** Coronal view of NAcc lesion. **e** Axial view of cingulotomy. **f** Coronal view of cingulotomy

15.4.2 Deep Brain Stimulation

Deep brain stimulation (DBS) has been considered as an effective treatment for a variety of neurological and psychotic disorders refractory to normal therapy, including Parkinson's disease (PD), dystonia, tremor, and obsessive-compulsive disorder (OCD) [56–59]. Deep brain stimulation (DBS) is a neurosurgical treatment involving implantation of electrodes that send electrical impulses to specific locations in the brain. Unlike ablative procedures, DBS is a reversible intervention that causes less damage to neural tissue. Furthermore, most side effects are reversible and can be managed by adjusting stimulation parameters.

DBS is an innovative and promising approach for the treatment of patients with treatment-refractory reward-related psychiatric disorders, DBS targets, such as the NAcc, the ventral capsule/ventral striatum (VC/VS), and SCC, have been used in the treatment of OCD, addiction, MDD, and AN. We demonstrated the efficacy of DBS for AN, as DBS targeting the NAcc reduced excessive hypermetabolism in the frontal lobe, hippocampus, and lentiform nucleus. These findings suggest that DBS can reduce maladaptive activity and connectivity in the stimulated region and restore diseased neural networks to a healthy state [31].

To date, there are few publications regarding the effects of DBS on AN. The first study (a case series) of DBS in AN was conducted by Wu et al. [55] in Shanghai. Four adolescent patients with AN treated with DBS of the NAcc exhibited an average 65 % increase in body weight (average baseline BMI: 11.9 kg/m^2; average follow-up BMI: 19.6 kg/m^2) at a 38-month follow-up examination, and menstrual cycles were restored within 11 months for all these patients. At the final follow up, where DBS systems are explanted 1 year after the battery has fully discharged, no recurrence of symptoms was observed; thus patients were in remission according to Diagnostic and Statistical Manual of Mental Disorders-IV (DSM-IV) criteria. Wang et al. [60] report that ablation (6 AN patients) or DBS (2 patients) of the NAcc resulted in restoration of menstruation within 9 months of surgery, and a recovery in BMI to within a normal range (>18 kg/m^2) within 12 months. These two preliminary studies demonstrate that DBS is a viable option for weight restoration in AN.

Recently, Lipsman et al. [32] published the results of a phase 1 pilot trial of subcallosal cingulate (ACC) DBS in 6 adult patients with treatment-refractory AN. They observed that DBS was relatively safe in this population and resulted in improvements in mood, anxiety, affective regulation, and anorexia-related obsessions and compulsions in 4 patients. At 9-month follow-up examinations, only 3 patients exhibited improved BMI's relative to estimated historical baselines; menstruation status was not noted.

Given the similarities in symptomatology and associated neurocircuitry between OCD and AN, and the established efficacy of DBS for OCD [50, 51], we hypothesize that DBS of the NAcc and other areas associated with reward, might be effective in patients with chronic, treatment refractory AN, providing not only weight restoration, but also significant and sustained improvements in core AN symptoms and associated comorbidities and complications.

15.4.3 Ablative Procedures

As mentioned previously, not all treatment-refractory AN patients experience beneficial effects from DBS, especially the binging-purging subtype, and those with long term (>10 years) AN. In these cases, lesion procedures, such as capsulotomy and cingulotomy, should be considered, as discussed below.

15.4.3.1 Anterior Capsulotomy

Anterior capsulotomy is a stereotactic ablative procedure that involves specific lesions to disconnect limbic circuits involved in different psychiatric disorders, such as OCD, MDD, and addiction. Most patients exhibit relief of certain symptoms and improved cognitive function, without experiencing alterations in personality [61–64].

Anterior capsulotomy involves ablation of the anterior limb of the internal capsule to disconnect the prefrontal cortex and subcortical nuclei (including the dorsomedial thalamus), and is a widely used psychosurgical procedure. Ablations are performed by thermal coagulation or focal gamma radiation guided by computed tomography (CT) or magnetic resonance imaging (MRI). MRI is considered the best modality for locating the anterior capsule because of the large inter-individual differences in this structure. Targets are first identified by visualization of the internal capsule on stereotactic MRIs. Two bilateral trepanations are then performed immediately behind the coronal suture and a lesion is created by thermo-coagulation using radiofrequency probes reaching 80 °C for approximately 60 s. Lesions are typically 4 mm in diameter and 10 mm in length along the contoured target.

A recent study reported the results of 1 patient with OCD comorbid with AN who received bilateral anterior capsulotomy. The patient experienced significant weight gain and improvement in OCD symptoms at a 3 month follow-up examination [53]. In our institution, of the 150 patients who underwent capsulotomies during October 2005 to December 2013, 85 % experienced an improvement in symptoms, and menstruation resumed in all female patients. The results suggest that this is a very promising procedure for treatment of AN. In contrast to DBS, bilateral capsulotomy can cause short-term side effects including incontinence, disorientation, sleep-disorders, and refeeding syndrome. These symptoms usually resolve within 1 month of the operation. A few patients (<5 %) experience long-term side effects including memory loss, fatigue, excessive weight gain, and personality changes.

15.4.3.2 Anterior Cingulotomy

Anterior cingulotomy is one of the most popular psychosurgical procedures currently performed in the US [65, 66]. Clinicians based at Massachusetts General Hospital have significant experience with cingulotomies for treatment of OCD or MDD, and

report very positive outcomes [66, 67]. Typically lesions are created by thermo-coagulation through radiofrequency probes reaching 80–85 °C for 90 s. The electrode is then withdrawn by 1.0 cm and the lesion is enlarged superiorly using the same lesion parameters. These steps are repeated for the opposite hemisphere. This produces symmetrical bilateral lesions of the ACC.

Cingulotomy is a relatively safe procedure with a lower incidence of adverse events than anterior capsulotomy. Immediate, transient symptoms include headache, confusion, and urinary incontinence. In our institution, anterior cingulotomies are performed on AN patients only after a bilateral capsulotomy has failed for at least 1 year, and approximately half of these patients experience positive clinical outcomes with this procedure.

15.4.3.3 Lesioning of the Nucleus Accumbens

Dysfunctions of the primary reward system are a central feature of AN. The NAcc is a key component of this reward system, and may be important for progression of AN. NAcc DBS has been successfully used for treatment of OCD, drug addiction, MDD, and AN. Wang et al. [60] reported the results of 6 AN patients treated with NAcc lesioning. One year after the operation patients exhibited improved basic vital signs and BMI, restoration of menstruation, and improvements in the symptoms of depression, anxiety, and OCD. Although data were obtained from a limited number of cases, considering the successful reports of NAcc DBS, lesioning of the NAcc should be considered as a potential procedure for treatment of refractory AN.

15.4.3.4 Combined Surgical Procedures

As stated above, the majority of AN patients present with psychiatric comorbidities including OCD, MDD, or anxiety disorders. Personality disorders and alcohol or substance abuse may also be present among those with the binging-purging subtype of AN. These parallel symptoms indicate that there is a considerable overlap in reward system neurocircuitry between these psychiatric disorders and eating disorders. For some chronic, refractory AN patients, if the first surgical procedure has failed, a second surgery targeting areas including the NAcc, the anterior internal capsule, and the ACC, should be considered, which can lead to improvements in both core AN symptoms and associated comorbidities and complications.

NAcc DBS Combined with Anterior Capsulotomy

Animal experiments suggest that DBS of the NAcc is a potential treatment option for AN either alone or in combination with an anterior capsulotomy [68]. In our first series, of 15 AN patients treated with NAcc DBS, 12 cases experienced treatment failure and thus bilateral anterior capsulotomies were performed at a second surgery. All these patients achieved a significant improvement in both eating behaviors and psychiatric symptoms [54]. NAcc DBS combined with a bilateral or unilateral anterior capsulotomy is therefore a viable treatment option for severe, treatment-refractory AN patients.

Anterior Capsulotomy Combined with Anterior Cingulotomy

Given the successful results of anterior cingulotomy in OCD and anxiety, this procedure should be considered as a potential second surgery for AN patients experiencing symptoms of OCD, depression, or anxiety, following failure of the initial bilateral anterior capsulotomy. Notably, of 12 patients at our institution in whom bilateral anterior capsulotomies failed, an additional anterior cingulotomy resulted in further improvements in about half of these patients.

15.5 Grading of Anorexia Nervosa and Surgical Options

Patients with AN have elevated rates of lifetime diagnoses of anxiety disorders, MDD, OCD, personality disorders, and substance abuse disorders. Severe comorbidities and longer disease duration contribute to less favorable outcomes for AN. Based on data obtained from 180 cases of surgical

treatment for AN, we categorize AN into 4 grades depending on clinical characteristics, which in turn guide the selection of treatment options.

15.5.1 Grading of AN According to Clinical Features

Grade I: Dieting and/or excessive exercise.

Grade II: Dieting and at least one psychiatric symptom such as OCD, anxiety, or depression.

Grade III: Binge-eating and/or purging behaviors (self-induced vomiting or the misuse of laxatives, diuretics), accompanied by psychiatric symptoms including OCD, anxiety, or depression.

Grade IV: Binge-eating and/or purging behaviors, accompanied by at least one of the following severe psychiatric disorders: substance abuse, kleptomania, promiscuity, self-injurious behavior, or a personality disorder.

Note that if AN disease duration is longer than 6 years, the patient will be graded one level higher.

15.5.2 Selection of Surgical Treatment

Patient treatment options depend on the grade of AN, as follows.

Grade I: Psychotherapeutic interventions and pharmacological therapies.

Grade II: Psychotherapeutic interventions/pharmacological therapies or/and bilateral NAcc DBS.

Grade III: Bilateral anterior capsulotomy or bilateral NAcc ablation.

Grade IV: Bilateral anterior capsulotomy combined with bilateral anterior cingulotomy.

15.6 Indications and Patient Selection Criteria

Since there are few publications regarding patient selection criteria and limited data are available, there are no definite guidelines on AN patient selection criteria. However, the general consensus regarding selection criteria for surgery in our institution is as follows:

1. Patients must exhibit a consistent diagnosis of AN, either the restricting or binge-purging subtype, as defined by DSM-IV criteria and based on a psychiatric interview.
2. Patients must be confirmed as treatment-refractory AN. In our center, treatment-refractory AN is defined as follows. Firstly, patients must have been treated with an appropriate therapy for more than 3 years. Secondly, at least two types of therapy (including pharmacological treatment, behavioral therapy, and psychotherapy) must have been applied with no response. Lastly, patients must have experienced a rapid decrease in body weight over a short time period, which could be life threatening without effective intervention.
3. AN must be of disabling severity with substantial functional impairment according to DSM-IV criterion C, and patients must exhibit a global assessment of functioning (GAF) score of 45 or less for at least 2 years.
4. Patient weight must be <85 % of ideal body weight (and/or BMI < 17.5).
5. Patients or their representatives must be willing to give informed consent for treatment and any subsequent follow-up study.
   Exclusion criteria are as follows:
1. Unstable physical condition (severe electrolyte disturbances, cardiac failure, or other physical contraindications for surgery/anesthesia).
2. Patients with obvious encephalotrophy caused by Alzheimer's disease, tumor, or trauma, as confirmed by MRI.
3. Patients with any contraindication to MRI (pregnancy, pacemakers, or metal implants contraindicated for MRI, not including the DBS implant and the stimulator itself).
4. Patients with severe heart disease or other organic problems contraindicated for neurosurgery.
5. Patients younger than 14 years.
6. Refusal to sign the patient information and consent form.

15.7 Perioperative Patient Management

Considering the wide range of physiological abnormalities observed in AN, careful perioperative management is required.

15.7.1 Preoperative Management

As a result of long-term malnutrition, most AN patients have an unstable physical condition which is contraindicated for surgery or anesthesia. These conditions include severe electrolyte disturbances, cardiac failure, abnormal liver function, and coagulation abnormalities, amongst others. Therefore, more detailed preoperative screening examinations such as electrocardiograms and appropriate blood tests (disseminated intravascular coagulation tests, blood biochemical examinations, routine blood tests, blood glucose tests) are essential to assess potential medical risks.

According to our experiences, hypokalemia and hypoalbuminemia are the most common electrolyte disorders, which should be restored to normal conditions before surgery. In addition, most patients with AN exhibit comorbidities such as OCD, depression, and anxiety. The mental status of AN patients is often unstable and patients frequently present with irritation and deep depression. Thus, patients must be closely monitored throughout the entire procedure.

15.7.2 Intraoperative Management

Local anesthesia is recommended during the lesioning procedure to avoid hypervolemia and excessive dilution of electrolytes. For AN patients receiving DBS treatment, local and general anesthesia are required. Considering the potential anesthetic complications, a thorough preoperative anesthetic assessment and evaluation is required. In addition, doses of most (anesthetic) drugs should be adjusted for weight, and during the operation, electrocardiographic changes and potassium levels should be monitored carefully to minimize the risk of arrhythmias.

Specific caution must be taken during the burr hole procedure because the skull of AN patients is usually very thin; excessive pressure to the dura may cause epidural hematomas. To avoid cerebrospinal fluid overflow during the operation, fibrin glue should be applied immediately after opening the dura. Furthermore, a warm air blower is necessary during the operation to maintain normal body temperature. Lastly, the operation should be completed in a timely manner and appropriate soft mats should be applied to avoid bedsores.

15.7.3 Postoperative Management

Since patients with AN exhibit a very low body weight, strict control of rehydration fluids should be observed after surgery. According to our experience, mannitol should not be administered considering the risk of intracranial hemorrhage. Blood tests should also be monitored closely to avoid fluid and electrolyte disturbances. Pharmacological therapies should be administered on the second day after surgery, but dosage should be adjusted based on the patients' symptoms; psychotherapeutic interventions can be initiated 2 weeks after surgery.

15.8 Adverse Events Associated with Surgery for Anorexia Nervosa

Complications of stereotactic surgery in AN patients can be classified into the following subtypes.

15.8.1 Operative Complications

Intracranial hematomas are a severe complication of stereotactic surgery. In 216 cases of stereotactic surgery at our institution, four cases of epidural hematoma were observed; three recovered after surgery and 1 patient died as a result of disseminated intravascular coagulation. Hematomas occur more frequently in AN patients than in other disorders treated with stereotactic surgery, such as Parkinson's disease, dystonia, OCD, and others, likely as a result of the serious condition of patients with AN.

Wound infections are more common after DBS treatment than lesioning procedures as a result of subcutaneous hydrops and subcutaneous hematomas in DBS. In our center, the rate of wound infections is about 2 %, which is similar to other medical centers.

15.8.2 Neuropsychological Complications

Neuropsychological complications can be divided into short-term and long-term complications. Short-term side effects include incontinence, disorientation, sleep disorders, and headache. These symptoms usually resolved within 1 or 2 months of the operation. A number of patients experience long-term side effects including memory loss, fatigue, excessive weight gain, and personality changes.

15.8.3 DBS System-Associated Complications

In addition to surgical complications, hardware problems with the DBS system, including lead or wire fracture, hardware rejection, malfunction of the implantable pulse generator, and lead migration, can occur. Bhatia et al. reviewed a total of 191 patients who received 330 electrode implants and found that the overall incidence of hardware-related problems was 4.2 %, based on the total number of systems implanted. The mean duration between implantation and complication was 1.8 years [69]. Similar results were observed in our institution.

15.9 Conclusions and Future Outlook

AN is a complex and severe, sometimes life-threatening, psychiatric disorder with a high rate of relapse under current therapies. Stereotactic surgery provides a viable option for treatment of refractory AN. Although positive outcomes have been reported for psychosurgery of refractory AN, limited data on the surgical management of AN patients are available, particularly in the context of experimental trials, and the safety and efficacy of psychosurgery remains under investigation. Several concerns must be addressed to further the application of stereotactic surgery for AN. First, a deeper understanding of the exact etiology and neural circuit of AN must be elucidated. Second, a continuing evolution of stereotactic and functional techniques should be maintained to reduce the unnecessary damage to the brain. Finally, more specific psychometric testing methods should be used to better define the disorder and evaluate surgical outcomes.

Optimum indications for performing these procedures are conditions suitable for the creation of localized lesions capable of disconnecting specific limbic system circuits. We have made appreciable progress along this path, and both stimulation of different brain centers and disconnection of interconnecting pathways hold great potential for solving a significant proportion of psychiatric illnesses that do not respond to pharmacological therapy. Specifically, for OCD there is sufficient evidence to support the view that stereotactic surgery via ablation or radiosurgery is a safe and efficacious option for treating cases refractory to medication and cognitive therapy. As is the case with other surgical procedures, adverse effects and complications are gradually decreasing, and these lesioning techniques are gaining increasing acceptance in psychiatry. The outcomes achieved, in particular the improved quality of life of patients, are especially noteworthy.

Conflict of Interest Statement The authors declare that there are no conflicts of interest.

References

1. Steiner H, et al. Risk and protective factors for juvenile eating disorders. Eur Child Adolesc Psychiatry. 2003;12(Suppl 1):i38–46.
2. Yager J, Andersen AE. Clinical practice. Anorexia nervosa. N Engl J Med. 2005;353(14):1481–8.
3. Keski-Rahkonen A, et al. Epidemiology and course of anorexia nervosa in the community. Am J Psychiatry. 2007;164(8):1259–65.
4. Hoek HW, van Hoeken D. Review of the prevalence and incidence of eating disorders. Int J Eat Disord. 2003;34(4):383–96.
5. Berkman ND, Lohr KN, Bulik CM. Outcomes of eating disorders: a systematic review of the literature. Int J Eat Disord. 2007;40(4):293–309.
6. Forcano L, et al. Suicide attempts in anorexia nervosa subtypes. Compr Psychiatry. 2011;52(4):352–8.
7. Norrington A, et al. Medical management of acute severe anorexia nervosa. Arch Dis Child Educ Pract Ed. 2012;97(2):48–54.
8. Herpertz-Dahlmann B. Adolescent eating disorders: definitions, symptomatology, epidemiology and comorbidity. Child Adolesc Psychiatr Clin North Am. 2009;18(1):31–47.
9. Treasure J, Claudino AM, Zucker N. Eating disorders. Lancet. 2010;375(9714):583–93.
10. Bulik CM, et al. Alcohol use disorder comorbidity in eating disorders: a multicenter study. J Clin Psychiatry. 2004;65(7):1000–6.
11. Strober M, Freeman R, Morrell W. The long-term course of severe anorexia nervosa in adolescents: Survival analysis of recovery, relapse, and outcome predictors over 10–15 years in a prospective study. Int J Eat Disord. 1997;22(4):339–60.
12. Steinhausen HC. The outcome of anorexia nervosa in the 20th century. Am J Psychiatry. 2002;159(8):1284–93.
13. Herzog DB, et al. Recovery and relapse in anorexia and bulimia nervosa: a 7.5-year follow-up study. J Am Acad Child Adolesc Psychiatry. 1999;38(7):829–37.
14. Connan F, et al. A neurodevelopmental model for anorexia nervosa. Physiol Behav. 2003;79(1):13–24.
15. Clarke TK, Weiss AR, Berrettini WH. The genetics of anorexia nervosa. Clin Pharmacol Ther. 2012;91 (2):181–8.
16. Noordenbos G, Seubring A. Criteria for recovery from eating disorders according to patients and therapists. Eat Disord. 2006;14(1):41–54.
17. Kaye WH, et al. Neurocircuity of eating disorders. Curr Top Behav Neurosci. 2011;6:37–57.
18. Kaye WH, Fudge JL, Paulus M. New insights into symptoms and neurocircuit function of anorexia nervosa. Nat Rev Neurosci. 2009;10(8):573–84.
19. Frank GK, et al. Increased dopamine D2/D3 receptor binding after recovery from anorexia nervosa measured by Positron emission tomography and [11C] raclopride. Biol Psychiatry. 2005;58 (11):908–12.
20. Kaye WH, et al. Nothing tastes as good as skinny feels: the neurobiology of anorexia nervosa. Trends Neurosci. 2013;36(2):110–20.
21. Friederich HC, et al. Neurocircuit function in eating disorders. Int J Eat Disord. 2013;46(5):425–32.
22. Kaye WH, et al. Abnormalities in CNS monoamine metabolism in anorexia nervosa. Arch Gen Psychiatry. 1984;41(4):350–5.

23. Bergen AW, et al. Association of multiple DRD2 polymorphisms with anorexia nervosa. Neuropsychopharmacology. 2005;30(9):1703–10.
24. Friederich HC, et al. Differential motivational responses to food and pleasurable cues in anorexia and bulimia nervosa: a startle reflex paradigm. Psychol Med. 2006;36(9):1327–35.
25. Halford JC, Cooper GD, Dovey TM. The pharmacology of human appetite expression. Curr Drug Targets. 2004;5(3):221–40.
26. Nunn K, et al. The fault is not in her parents but in her insula–a neurobiological hypothesis of anorexia nervosa. Eur Eat Disord Rev. 2008;16(5):355–60.
27. Phillips ML, et al. Neurobiology of emotion perception II: Implications for major psychiatric disorders. Biol Psychiatry. 2003;54(5):515–28.
28. Phillips ML, et al. Neurobiology of emotion perception I: the neural basis of normal emotion perception. Biol Psychiatry. 2003;54(5):504–14.
29. Shin LM, Liberzon I. The neurocircuitry of fear, stress, and anxiety disorders. Neuropsychopharmacology. 2010;35(1):169–91.
30. Giel KE, et al. Attentional processing of food pictures in individuals with anorexia nervosa–an eye-tracking study. Biol Psychiatry. 2011;69(7):661–7.
31. Zhang H-W, et al. Metabolic imaging of deep brain stimulation in anorexia nervosa: a 18F-FDG PET/CT study. Clin Nucl Med. 2013;38(12):943–8.
32. Lipsman N, et al. Subcallosal cingulate deep brain stimulation for treatment-refractory anorexia nervosa: a phase 1 pilot trial. Lancet. 2013;381(9875):1361–70.
33. Frank GK. Altered brain reward circuits in eating disorders: chicken or egg? Curr Psychiatry Rep. 2013;15(10):396.
34. Focker M, Knoll S, Hebebrand J. Anorexia nervosa. Eur Child Adolesc Psychiatry. 2013;22:S29–35.
35. Guarda AS. Treatment of anorexia nervosa: insights and obstacles. Physiol Behav. 2008;94(1):113–20.
36. Wade TD, Treasure J, Schmidt U. A case series evaluation of the Maudsley model for treatment of adults with anorexia nervosa. Eur Eat Disord Rev. 2011;19(5):382–9.
37. Bulik CM, et al. Anorexia nervosa treatment: a systematic review of randomized controlled trials. Int J Eat Disord. 2007;40(4):310–20.
38. Brewerton TD. Antipsychotic agents in the treatment of anorexia nervosa: neuropsychopharmacologic rationale and evidence from controlled trials. Curr Psychiatry Rep. 2012;14(4):398–405.
39. McKnight RF, Park RJ. Atypical antipsychotics and anorexia nervosa: a review. Eur Eat Disord Rev. 2010;18(1):10–21.
40. Wilson GT, Shafran R. Eating disorders guidelines from NICE. Lancet. 2005;365(9453):79–81.
41. Couturier J, Lock J. What is recovery in adolescent anorexia nervosa? Int J Eat Disord. 2006;39 (7):550–5.
42. Drury MO. An emergency leucotomy. Br Med J. 1950;2(4679):609.

43. Crisp AH, Kalucy RS. The effect of leucotomy in intractable adolescent weight phobia (primary anorexia nervosa). Postgrad Med J. 1973;49(578):883–93.
44. Morgan JF, Crisp AH. Use of leucotomy for intractable anorexia nervosa: a long-term follow-up study. Int J Eat Disord. 2000;27(3):249–58.
45. Birley JL. Modified frontal leucotomy: a review of 106 cases. Br J Psychiatry. 1964;110:211–21.
46. Carmody JT, Vibber FL. Anorexia nervosa treated by prefrontal lobotomy. Ann Intern Med. 1952;36 (2:2):647–52.
47. Kay DW. Anorexia nervosa: a study in prognosis. Proc R Soc Med. 1953;46(8):669–74.
48. Sargant W. Leucotomy in psychosomatic disorders. Lancet. 1951;2(6673):87–91.
49. Sifneos PE. A case of anorexia nervosa treated successfully by leucotomy. Am J Psychiatry. 1952;109(5):356–60.
50. Zamboni R, et al. Dorsomedial thalamotomy as a treatment for terminal anorexia: a report of 2 cases. Acta Neurochirurgica. 1993;34–35.
51. Kelly D, Mitchell-Heggs N. Stereotactic limbic leucotomy—a follow-up study of thirty patients. Postgrad Med J. 1973;49(578):865–82.
52. Mitchell-Heggs N, Kelly D, Richardson A. Stereotactic limbic leucotomy–a follow-up at 16 months. Br J Psychiatry. 1976;128:226–40.
53. Barbier J, et al. Successful anterior capsulotomy in comorbid anorexia nervosa and obsessive-compulsive disorder: case report. Neurosurgery. 2011;69(3): E745–51; discussion E751.
54. Bomin S, Li D, Zhan S (2007) DBS for anorexia nervosa. The eighth world congress of International Neuromodulation Society. Acapulco, Mexico.
55. Wu H, et al. Deep-brain stimulation for anorexia nervosa. World Neurosurg. 2012;80(3-4):S29 e1–10.
56. Deuschl G, et al. A randomized trial of deep-brain stimulation for Parkinson's disease. N Engl J Med. 2006;355(9):896–908.
57. Mueller J, et al. Pallidal deep brain stimulation improves quality of life in segmental and generalized dystonia: results from a prospective, randomized sham-controlled trial. Mov Disord. 2008;23(1):131–4.
58. O'Sullivan D, Pell M. Long-term follow-up of DBS of thalamus for tremor and STN for Parkinson's disease. Brain Res Bull. 2009;78(2–3):119–21.
59. Goodman WK, Alterman RL. Deep brain stimulation for intractable psychiatric disorders. Annu Rev Med. 2011;63:511–24.
60. Wang J, et al. Treatment of intractable anorexia nervosa with inactivation of the nucleus accumbens using stereotactic surgery. Stereotact Funct Neurosurg. 2013;91(6):364–72.
61. Zhan S, et al. Long-term follow-up of bilateral anterior capsulotomy in patients with refractory obsessive-compulsive disorder. Clin Neurol Neurosurg. 2014;119:91–5.
62. Zuo C, et al. Metabolic imaging of bilateral anterior capsulotomy in refractory obsessive compulsive

disorder: an FDG PET study. J Cereb Blood Flow Metab. 2013;33(6):880–7.

63. Christmas D, et al. Long term outcome of thermal anterior capsulotomy for chronic, treatment refractory depression. J Neurol Neurosurg Psychiatry. 2011;82 (6):594–600.

64. Hurwitz TA, et al. Bilateral anterior capsulotomy for intractable depression. J Neuropsychiatry Clin Neurosci. 2012;24(2):176–82.

65. Cosgrove GR, Rauch SL. Stereotactic cingulotomy. Neurosurg Clin N Am. 2003;14(2):225–35.

66. Dougherty DD, et al. Prospective long-term follow-up of 44 patients who received cingulotomy for treatment-refractory obsessive-compulsive disorder. Am J Psychiatry. 2002;159(2):269–75.

67. Baer L, et al. Cingulotomy for intractable obsessive-compulsive disorder. Prospective long-term follow-up of 18 patients. Arch Gen Psychiatry. 1995;52 (5):384–92.

68. van der Plasse G, et al. Deep brain stimulation reveals a dissociation of consummatory and motivated behaviour in the medial and lateral nucleus accumbens shell of the rat. PLoS One. 2012;7(3):e33455.

69. Bhatia S, et al. Surgical complications of deep brain stimulation. Stereotact Funct Neurosurg. 2008;86 (6):367–72.

Neurosurgery for the Treatment of Refractory Schizophrenia

16

Bomin Sun, Wei Liu, Shikun Zhan, Qianqian Hao, Dianyou Li, Yixin Pan, Yongchao Li and Guozhen Lin

Abstract

Schizophrenia is a chronic, severe, and disabling psychiatric disease that is characterized by perturbations in cognition, affect, and behavior. Of the many available treatments, pharmaceutical interventions remain as first choice-treatments. However, about 20 % of patients with schizophrenia exhibit refractory schizophrenia that does not respond well to pharmaceutical treatments. As a result, neurosurgery performed for the treatment of refractory schizophrenia, also called psychosurgery, is an alternative treatment that has a long history. With the refinement and improved accuracy of neuroimaging techniques, modern psychosurgery has greater success with fewer risks. Nevertheless, these procedures are still invasive methods and the resulting lesions are irreversible. Therefore, we must keep in mind that surgical therapy should only be considered as a supplementary part of the comprehensive treatment of schizophrenia and the inclusion criteria for surgery must be strict.

16.1 Introduction

Schizophrenia, which was also called "dementia praecox" by Emil Kraepelin, a German psychiatrist in the late nineteenth and early twentieth century, is a chronic, severe, and disabling mental disorder characterized by perturbations in cognition, affect, and behavior. It is diagnosed on the basis of a series of clinical psychiatric symptoms such as auditory hallucinations, paranoia, or disorganized speech and thinking. Symptoms of schizophrenia typically emerge in adolescence and early adulthood, with a global lifetime prevalence of about 0.30–0.66 % [1]. Schizophrenia does not only affect mental health, but also negatively impacts physical health, shortening the life expectancy of patients with schizophrenia by 12–15 years compared to the general population; this gap has also widened over recent decades [2]. Therefore, schizophrenia causes more loss of life than most cancers and physical illnesses. Furthermore, it is one of the most burdening and costly illnesses worldwide [3–5].

B. Sun (✉) · W. Liu · S. Zhan · Q. Hao · D. Li · Y. Pan
Department of Functional Neurosurgery, Ruijin Hospital, School of Medicine, Shanghai Jiao Tong University, Shanghai, China

Y. Li · G. Lin
Department of Psychiatry, Ruijin Hospital, School of Medicine, Shanghai Jiao Tong University, Shanghai, China

B. Sun and A. De Salles (eds.), *Neurosurgical Treatments for Psychiatric Disorders*,
DOI 10.1007/978-94-017-9576-0_16
© Shanghai Jiao Tong University Press, Shanghai and Springer Science+Business Media Dordrecht 2015

The exact mechanisms underlying schizophrenia are still unclear. However, scientists have long known that genetic factors play an important role in the development of schizophrenia. The illness occurs in less than 1 % of the general population, but, interestingly, it occurs in about 10 % of people who have a first-degree relative with the disorder. Monozygotic twins have a concordance rate of about 50 % [6]. Besides genetic susceptibility, many environmental factors may be involved in the development of schizophrenia, such as exposure to viruses, difficulties during birth, and other unknown psychosocial factors. Therefore, most researchers believe that interactions between genes and the environment are necessary for the development of schizophrenia.

There are many hypotheses to explain the underlying mechanisms of schizophrenia. Rossum [7] first presented the dopamine (DA) hypothesis of schizophrenia based on the observation that antipsychotics may block DA receptors. Subsequently, accumulating evidence supported the idea that schizophrenia is associated with frontal-subcortical neuronal circuits, especially the orbito-frontal and anterior cingulate circuits [8–11]. The orbito-frontal circuit projects to the ventromedial caudate nucleus and the anterior cingulate circuit sends fibers to the ventral striatum, which includes the ventromedial caudate, ventral putamen, nucleus accumbens, and olfactory tubercle. These circuits primarily use DA as a neurotransmitter, and process cortical-subcortical emotional information. Disrupting these circuits can thus trigger the onset of schizophrenia's positive symptoms. Besides the DA hypothesis, it was reported that the serotoninergic system plays an important role in the negative symptoms of schizophrenia. Serotoninergic neurons from the dorsal and median raphe nucleus project to the prefrontal cortex (PFC), and the PFC sends projections back to the raphe nuclei providing feedback control of cortical serotonin release. Serotonin could stimulate 5-HT2A receptors in the PFC that inhibits the activity of dopaminergic neurons in this area.

At present, pharmaceutical treatment is the first option pursued in schizophrenia. The first-line drugs used in schizophrenia include: Haloperidol, Perphenazine, Chlorpromazine, Risperidone, Aripiprazole, Clozapine, and Olanzapine. Among these drugs, Haloperidol, Perphenazine, and Chlorpromazine are first-generation antipsychotics, while the remainder are second-generation antipsychotics. Although controversy remains over the higher rate of effectiveness of second-generation antipsychotics, the use of drugs such as Clozapine and Olanzapine has grown due to their inducing fewer side effects. Medication usually shows good results in the treatment of positive symptoms of schizophrenia while negative symptoms are generally less receptive to similar treatment. Besides medication, family therapy, supported employment, skills training, and other psychosocial interventions may be helpful in the treatment of schizophrenia [12–15]. However, approximately 20 % of schizophrenics remain non-responsive to any of the aforementioned treatments [16]. For refractory schizophrenia, psychosurgery, also called neurosurgery for mental disorders, is considered as a last resort. In this chapter, we briefly introduce the history, indications, optimal surgical target, surgical procedure, and surgical results of psychosurgery applied in schizophrenia.

16.2 A Brief History of Psychosurgery

Psychosurgery, including the lesion and stimulation techniques, has a long and storied history which can be traced back to ancient times. A skull with a trepanation hole identified in France has been carbon dated to the Neolithic period of the Stone Age, or approximately 5100 BC [17]. Signs of healing in the skull indicate a surgical rather than a traumatic origin of the wound. Literature on trephination for the relief of neuropsychiatric symptoms stemming from mental disorders can be dated back to 1500 BC [18].

In the modern era, the links between the brain and behavior was brought into cultural awareness through the famous account of Phineas P. Gage, a railroad worker in Vermont. Gage experienced a terrible explosion that caused severe head trauma. He miraculously survived, but his personality was profoundly altered [19]. The first psychosurgical procedure was performed in 1888 by Swiss psychiatrist Gottlieb Burckhardt, who contributed widely to the birth of modern psychosurgery. The process involved the excision of cerebrum at multiple foci in frontal, parietal, and temporal cortices. The results of six cases ranged from success (in three patients) to failure (in one fatal case) [20]. Almost 50 years later, the Portuguese neurologist Egas Moniz, who is often regarded as the founder of psychosurgery, performed the first prefrontal lobotomy in 1935 with the help of neurosurgeon Almeida Lima. Different from the psychosurgical interventions performed by Burckhardt, Moniz's surgery focused on the white matter of the brain and garnered great attention worldwide. He won the Nobel Prize for Medicine in 1949, which is still highly controversial today. In the United States, Freeman and Watts introduced the prefrontal lobotomy in 1942. There was an upsurge in surgical interventions between 1943 and 1954 because of the lack of effective psychopharmacological agents and the large social and financial burdens of psychiatric illness.

However, with the introduction of newer psychotropic medications, such as chlorpromazine, and the growing realization of severe surgical side effects, psychosurgery lost its popularity as a treatment [21]. Although stereotactic and functional neurosurgery for alleviating psychiatric disorders was maturing due to the development of stereotactic neurosurgical devices and neuroimaging, it is approved only in specific circumstances and performed only in a few specialized centers across the globe, largely as a precaution against widespread abuse similar to that of the prefrontal lobotomy. Several procedures including anterior capsulotomy, anterior cingulotomy, amygdaloidotomy, subcaudate tractotomy, and limbic leucotomy have been sparingly applied in schizophrenia patients [18, 22–26]. Different from the interventions used in the past, most procedures today are performed with the help of CT or MRI guidance. The high-resolution of MRI provides the exact location of the target, which has reduced the severe adverse effects. These procedures are relatively safe, minimally invasive, effective, and have fewer side effects and complications compared to the prefrontal lobotomy.

16.3 Patient Selection Criteria

Patient selection criteria are strict for treating refractory schizophrenia (TRS). A general consensus about the selection criteria for TRS surgery in our center is summarized below:
1. Patients diagnosed with schizophrenia in the Department of Psychiatry by independent psychiatrists according to the DSM-IV.
2. Refractory schizophrenia patients confirmed by a team of psychiatrists, neurosurgeons, and neurologists and proposed for neurosurgical treatment. In our center, refractory schizophrenia is defined as follows:
    (I) Illness severity with a score of ≥35 on the 18-item Brief Psychiatric Rating Scale (BPRS, scored 1–7) and a clinical global impression (CGI) >4.
    (II) At least three periods of treatment in the three preceding years with neuroleptic agents (at least two different chemical classes) at dosages equivalent to or greater than 500 mg/d of Chlorpromazine for a period of 8 weeks, each without significant symptomatic relief.
    (III) Duration of mental disorder >3 years and no period of good function.
3. Patients or their representatives must be able and willing to give informed consent and have the support of their family.
4. Patients are between the ages of 18 and 60 years old.
5. Pregnant women are excluded.

6. Patients are considered for psychosurgery only if there are no contraindications, such as severe organic brain damage.

16.4 Surgical Treatment

The advent of stereotactic and functional neurosurgery reemerged as an option for the most severe, chronic, and refractory schizophrenia patients after the decline of the classical lobotomy. As I mentioned above, the most common procedures have included anterior cingulotomy, subcaudate tractotomy, limbic leucotomy, anterior capsulotomy, and amygdaloidotomy. In our center, anterior capsulotomy and anterior cingulotomy are the most performed surgeries. They are described in more detail below.

16.4.1 Anterior Capsulotomy

In this procedure, lesions are made within the anterior limb of the internal capsule to cut the connective fibers between prefrontal cortex and subcortical nuclei (dorsomedial thalamus included). The lesions may be produced by thermal coagulation or focal gamma radiation guided by CT or MRI. Because of the large individual differences in the anterior capsule, MRI targeting became the best modality to identify the location of the structures. The target is identified with the visualization of the internal capsule on stereotactic MRIs. Usually, the target lies 15–17 mm anterior to the AC, 15–17 mm lateral to the midline, and 2–4 mm under the AC-PC line. Two bilateral trepanations are made immediately behind the coronal suture and the lesion is created by thermo-coagulation through radiofrequency probes reaching 80 °C for approximately 60 s. The first lesion is located 3–4 mm below the AC-PC line and extends up to 10-mm above the AC-PC line. During lesioning, neurological testing is carried out to ensure no impairment of motor or sensory functions. After adequate cooling, the electrode is withdrawn 2 mm and the ablation procedure is repeated 4–5 times to ensure the complete ablation of the target. Finally, a lesion 4-mm in diameter and 10-mm in length along the contoured target is produced [27] (Fig. 16.1).

16.4.2 Anterior Cingulotomy

In the U.S., anterior cingulotomy is currently one of the most widely used psychosurgical procedures [28]. In our center, cingulotomy is usually performed together with capsulotomy to control the symptoms of some very severely refractory schizophrenia patients. In this procedure, MRI is also used to identify the location of the target structures. The initial targets are located 0.7 cm lateral to the midline bilaterally, 2 cm posterior to the most anterior portions of the frontal horns,

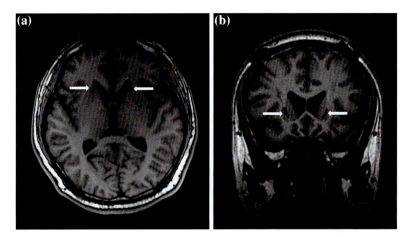

Fig. 16.1 MRI slices showing a typical lesion in the mid-third portion of the bilateral ALIC (*arrows*). **a** Axial view. **b** Coronal view

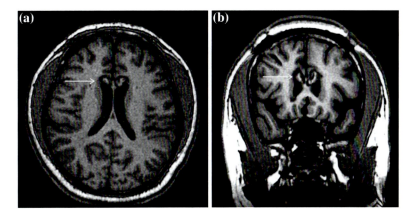

Fig. 16.2 MRI slices showing a typical lesion in the bilateral anterior cingulate gyrus (*arrows*). **a** Axial view. **b** Coronal view

and 1-mm above the roof of the ventricles. Typically, lesions are created by thermo-coagulation through radiofrequency probes reaching to 80–85 °C for 90 s. The electrode is then withdrawn 1 cm and the lesion is enlarged superiorly using the same lesion parameters. These steps are repeated for the opposite hemisphere. This produces bilateral symmetrical lesions in the anterior cingulate cortices [29] (Fig. 16.2).

16.5 Surgical Outcomes

The prognosis of schizophrenia in patients undergoing different types of psychosurgery varies widely. Frontal lobotomy was the most common psychosurgery; between the 1940s and the 1950s, over 40,000 Americans were lobotomized. If the surgery was performed before the development of severe schizophrenia, Freeman found that lobotomy reduced the likelihood of disease progression [30]. In contrast to the findings of Freeman, Dynes found that some patients remained hospitalized for more than a decade even after classical lobotomy [31]. Miller and Cummings [32] believed that psychosurgery should be applied in a limited fashion for more problematic and intractable psychological disorders considering the improvements found in violent behavior in schizophrenia patients. Some reviews have also focused on the role of lobotomy in the treatment of schizophrenia. By investigating more than 7,500 patients who received a frontal lobotomy in England from 1942 to 1952, Tooth and Newton found that only 18 % of patients showed signs of improvement [33]. Da Costa reported that frontal lobotomy reduced aggression and/or produced a marked to slight improvement in 16 schizophrenia patients.

Stereotactic and functional neurosurgery including anterior cingulotomy, subcaudate tractotomy, limbic leucotomy, anterior capsulotomy, and amygdaloidotomy were introduced later as an alternative treatment for refractory schizophrenia patients. Compared with lobotomy, these procedures are demonstrated to be relatively safe and have better outcomes. Among these modern procedures, patients who underwent cingulotomy had the best reported outcomes [34]. In 1987, Ballantine et al. reported a study involving 11 patients with schizophrenia who underwent anterior cingulotomy with a long-term follow-up, in which 4 of 11 patients experienced considerable improvement without deficits in intellectual or emotional function. In our center, cingulotomy is performed only on patients who do not respond well to treatment with capsulotomy. In our experience, the combination of cingulotomy and capsulotomy usually control the symptoms of severely refractory schizophrenia patients in spite of more complications. Similar to cingulotomy, stereotactic subcaudate tractotomy also has little impact on schizophrenia [35]. According to the studies of Talairach and Herner, the initial outcomes of anterior capsulotomy for the treatment of schizophrenia were disappointing, with only

27 % of patients having a positive response. However, we find better results with anterior capsulotomy in our schizophrenia patients. In our center, 100 refractory schizophrenia patients who met the inclusion criteria (see **Patient Selection Criteria** above) were treated with capsulotomy guided by MRI; 74 % of such patients demonstrated improvements. The accurate target localization with the help of MRI greatly contributes to the improved outcomes of capsulotomy. Amygdaloidotomy is usually used in schizophrenia patients with severely aggressive behavior and a large percentage of cases showed a marked reduction in aggressive behavior [36]. In our center, amygdaloidotomy is restricted to refractory schizophrenia patients with severely aggressive behavior. The results are consistent with the aforementioned study. Besides our center, many neurosurgeons in China have also applied stereotactic surgery in schizophrenia patients (see Table 16.1).

16.6 Complications

The classical lobotomy had a high rate of complications [18, 37–39]. The short-term complications included confusion, frailty, and languor. The long-term sequelae, which were known as "frontal lobe syndrome", included inertia, apathy, social withdrawal, and attention deficits. Furthermore, some patients developed epilepsy postoperatively and hemorrhage was another severely adverse effect, which was sometimes fatal. As a consequence, most neurosurgeons agreed that frontal lobotomy was not a beneficial intervention. With the introduction of stereotactic and functional neurosurgery, complications have been greatly reduced and capsulotomy is considered the safest procedure. Rare complications including fatigue, loss of initiative, memory deficits, weight gain, and intracranial hemorrhage have been reported following anterior capsulotomy. In our experience, fatigue, loss of initiative, and memory deficits are observed postoperatively and recover in a few months, while intracranial hemorrhage and epilepsy are rarely seen

after the surgery. Cingulotomy is also quite safe and no severe complications such as hemiplegia, aphasia, or death directly caused by cingulotomy have been reported [40]. Teuber et al. [41] reviewed the results of cingulotomy in a wide range of patients and found a small incidence of permanent cognitive deficits. Similar to cingulotomy, stereotactic subcaudate tractotomy does not produce deficits in intellectual or emotional function [42, 43].

16.7 New Developments

Deep brain stimulation (DBS) is a new form of neurosurgery that was originally developed to treat Parkinson's disease (PD) and is emerging as a potential treatment for some mental disorders. Compared to ablative neurosurgery, DBS has the advantage of reversibility and adjustability; the parameters of the stimulation can be changed and the electrodes can be removed from the brain. DBS has been applied in obsessive and compulsive disease (OCD), and major depression [44–48]. To the best of our knowledge, there are no published articles focused on the application of DBS in schizophrenia patients. Importantly, DBS testing using schizophrenia animal models is increasing. Perez et al. [49] provided initial preclinical evidence demonstrating the feasibility of hippocampal DBS as a potential novel approach for the treatment of schizophrenia by implanting the electrodes in the ventral hippocampus in a rodent model of schizophrenia. Similar results were found by Ewing et al. [50]. Besides the hippocampus, the mediodorsal thalamic nucleus and nucleus accumbens are also considered potential targets of DBS in the treatment of schizophrenia [51, 52]. Furthermore, a clinical study of DBS application in schizophrenia in humans aimed at the nucleus accumbens/ ventral striatum and ventral tegmental area has already been registered (ClinicalTrials.gov Identifier: NCT01725334). As in the development of neuroimaging, the improved targeting efficiency of DBS in schizophrenia now deserves increased attention.

Table 16.1 Summary of the stereotactic neurosurgery in schizophrenia patients in China

Series (ref. no.)	No. of patients	Target area	Follow-up period	Patients with improvement	Complications
Liu Weiqin et al. (2002)	118	Bilateral arterial limb of internal capsule + bilateral cingulate gyrus + amygdaloid nucleus	6 months	Improvement: 108; No improvement: 10	Hallucinations, mania: 16; Urinary incontinence: 6; Hemiplegic paralysis: 2
	13	Bilateral arterial limb of internal capsule + bilateral cingulate gyrus		Improvement : 6; No improvement: 7	
	7	Bilateral anterior limb of internal capsule + bilateral cingulate gyrus + amygdaloid nucleus + hippocampus		Improvement: 7	
Wang Xiaofeng et al. (2002)	51	Bilateral anterior limb of internal capsule + cingulated gyrus + amygdaloid nucleus	6 months	PANSS evaluation P: $p < 0.01$; N: $p < 0.01$; G: $p < 0.01$	[a]
Xu Zhiju et al. (1996)	18	Cingulated gyrus	10 years	Improvements: 9; No improvements: 9	[a]
Chen Chengyu et al. (2002)	25	Amygdaloid nucleus	6 months	Obvious improvements: 12; Improvements: 13; No improvements: 2	Aphthy: 8; Urinary incontinence: 3; Hypererosia: 1; Cerebral hemorrhage: 1; Cerebrospinal leak: 1
Zhou Jianyun et al. (2005)	11	Cingulated gyrus + amygdaloid nucleus + anterior limb of internal capsule + caudate	6 months	Obvious improvements: 6; Improvements: 2; No improvements: 3	Aphthy: 2; Urinary incontinence: 3; Temporary hypomnesia: 2
Wu Shengling et al. (1992)	23	Bilateral anterior cingulated gyrus	5 years	Obvious improvements: 2; Improvements: 11; No improvement: 10	Mild personality changes: 1; Mild intelligent down: 1; Suicide: 1
	27	Bilateral anterior cingulated gyrus + bilateral amygdaloid nucleus	3 years	Obvious improvements: 4; Improvements: 12; No improvements: 11	Mild personality changes: 1; Mild intelligent down: 4; Suicide: 1

(continued)

Table 16.1 (continued)

Series (ref. no.)	No. of patients	Target area	Follow-up period	Patients with improvement	Complications
Huang Heqing et al. (1995)	52	Bilateral amygdaloid nucleus + anterior limb of internal capsule	1 year	Obvious improvements: 17 Improvements: 15 No improvements: 15 Recurrence: 5	Urinary incontinence: 30 Hiccup: 31 Fecal incontinence: 2 Hyperactivity: 6 Hypererosia: 3 Hemiplegic paralysis: 3 Aphasia: 1
Dou Changwu (1992)	5	Bilateral cingulated gyrus + amygdaloid nucleus	7 months	Obvious improvements: 2 Improvements: 3 No improvements: 0 Miss: 1	Urinary incontinence: 2
	1	Right cingulated gyrus + amygdaloid nucleus			
Wang Yifang et al. (2006)	17	Amygdaloid nucleus + anterior limb of internal capsule + bilateral medial septum	6 months	Obvious improvements: 13 Improvements: 3 No improvements: 1	[a]
Du Xiaopei et al. (1992)	10	Unilateral amygdaloid nucleus + anterior limb of internal capsule (n = 3) Unilateral cingulated gyrus (n = 3) Anterior limb of internal capsule + mediodorsal thalamic nucleus (n = 1) Unilateral anterior limb of internal capsule (n = 2) Amygdaloid nucleus + cingulated gyrus (n = 1)	1 year	Obvious improvements: 2 Improvements: 6 No improvements: 2	[a]

(continued)

Table 16.1 (continued)

Series (ref. no.)	No. of patients	Target area	Follow-up period	Patients with improvement	Complications
Yao Xuefeng et al. (2010)	32	Bilateral cingulated gyrus + anterior limb of internal capsule + amygdaloid nucleus + bilateral medial septum (For PS)[b] + bilateral caudate nucleus (For NS)[b]	4 weeks	Obvious improvements: 17 Improvements: 11 No improvements: 4	Fever: 6 Urinary incontinence: 15 Focal cerebral hemorrhage: 8 Temporarily muscle weakness: 3
Liu Jianxin et al. (2003)	25	Medial septum + amygdaloid nucleus + cingulated gyrus	4 weeks	Obvious improvements: 15 Improvements: 10	Fever: 2 Urinary incontinence: 3 Epilepsy: 1
Li Zhibang et al. (1998)	18	Bilateral anterior cingulated gyrus + amygdaloid nucleus (n = 16) Bilateral anterior cingulated gyrus + anterior limb of internal capsule (n = 1) Bilateral amygdloid nucleus + anterior red nucleus	6 years	Obvious improvements: 4 Improvements: 7 No improvements: 7	Urinary incontinence: 5 Hemiplegic paralysis: 2 Anosmia: 2 Dead: 1
Li Shuande et al. (2002)	35	Amygdaloid nucleus + anterior cingulated gyrus	1 years	Obvious improvements: 21 Improvements: 13 No improvements: 1	[a]
Nan Wu et al. (2004)	6	Bilateral amygdaloid nucleus + anterior limb of internal capsule + callosal gyrus	6 months	Obvious improvements: 5 Improvements: 1	Drowsiness: 1 Urinary incontinence: 1
Shi Qingfeng et al. (1994)	20	Mediodorsal thalamic nucleus (n = 9) Unilateral mediodorsal thalamic nucleus + bilateral amygdaloid nucleus (n = 9) Unilateral mediodorsal thalamic nucleus + Unilateral amygdaloid nucleus (n = 2)	4 weeks	Obvious improvements: 2 Improvements: 14 No improvements: 4	Urinary incontinence: 4 Bulimia: 4 Hemiplegic paralysis: 1

(continued)

Table 16.1 (continued)

Series (ref. no.)	No. of patients	Target area	Follow-up period	Patients with improvement	Complications
Kuang Weiping et al. (2010)	126	Nucleus accumbens	4 weeks	Obvious improvements: 78 Improvements: 36 No improvements: 12	Urinary incontinence: 25 Hemiplegic paralysis: 3 Drowsiness: 61 Sweaty: 44
Gan Jingli et al. (2005)	32	Amygdaloid nucleus + cingulaged gyrus	1 years	Obvious improvements: 20 Improvements: 11 No improvements: 1	Fever: 26 Urinary Incontinence: 10 Epilepsy: 1 Silence: 2
Fu Xianming et al. (2004)	39	Bilateral amygdaloid nucleus + cingulated gyrus (n = 24) Bilateral cingulated gyrus + anterior limb of internal capsule (n = 5) Bilateral amygdaloid nucleus + anterior limb of internal capsule (n = 4) Bilateral cingulated gyrus + anterior limb of internal capsule + amygdaloid nucleus (n = 4) Bilateral cingulated gyrus + anterior limb of internal capsule + right amygdaloid nucleus (n = 1)	4 weeks	Obvious improvements: 21 Improvements: 14 No improvements: 4	Fever: 5 Urinary Incontinence: 6 Hypererosia: 1 Bad memory: 1 Involuntary movement: 2
Pan Yixin et al. (2011)	20	Anterior limb of internal capsule	3 years	Obvious improvements: 12 Improvements: 5 No improvements: 3	Urinary incontinence: 3 Confusion: 1 Bad memory: 1 Obesity: 2 Apathetic: 4 Personality change: 2

(continued)

Table 16.1 (continued)

Series (ref. no.)	No. of patients	Target area	Follow-up period	Patients with improvement	Complications
Cao Tao et al. (1992)	16	Bilateral cingulated gyrus + amygdala	4 weeks	Recovery: 2; Obvious improvements: 3; Improvements: 6; No improvements: 5	Urine incontinence: 12; Mutism and fatigues: 6
Tang Yunlin et al. (1989)	106	Bilateral cingulated gyrus + amygdala	2 years	Obvious improvements: 51; Improvements: 38; No improvements: 17	Urine incontinence: 29; Hemiparesis: 1; Wound infection: 4
Yang Shaohai et al. (1992)	19	Bilateral cingulated gyrus	5 years	Obvious improvements: 9; Improvements: 10; No improvements: 19	[a]
	11	Bilateral cingulated gyrus + amygdala			
	6	Bilateral capsulotomy + amygdala			
	1	Bilateral cingulated gyrus + capsulotomy			
	1	Bilateral capsulotomy			

[a] No data presented
[b] *PS* positive syndrome; *NS* negative syndrome

16.8 Conclusion

Schizophrenia is usually accompanied by significant social or occupational dysfunctions that cause a heavy economic burden for both the patient's family and society as a whole. In the U.S., the cost of schizophrenia was estimated to be $62.7 billion in 2002 [4]. Therefore, there is a very urgent need to find a new method for the treatment of refractory schizophrenia. We propose that modern stereotactic neurosurgery (including capsulotomy and cingulotomy) may be a potential method for such treatment. However, these procedures are still invasive and the lesions created are irreversible. Therefore, we must keep in mind that surgical therapy should only be considered as a supplementary part of the comprehensive treatment of schizophrenia and the inclusion criteria must be strict. Close psychiatric follow-up is necessary not only to monitor improvement of symptoms, but also to assess potential adverse psychiatric consequences. Finally, to help the patients recover, surgery should be accompanied by an appropriate psychological rehabilitation plan and family-social support program.

References

1. Saha S, Chant D, McGrath J. A systematic review of mortality in schizophrenia: is the differential mortality gap worsening over time? Arch Gen Psychiatry. 2007;64:1123–31.
2. van Os J, Kapur S. Schizophrenia. Lancet. 2009;374:635–45.
3. Goeree R, Farahati F, Burke N, Blackhouse G, O'Reilly D, Pyne J, Tarride JE. The economic burden of schizophrenia in canada in 2004. Curr Med Res Opin. 2005;21:2017–28.
4. Wu EQ, Birnbaum HG, Shi L, Ball DE, Kessler RC, Moulis M, Aggarwal J. The economic burden of schizophrenia in the united states in 2002. J Clin Psychiatry. 2005;66:1122–9.
5. Zhai J, Guo X, Chen M, Zhao J, Su Z. An investigation of economic costs of schizophrenia in two areas of china. Int J Ment Health Syst. 2013;7:26.
6. Cardno AG, Gottesman II. Twin studies of schizophrenia: from bow-and-arrow concordances to star wars Mx and functional genomics. Am J Med Genet. 2000;97:12–7.
7. van Rossum JM. The significance of dopamine-receptor blockade for the mechanism of action of neuroleptic drugs. Arch Int Pharmacodyn Ther. 1966;160:492–4.
8. Goldman-Rakic PS, Selemon LD. Functional and anatomical aspects of prefrontal pathology in schizophrenia. Schizophr Bull. 1997;23:437–58.
9. Tekin S, Cummings JL. Frontal-subcortical neuronal circuits and clinical neuropsychiatry: an update. J Psychosom Res. 2002;53:647–54.
10. Volk DW, Lewis DA. Prefrontal cortical circuits in schizophrenia. Curr Top Behav Neurosci. 2011;4: 485–508.
11. Laviolette SR. Dopamine modulation of emotional processing in cortical and subcortical neural circuits: evidence for a final common pathway in schizophrenia? Schizophr Bull. 2007;33:971–81.
12. Rodrigues MG, Krauss-Silva L, Martins AC. Meta-analysis of clinical trials on family intervention in schizophrenia. Cad Saude Publica 2008;24:2203–18.
13. Pharoah F, Mari J, Rathbone J, Wong W. Family intervention for schizophrenia. Cochrane Database Syst Rev. 2006;CD000088(12).
14. Medalia A, Choi J. Cognitive remediation in schizophrenia. Neuropsychol Rev. 2009;19:353–64.
15. McGurk SR, Twamley EW, Sitzer DI, McHugo GJ, Mueser KT. A meta-analysis of cognitive remediation in schizophrenia. Am J Psychiatry. 2007;164:1791–802.
16. Smith T, Weston C, Lieberman J. Schizophrenia (maintenance treatment). Am Fam Physician. 2010; 82:338–9.
17. Alt KW, Jeunesse C, Buitrago-Tellez CH, Wachter R, Boes E, Pichler SL. Evidence for stone age cranial surgery. Nature. 1997;387:360.
18. Mashour GA, Walker EE, Martuza RL. Psychosurgery: past, present, and future. Brain Res Brain Res Rev. 2005;48:409–19.
19. Damasio H, Grabowski T, Frank R, Galaburda AM, Damasio AR. The return of Phineas gage: clues about the brain from the skull of a famous patient. Science. 1994;264:1102–5.
20. Joanette Y, Stemmer B, Assal G, Whitaker H. From theory to practice: the unconventional contribution of Gottlieb Burckhardt to psychosurgery. Brain Lang. 1993;45:572–87.
21. Feldman RP, Goodrich JT. Psychosurgery: a historical overview. Neurosurgery 2001;48:647–57; discussion 649–57.
22. Kelly D, Mitchell-Heggs N. Stereotactic limbic leucotomy–a follow-up study of thirty patients. Postgrad Med J. 1973;49:865–82.
23. Jimenez-Ponce F, Soto-Abraham JE, Ramirez-Tapia Y, Velasco-Campos F, Carrillo-Ruiz JD, Gomez-Zenteno P. Evaluation of bilateral cingulotomy and anterior capsulotomy for the treatment of aggressive behavior. Cir Cir 2011;79:107–13.
24. da Costa DA. The role of psychosurgery in the treatment of selected cases of refractory schizophrenia: a reappraisal. Schizophr Res. 1997;28:223–30.
25. Goktepe EO, Young LB, Bridges PK. A further review of the results of stereotactic subcaudate tractotomy. Br J Psychiatry. 1975;126:270–80.

26. Vaernet K, Madsen A. Stereotaxic amygdalotomy and basofrontal tractotomy in psychotics with aggressive behaviour. J Neurol Neurosurg Psychiatry. 1970;33:858–63.
27. Sun B, Krahl SE, Zhan S, Shen J. Improved capsulotomy for refractory Tourette's syndrome. Stereotact Funct Neurosurg. 2005;83:55–6.
28. Ballantine HT Jr, Bouckoms AJ, Thomas EK, Giriunas IE. Treatment of psychiatric illness by stereotactic cingulotomy. Biol Psychiatry. 1987;22:807–19.
29. Dougherty DD, Baer L, Cosgrove GR, Cassem EH, Price BH, Nierenberg AA, Jenike MA, Rauch SL. Prospective long-term follow-up of 44 patients who received cingulotomy for treatment-refractory obsessive-compulsive disorder. Am J Psychiatry. 2002;159:269–75.
30. Freeman W. Frontal lobotomy in early schizophrenia. Long follow-up in 415 cases. Br J Psychiatry. 1971;119:621–4.
31. Dynes JB. Lobotomy–twenty years later. Va Med Mon. 1918;1968(95):306–8.
32. Miller BL, Cummings JL. The human frontal lobes: functions and disorders. New York: Guilford Press; 2007. p. 505–17.
33. Tooth GC, Newton MP. Leucotomy in England and Wales 1942–1954. Reports on Public Health and Medical Subjects, No 104 Ministry of Health, London, UK: 1961; Her Majesty's Stationery Office.
34. Leiphart JW, Valone FH III. Stereotactic lesions for the treatment of psychiatric disorders. J Neurosurg. 2010;113:1204–11.
35. Bridges PK, Bartlett JR, Hale AS, Poynton AM, Malizia AL, Hodgkiss AD. Psychosurgery: stereotactic subcaudate tractomy. An indispensable treatment. Br J Psychiatry. 1994;165:599–611; discussion 593–612.
36. Kiloh LG, Gye RS, Rushworth RG, Bell DS, White RT. Stereotactic amygdaloidotomy for aggressive behaviour. J Neurol Neurosurg Psychiatry. 1974;37:437–44.
37. Elias WJ, Cosgrove GR. Psychosurgery. Neurosurg Focus. 2008;25:E1.
38. Robison RA, Taghva A, Liu CY, Apuzzo ML. Surgery of the mind, mood, and conscious state: an idea in evolution. World Neurosurg. 2013;80:S2–26.
39. Miller A. The lobotomy patient—a decade later: a follow-up study of a research project started in 1948. Can Med Assoc J. 1967;96:1095–103.
40. Cosgrove GR, Rauch SL. Psychosurgery. Neurosurg Clin N Am. 1995;6:167–76.
41. Teuber JL, Corkin S, Twitchell TE. Study of cingulotomy in man: a summary. Neurosurgical

treatment in psychiatry, pain, and epilepsy. Baltimore: University Park Press; 1977.
42. Poynton AM, Kartsounis LD, Bridges PK. A prospective clinical study of stereotactic subcaudate tractotomy. Psychol Med. 1995;25:763–70.
43. Ramamurthi B. Thermocoagulation for stereotactic subcaudate tractotomy. Br J Neurosurg. 1999;13:219.
44. Dettling M, Anghelescu IG. Subthalamic nucleus stimulation in severe obsessive-compulsive disorder. N Engl J Med. 2009;360:931 (Author reply 932).
45. Kapoor S. Subthalamic nucleus stimulation in severe obsessive-compulsive disorder. N Engl J Med. 2009;360:931–2 (Author reply 932).
46. Mallet L, Polosan M, Jaafari N, Baup N, Welter ML, Fontaine D, du Montcel ST, Yelnik J, Chereau I, Arbus C, Raoul S, Aouizerate B, Damier P, Chabardes S, Czernecki V, Ardouin C, Krebs MO, Bardinet E, Chaynes P, Burbaud P, Cornu P, Derost P, Bougerol T, Bataille B, Mattei V, Dormont D, Devaux B, Verin M, Houeto JL, Pollak P, Benabid AL, Agid Y, Krack P, Millet B, Pelissolo A. Subthalamic nucleus stimulation in severe obsessive-compulsive disorder. N Engl J Med. 2008;359:2121–34.
47. Saleh C. Are the anterior internal capsules and nucleus accumbens suitable DBS targets for the treatment of depression? Prog Neuropsychopharmacol Biol Psychiatry. 2010;35:310 (Author reply 311).
48. Cusin C, Dougherty DD. Somatic therapies for treatment-resistant depression: ECT, TMS, VNS, DBS. Biol Mood Anxiety Disord. 2012;2:14.
49. Perez SM, Shah A, Asher A, Lodge DJ. Hippocampal deep brain stimulation reverses physiological and behavioural deficits in a rodent model of schizophrenia. Int J Neuropsychopharmacol. 2012; 16:1331–9.
50. Ewing SG, Grace AA. Deep brain stimulation of the ventral hippocampus restores deficits in processing of auditory evoked potentials in a rodent developmental disruption model of schizophrenia. Schizophr Res. 2013;143:377–83.
51. Ewing SG, Puri B, Pratt JA. Deep brain stimulation of the mediodorsal thalamic nucleus yields increases in the expression of zif-268 but not c-fos in the frontal cortex. J Chem Neuroanat. 2013;52:20–4.
52. Ewing SG, Grace AA. Long-term high frequency deep brain stimulation of the nucleus accumbens drives time-dependent changes in functional connectivity in the rodent limbic system. Brain Stimul. 2013;6:274–85.

Surgical Management for Aggressive Behavior

17

Wei Wang and Peng Li

The etiology of human aggressive behavior has not been elucidated. In clinical practice, the definition of aggressive behavior is as follows: attack to property, others, or oneself with the deliberate intention of destruction. Organic psychosis, schizophrenia, mental retardation, emotional disorders, and personality disorders can be associated with aggressive behavior, and most frequently occur in the acute phase of mental illness [1]. In 1990, a regional epidemiological investigation for violent psychosis in the United States showed that the incidence of aggressive behavior in patients with psychiatric disorders was five times that of normal people. Moreover, 50 % of the patients with psychiatric disorders and 10 % of patients with schizophrenia have histories of making threats, agitation, and aggressive behavior [2]. This aggressive behavior causes serious threat to the safety of medical staff, the whole society, and even to patients themselves.

A variety of drugs have been recommended for the treatment of aggressive behavior, including typical and atypical antipsychotic drugs such as benzodiazepines, mood stabilizing drugs, beta blockers, selective 5-HT re-uptake inhibitors, etc. These drugs have different effects on brain neurotransmitter systems. At present, the knowledge of the etiology of aggressive behavior is limited.

Several chemical compounds are supposed to have influence to the aggressive behavior such as 5-HT, dopamine, y-aminobutyric acid (GABA), norepinephrine and other neurotransmitters [1]. However, the detailed mechanism underlying aggressive behavior is still unclear. Current neurophysiological research on the management of large numbers of patients with schizophrenia accompanied by agitated and aggressive behaviors is limited. Although improvement of aggressive behaviors with medication can be observed, the efficacy is still not ideal in many cases. Thus, surgical management may be a possible choice for carefully selected patients.

From 1935 to 1937, Moniz and Lima first reported successful results of bilateral frontal lobe lobotomies for the treatment of mental disorders. The main purpose of the treatment was to improve impulse, violence, and difficultly controlled behaviors. Based on their results, they proposed the "psychosurgical method" for treating certain cases of mental disorders [3, 4]. In 1947, with the help of the stereotactic technique, the mediodorsal thalamotomy was successfully completed by Wycis and Spiegel to treat patients with serious mental disorders. This new surgical approach resulted in smaller regions of damage, which helped to reduce the side effects of surgery. Moreover, patient disabilities and the number of mortalities were significantly reduced. In recent years, along with the development of clinical psychiatry, neurophysiology, neuroanatomy, imaging techniques, and functional

W. Wang (✉) · P. Li
West China Hospital of Sichuan University,
Chengdu, China

B. Sun and A. De Salles (eds.), *Neurosurgical Treatments for Psychiatric Disorders*,
DOI 10.1007/978-94-017-9576-0_17
© Shanghai Jiao Tong University Press, Shanghai and Springer Science+Business Media Dordrecht 2015

neurosurgery, more attention has been paid to psychosurgery by clinicians [5].

Mental and behavioral disorders associated with aggressive behavior can be observed in patients with schizophrenia, schizoaffective disorder, mental retardation, personality disorders, and other psychiatric illnesses. For serious medically refractive patients with aggressive behavior, inclusion criterion for surgical management may be suggested as: (1) confirmed diagnosis by more than two psychiatrists, (2) at least 6 weeks of failed medication with more than three kinds of drugs with normalized psychological management that cannot relieve symptoms, (3) more than 5 years of disease history, (4) patients between 18 and 75 years old (for stereotactic surgery or radiosurgery treatment). However, for patients with severe mental retardation, considering the serious influence on daily life and with behavioral training being conducted soon after the operation, surgery can be carefully considered when the patient is more than 10 years old. (5) Behavior has seriously influenced the patient's ability to lead a normal life and does harm to the patient and his/her family members, (6) families and patients can accept the risk of operation, and can keep up subsequent treatment and long-term follow-up.

The following patients should be excluded from receiving psychosurgery: (1) patients whose age does not conform to the inclusion criteria, (2) those with disease duration of less than 5 years, (3) those with lack of normative medication, psychological treatment, and/or hospitalization, (4) patients with some accompanying bodily disease such as: infectious disease, metabolic disease, frailness, seriously high blood pressure, heart disease, and/or severe pathological brain disease, (5) patients whose psychosurgical targets have been damaged, (6) those with other bodily reason that impedes proper implementation of the surgery, (7) those refusing treatment (with the exception of mental disorder without self-knowledge), (8) lack of good family support, since postoperative follow-up would not be guaranteed and post-surgical management would be difficult, (9) conflicts with the law, ethics, politics, and/or religion [6, 7].

For patients that meet the standards of psychosurgery, psychiatrists and neurological surgeons should again carefully evaluate the condition of the patients before the operation. This should include assessments of a patient's diagnosis and previous drug and psychological behavior treatment, judgment of patient and family expectations, status of support and supervision, and whether the procedure would comply with the country's ethics and laws. Relevant preoperative examination, neural electrophysiological, image and psychological measurement are also important for preparation of the operation. Good cooperation between doctors, patients, and their families helps to have better disease improvement.

The theoretical basis of modern psychosurgery considers that human mental processes are extremely complex. Although the specific anatomical structure related to mental disorders is yet to be clarified, the limbic system and its connected structures are thought to have close relationship with a human's mental activities. The anatomy and theoretical basis of modern psychosurgery mainly concentrate on three circuits of the human limbic system: the internal and lateral circuits, and the defense reaction circuit. These structures have complex connections to the basal ganglia and frontal lobe, which are closely related to mental activities such as emotion and motivation [8].

(1) The internal circuit of the limbic system, which was first reported by Papez in 1937, begins at the septal area and passes through the cingulate gyrus to the hippocampus, via the mammillary body. It then runs again from the mammillary body-thalamus access to the anterior nucleus of the thalamus, and then back to the cingulate gyrus.

(2) The lateral circuit of the limbic system, which was first reported by Yakovlev in 1948, contains fiber tracts that originate in the orbitofrontal cortex, the insular lobe, frontal temporal lobe, and amygdala. These fiber tracts project to the mediodorsal thalamic nucleus, and then run back to the orbitofrontal cortex.

(3) The defense reaction circuit of the limbic system, which was reported by Kelly,

originates from the hypothalamus via the stria terminalis and runs from the septal area to the amygdala before returning to the hypothalamus [5].

Lesions to the structures of these three circuits and related structures may change brain neurotransmitters, thus achieving the purpose of improving and controlling psychiatric disorders. Operations can be completed under local or general anesthesia. Stereotactic radiofrequency thermocoagulation, stereotactic radiosurgery, and deep brain stimulation are the most popular surgical procedures used to treat psychiatric disorders.

Common surgical targets include the anterior limb of the internal capsule, amygdaloid nucleus, and medial septal area [8–10].

(1) The anterior limb of the internal capsule contains the efferent fiber tracts of the anterior nucleus of the thalamus and frontal lobe, the frontopontine tract, and the tracts between the orbitofrontal cortex and hypothalamus. Lesions to the anterior limb of the internal capsule aim to cut off the fiber tracts between the thalamus and the prefrontal cortex, which serve to partially interrupt communication between the nucleus medialis thalami and the frontal lobe. An anterior internal capsulotomy has been reported to be an effective treatment option for obsessive-compulsive disorder, anxiety, and phobia in selected patients.

(2) The amygdaloid nucleus, also known as the amygdala complex, receives afferent fibers from the olfactory bulb and anterior olfactory nucleus, via the lateral olfactory stria. The fibers from the piriform area and diencephalon end in the basolateral amygdaloid nucleus. In addition, the amygdaloid nucleus receives fibers from the hypothalamus, thalamus, brainstem reticular formation, and neocortex. The afferent fibers of the amygdaloid nucleus pass through the terminal stria and septal area, medial preoptic nucleus, anterior part of the hypothalamus, preoptic area, and the anterior commissure. Thus, a portion of the fibers end in the hypothalamus, dorsomedial nucleus of the thalamus,

and the midbrain reticular formation, while the other fibers end in the rein nuclear via the stria terminalis. The amygdaloid nucleus still has complex connection to the prefrontal cortex, cingulate gyrus, anterior part of the temporal lobe, and ventral insula. Thus, lesions to the amygdaloid nucleus result in behavior that is mild and calm, with lack of initiative and will. Obvious improvement has been reported following amygdalohippocampectomy for the treatment of mania, aggressive and destructive behavior, and impulsive mood.

(3) Medial septal area: The nucleus accumbens is located in the septal area, which is divided into interior and lateral part. The interior part is located anterior to the anterior commissure and the lateral part is located posterior to the anterior commissure. The nucleus accumbens is a key part of the Papez circuit and comprises the lateral circuit of the basal limbic system. It is considered by many researchers to be a "relay station" of the limbic system, and has close fiber connections with many structures such as the hypothalamus, mammillary bodies, cingulate gyrus, amygdala, and hippocampus. Lesions to the interior part of the nucleus accumbens have been used to treat behaviors associated with vandalism, associability tension, irritability, and other symptoms. The optimal targets for patients with psychiatric disorders associated with mania, impulsiveness, aggression, self-injury, compulsion, and destruction, are the amygdaloid nucleus, anterior limb of the internal capsule, and medial septal area. Additionally, for the above target behaviors, the nucleus accumbens, cingulate gyrus, and caudate nucleus can be targeted in select patients.

Multiple bilateral target lesions are commonly used during operation. According to the condition of the individual patient and the experience of the surgeons, optimal basic targets and additional targets can be used. Secondary operation could be considered to expand the lesion foci or add new targets if the first surgery has failed. However, a second operation should be conducted with caution if multiple bilateral targets were used during the first surgery. Usually, there should be at least a 6-month interval between two operations. For select patients, deep brain stimulation could be used as initial or supplemental treatment.

Psychological assessment at different treatment periods should be carried out. These periods include pre-operation, 1 week, 3 months, 6 months, 1 year, and 2 years after surgery. There are several psychological assessment tools that can be used to evaluate the condition of patients before and after surgery. Such tools include the BRMS, forced to scale, WIS, WMS, BPRS, SCL-90, SDS and SAS, WAIS, WMS, GAS, MMPI, PAN, SS, SDSS-r, quality of life scale, tic disorders scale, adult intellectually evaluation form or simple intelligence assessment, sexual function and menstrual scale, etc. Psychiatric diagnosis and assessment should be independently carried out by a psychiatrist with the help of the above assessment tools. In addition, cognitive and brain function examination are suggested according to the conditions of the hospital [7].

Postoperative medication, rehabilitation, and follow-ups by psychiatrists and neurosurgeons are important. Guidance after discharge should be drawn up by physicians together with the patients' family members. Patients are suggested to have monthly follow-ups during the first 3 months after discharge. After that, continuous follow-up with an interval of 3–6 months is recommended.

We recommend a five level scale to evaluate the efficacy of treatment. Level I (restoration): characterized by a complete resolution of symptoms, normal psychiatric function, successful adaptation to daily life, no need of additional treatment, and a reduction in clinical scale score of more than 95 %. Level II (remarkable improvement): characterized by almost a complete resolution of symptoms, nearly normal function, adaptation to life without any treatment, and a reduction in clinical scale score of more than 70 %. Level III (partial improvement): characterized by partial symptom improvement, psychiatric function defects, some difficulty in adapting to daily life or reaching to a

standard level of II under large amounts of drug treatment, and a reduction in clinical scale score of more than 20 %. Level IV (no effect): no change in clinical symptoms, reduction in clinical scale score of less than 20 %. Level V (exacerbation): the clinical symptoms are aggravated, and there is an increase in clinical scale score of >10 %. Levels I, II, and III can be regarded as effective, while levels IV and V indicate treatment failure [7].

The most frequent complications of psychosurgery include incontinence, fever, silence, sleep, memory disorders, weight change, cognitive disorders, personality disorders, eroticism, fumbling, and suicide. Complications related with the neurological surgery itself include intracranial hematoma, pneumocrania, hemiplegia, infections, etc.

In 1990, Zheng Chun Ma reported the successful treatment of 17 out of 25 patients with schizophrenia who were accompanied by aggressive behavior. These patients had undergone stereotactic bilateral cingulotomy and amygdalotomy [11]. In 2004, 39 patients with schizophrenia and behavior disorder underwent surgical treatment by Ping Li, and the effective rate was reported to be 89.7 %. In 2008, Qingfen Wu reported a cohort of 16 surgically treated patients of mental retardation with aggressive behavior. All patients underwent cingulotomy and additional lesions of two or more targets, including the amygdala, interior part of the accumbens, anterior limb of the internal capsule, mediodorsal thalamic nucleus, and caudate nucleus. Obvious effects were reported in 14 out of 16 patients in this study [12]. In 2012, Fiacro Jimenez treated 10 patients with aggressive behavior by bilateral capsulotomy and cingulotomy. Their OAS and GAF scores decreased significantly after the procedure at the 6-month and 4-year follow-ups. Moreover, four patients showed mild and transitory postsurgical complications (hyperphagia and somnolence) [13, 14]. The studies that have been reported since 2000 are listed in Table 17.1.

A 16-year-old girl with mental retardation and symptoms of self-mutilation underwent bilateral capsulotomy and amygdalotomy. Her symptoms of aggressive behavior improved significantly.

Table 17.1 Studies in recent years

Year	Authors	Number of cases	Follow-up time	Treatment approach	Improved cases
2012 [13]	Fiacro Jiménez	10	4 years	Bilateral capsulotomy and cingulotomy	–
2008 [15]	Kim MC	2	8 years	Bilateral amygdalotomy and subcaudate tractotomy	1
2007 [16]	Fountas KN	1	–	Bilateral amygdalotomy	1
2005 [17]	Franzini A	2	1 year	Posterior hypothalamus stimulation	2
2001 [18]	Price BH	5	31.5 months	Limbic leucotomy	4
2009 [19]	Yang KJ	1	–	Bilateral nucleus accumbens lesion	1
2007 [20]	Wang Lianzhong	3	–	Bilateral capsulotomy, cingulotomy, and amygdalotomy	3
2008 [12]	Wu Qingfen	16	18 months	Bilateral capsulotomy, cingulotomy amygdalotomy, nucleus accumbens lesion, and subcaudate tractotomy	14

The follow-up magnetic resonance (MR) images are shown in Figs. 17.1, 17.2, 17.3, 17.4, 17.5, 17.6 and 17.7.

Based on the limited results of previous studies, psychosurgery for patients with positive clinical psychiatric symptoms such as aggressive behavior could not only effectively alleviate a patient's symptoms, but could also facilitate post-surgical behavioral therapy. On the other hand, effective surgical procedures could prevent patients from doing harm to themselves and others.

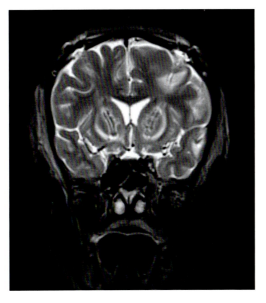

Fig. 17.1 Coronal MR image 1 week after bilateral capsulotomy

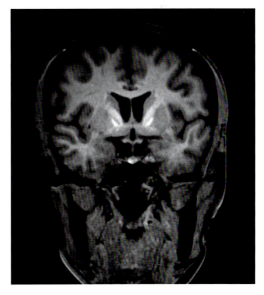

Fig. 17.2 Coronal MR image 3 months after bilateral capsulotomy

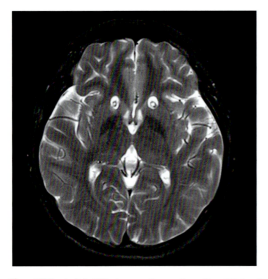

Fig. 17.3 Axial MR image 3 months after bilateral capsulotomy

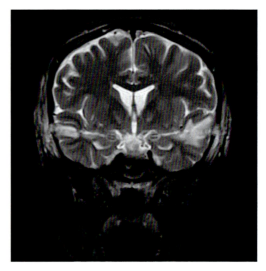

Fig. 17.5 Coronal MR image 1 week after bilateral amygdalotomy

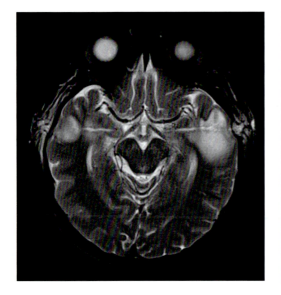

Fig. 17.4 Axial MR image 1 week after bilateral amygdalotomy

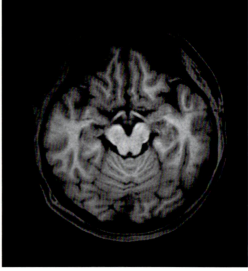

Fig. 17.6 Axial MR image 3 months after bilateral amygdalotomy

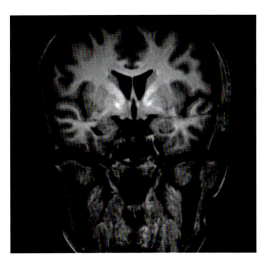

Fig. 17.7 Coronal MR image 3 months after bilateral amygdalotomy

References

1. Campbell M, Gonzalez NM, Silva RR. The pharmacologic treatment of conduct disorders and rage outbursts. Psychiatr Clin North Am. 1992;15(1):69–85.
2. Sramka M, Pogady P, Csolova Z, et al. Long-term results in patients with stereotaxic surgery for psychopathologic disorders. Bratisl Lek Listy. 1992;93(7):365–6.
3. Kopell BH, Rezai AR. Psychiatric neurosurgery: a historical perspective. Neurosurg Clin N Am. 2003;14(2):181–97.
4. Diering SL, Bell WO. Functional neurosurgery for psychiatric disorder: a historical persoective. Stereotact Funct Neurosurg. 1991;57(4):175–99.
5. Fedlman RP, Alterman RL, Goodrich JT. Contemporary psychosurgery and a look to the future. J Neurosurg. 2001;95(6):944–56.
6. Li P, Fu X, Wang Y. Targets, mechanism, efficacy and future expectation of stereotactic psychosurgery. Chin J Stereotact Funct Neurosurg. 2007;20(5):313–7.
7. Neurosurgery Branch of Chinese Medical Doctor Association. Clinical guidelines of psychosurgery. Chin J Nerv Psychiatr Dis. 2009;35(8):449–50.
8. Byrum J, Ahearn EP, Krishnan KR. A neuroanatomic model for depression. Prog Neuropsychopharmacol Biol Psychiatry. 1999;23:175–93.
9. Modell JC, Mountz JM, Curtis GC, et al. Neurophysiologic dysfunction in basal ganglia/limbic striatal and thalamocortical circuits as a pathogenetic mechanism of obsessive compulsive disorder. Clin Neurosic. 1989;1(1):27–9.
10. Li J, Wang X. The role of different intracranial structures in stereotactic surgery. Chin J Stereotact Funct Neurosurg. 2009;22(1):55–7.
11. Ma Z, Dou Y, Sun Y, et al. Preliminary observation of 25 patients with schizophrenia treated by stereotactic surgery. Chin J Stereotact Funct Neurosurg. 2004;17(6):321–4.
12. Wu Q, Liu C, Zhang W. Multi-target treatment of mental retardation by stereotactic techniques-a study of 16 cases. J Xinjiang Med Univ. 2008;31(11):1578–9.
13. Jiménez F, Soto JE, Velasco F. Bilateral cingulotomy and anterior capsulotomy applied to patients with aggressiveness. Stereotact Funct Neurosurg. 2012;90:151–60.
14. Jimenez-Ponce F, Soto-Abraham JE, Ramirez-Tapia Y, Velasco-Campos F, Carrillo-Ruiz JD, Gomez-Zenteno P. Evaluation of bilateral cingulotomy and anterior capsulotomy for the treatment of aggressive behavior. Cir Cir. 2011;79(2):107–13.
15. Kim MC, Lee TK. Stereotactic lesioning for mental illness. Acta Neurochir Suppl. 2008;101:39–43.
16. Fountas KN, Smith JR, Lee GP. Bilateral stereotactic amygdalotomy for self-mutilation disorder. Case report and review of the literature. Stereotact Funct Neurosurg. 2007;85:121–8.
17. Franzini A, Marras C, Ferroli P, Bugiani O, Broggi G. Stimulation of the posterior hypothalamus for medically intractable impulsive and violent behavior. Stereotact Funct Neurosurg. 2005;83:63–6.
18. Price BH, Baral I, Cosgrove GR, Rauch SL, Nierenberg AA, Jenike MA, Cassem EH. Improvement in severe self-mutilation following limbic leucotomy: a series of 5 consecutive cases. J Clin Psychiatry. 2001;62(12):925–32.
19. Kaijun Y, Songtao Q, Kewan W, et al. Operative technique and electrophysiologic monitoring of stereotactic accumbensotomy. Chin J Stereotact Funct Neurosurg. 2009;22(3):129–33.
20. Wang LZ, Yin ZM, Wen H, Jiang XL, Wang L. Stereotactic multi-target operation for patients with affective disorder. Chin J Surg. 2007;45(24):1676–8.

Deep Brain Stimulation in Aggressive Behavior

18

Giuseppe Messina, Giovanni Broggi, Roberto Cordella and Angelo Franzini

18.1 Introduction

Deep-brain stimulation (DBS) of the posterior hypothalamic region was originally introduced to treat trigeminal autonomic cephalalgias (TACs), which are thought to result from hyper-activation of the posterior hypothalamic region (pHr) occurring during bouts pain bouts in these pathologies [4, 10]. In fact, patients experiencing chronic luster headache attacks often exhibit aggressive bouts during such episodes [19]. In the past, the posterior hypothalamic region (pHr) was used as a lesional target in patients with aggressive behavior, epilepsy and, mental retardation [1, 2, 12–17]. Furthermore, disruptive behavior was found to be induced by acute electrical stimulation within the so-called "triangle of Sano" in a Parkinsonian patient [2]. The known interconnections between the pHr, the amygdala, and the overall so called "Papez circuit" [18] may explain the role of the pHr in the development of disruptive behavior. The choice of targeting the pHr for this pathology is determined by the crucial role of pHr within the limbic circuits, which appear to be dysregulated according to several clinic and experimental data

[5, 9, 13–16]. We chose to use DBS to severely impaired patients affected by refractory aggressive behavior and mental retardation. The first surgery was performed in 2002 [5]. We here describe our technique and long-term follow-up in seven patients.

18.2 Methods

Since 2002, we have administered DBS of the pHyp region to seven patients (ages 20–68 years; one female) affected by refractory aggressive behavior. The lack of cooperation from all patients, which was attributable to the severity of both the disruptive behavior and of the most prominent comorbid condition (mental retardation) prevented us from performing specific neuropsychologic assessments; the only evaluation scales we used were IQ and the Overt Aggression Scale. These scores are summarized in Table 18.1. All patients were of below average IQ. Two patients had refractory generalized multifocal epilepsy. The pathologic conditions associated with their disruptive behavior were: (1) posttraumatic bilateral damage of the temporomesial structures in one case; (2) congenital (unknown origin) in four cases; (3) congenital toxoplasmosis (the findings of magnetic resonance imaging [MRI] of the brain were normal in these patients); and (4) brain ischemia attributable to cardiac arrest in one case (findings from MRI demonstrated only diffuse damage of frontal cortex).

G. Messina (✉) · R. Cordella · A. Franzini
Functional Neurosurgical Unit, Fondazione IRCCS
Istituto Neurologico "Carlo Besta", Milan, Italy
e-mail: ghroggi@gmail.com

G. Broggi
Neurosurgical Division, Functional Neurosurgery
Unit, Istituto Galeazzi IRCCS, Milan, Italy

Table 18.1 General patient data, with a comparison between preoperative and postoperative OAS scores

Patient	1	2	3	4	5	6	7
Age at surgery, years	26	34	21	64	37	20	43
Etiology	Idiopathic	Perinatal toxoplasmosis	Idiopathic	Post-anoxia	Post-traumatic	Idiopathic	Idiopathic
Previous treatments	Chlorpromazine, Thoiridazine, Clotiapine, Carbamazepine, Clonazepam, Valproate	Chlorpromazine Quetiapine	Chlorpromazine Clotiapine Bromazepam Haloperidol	Promazine Clonazepam	Clonazepam Diazepam Promazine Haloperidol	Promazine Chlorpromazine Clonazepam	Promazine Lorazepam Haloperodol
Bran MRI	Normal	Normal	Normal	Bilateral frontal cortical atrophy	Bilateral temporal poroencephaly	Normal	Normal
IQ	20	20	40	30	20	30	20
Pre-op DAS	10	8	10	9	8	10	10
Post-op DAS	1	3	3	9	3	0	4
Follow-up, years	10	9	6	5	5	4	2

The Ethical Committee of our institution approved the surgical procedure in all of the patients, taking into account the chronicity and severity of the condition, the related burden to families, and the refractoriness to conservative treatments. The relatives of all of the patients provided their written consent after a detailed explanation of its hypothetical rationale and of the surgical risks was given. The stereotactic implantation was performed with the Leksell frame (Eleckta, Stockholm, Sweden) under general anesthesia in all patients. Preoperative antibiotics were administrated to all patients. A preoperative MRI (brain axial volumetric fast spin echo inversion recovery and T2 images) was used to obtain high-definition images for the precise determination of both anterior and posterior commissures and midbrain structures below the commissural plane, such as the mammillary bodies and the red nucleus. MRIs were fused with 2-mm thick computed tomography (CT) slices that were obtained under stereotactic conditions by the use of an automated technique that is based on a mutual-information algorithm (Frame-link 4.0, Sofamor Danek Steathstation; Medtronic, Minneapolis, Minnesota, USA).

The workstation also provided stereotactic coordinates of the target: 3 mm behind the mid-commissural point, 5 mm below this point, and 2 mm lateral from the midline.

A possible error in this intervention could be attributable to the anatomical individual variability of the angle between the brainstem and the commissural plane. To correct this possible error, we introduced a third anatomical landmark, which allowed final target registration. We called this landmark the "interpeduncular nucleus" or "interpeduncular point," and it is placed in the apex of the interpeduncular cistern 8 mm below the commissural plane at the level of the maximum diameter of the mammillary bodies [6]. The Y value of the definitive target (anteroposterior coordinate to the mid-commissural point in the classical mid-commissural reference system) was corrected in our patients, and the definitive target coordinate was chosen 2 mm posterior to the interpeduncular point instead of 3 mm posterior to the mid-commissural point. A dedicated program

and atlas has been developed and is freely available on the internet to get the proper coordinates of the target (www.angelofranzini.com/BRAIN.htm).

During the surgical session, all patients received general anesthesia. Target control infusion was used. This method of intravenous infusion of anesthetic drugs has been studied for its ability to achieve targeted blood or effect-site concentration for selected drugs. Maintaining a constant plasma or effect compartment concentration of an intravenous anesthetic requires continuous adjustment of the infusion rate according to the pharmacokinetic properties of the drugs, which can be achieved by commercially available target controlled infusion pumps (in our study, we used Injectomat Agilia, Fresenius Kabi, France).

A rigid cannula was inserted through a 3-mm, coronal, paramedian twist-drill hole and placed up to 10 mm from the target. This cannula was used as both a guide for microrecording and for the placement of the definitive electrode (Quad 3389; Medtronic).

As far as microrecording is concerned, in two patients spontaneous neuronal activity was recorded along four trajectories (two in each patient). Along the trajectories, it was possible to identify several types of firing discharge rates and patterns. Of the several recorded neurons, a total of 14 cells located within the posterior hypothalamus were further analyzed. None showed either activation or inhibition after tactile and pinprick stimulation. The average firing rate for these cells was 13 Hz, although nine cells (64 %) showed a low-frequency discharge at around 5 Hz, and the remaining five cells (36 %) discharged at greater frequencies (26 Hz). Several firing patterns have been noticed: four cells exhibited tonic regular discharge, four cells exhibited tonic irregular discharge, four exhibited a bursting discharge, and two had a sporadic firing. Periodicity was described in five units (four bursting and one regular), but the remaining one randomly fired [3]. Microrecordings within the pHyp were performed within 2 mm of the stereotactic coordinates (specifically, as stated previously, 2 mm lateral to the commissural line, 3 mm posterior to the mid-commissural point, and 5 mm below the commissural line).

It is important to note that there is no clear evidence of the neurophysiologic characteristics of either the superior or inferior borders of the nucleus. However, the presence of greater firing rates more than 5 mm from the target may suggest that the microelectrode is passing through the thalamus, whereas the lack of neuronal activity at the target site and beyond may indicate that the microelectrode is not in the pHyp but in adjacent structures (that is, the interpeduncular cistern at the inferior border).

No vegetative responses or cardiovascular effects were elicited by intraoperative macrostimulation at therapeutic parameters (185 Hz, 80 µs, from 1 to 3 V). At increasing charge density above this level, internal gaze deviation was observed in all cases. When side effects were ruled out at the standard parameters of stimulation, the guiding cannula was removed and the electrode secured to the skull with microplates.

Postoperative stereotactic CT was performed to assess the positioning of the electrode and rule out complications (Fig. 18.1).

A bilateral implantable pulse generator (IPG; Soletra; Medtronic.) was placed in the subclavicular pocket and connected to the brain electrode for chronic electrical stimulation.

The parameters of chronically delivered electrical currents were 185 Hz, 60–90 µs, and 1–3 V in unipolar configuration with case positive. The current amplitude was progressively increased until the impairment of ocular movements, as side effect, was reached in all cases.

18.3 Results

Follow-up cases ranged from 1 to 9 years of age. Case 1's self-aggression promptly stopped, and bursts of uncontrolled violence became less frequent, disappearing completely within 3 weeks. The patient returned to family and began to attend a therapeutic community for mentally impaired patients. Generalized epileptic seizures disappeared, and partial seizures and absences were reduced 50 %. Antiepileptic drug therapy was continually checked and was reduced to 30 %.

Case 2 had an immediate disappearance of violence bursts and was discharged from the institution where he had been hospitalized for a long time. Forced bed contention was withdrawn, and he was charged to a therapeutic community for mentally disabled patients. Three years later, after the IPG was temporary turned off for knee surgery, the patient's violent behavior relapsed, and when the chronic stimulation was restored, the therapeutic effect resulted considerably reduced despite the increase in current amplitude, which could not be set greater than 2 V because of the appearance of side effects. The psychiatrists who had the patient in their charge suggested a possible evolution of the original disease to explain the loss of the therapeutic effect.

With the IPG turned on, the burst of violence are still less frequent and less intense than in the absence of stimulation. And duration of the violence attacks only when the amplitude of stimulation was set to 1.8 V few months after surgery. This patient is still quiet, and her social activities have improved consistently. Now she is able to attend a psychiatric rehabilitation center and her family integration is good. Violence bursts may appear only if the patient is provoked by adverse events.

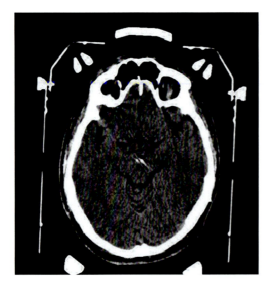

Fig. 18.1 Postoperative computed tomography scan showing the electrode tips at the level of the posterior hypothalamic region, bilaterally

18.4 Discussion

Case 4 had only an improvement in sleep habits (before surgery, he slept only 2 h per night, and after surgery he sleep more than 6 h per night). His behavior was not affected by the stimulation despite the electrical current increased to 2 V' amplitude.

Two years after surgery, the stimulator was turned off but the improvement of sleep was not reverted to the preoperative condition, and at 3 years follow-up, the patient still sleeps more than 6 h per night. The same patient had a stable decrease of arterial pressure, and all antihypertensive drugs could be withdrawn; this effect is still persists despite the IPG being turned off.

Case 5 had a prompt, marked improvement of aggressive behavior, and care by the family became consistently easier. The therapeutic effect persisted at 1-year follow-up, but when both IPGs were turned off, the violent behavior reappeared within a few hours. The left IPG had been removed because of skin erosion (but has been subsequently reimplanted) and the therapeutic effects seemed to be sustained only by the right-side stimulation of the pHyp; the reimplantation of the left IPG anyway led to further reduction of the frequency of violent outbursts.

At 1-year follow-up, in case 6 the rate of epileptic seizures decreased to 50 % of the pre-operative condition just during the early post-operative weeks. In this patient the insertion of the second electrode at the target was immediately followed by the disappearance of interictal epileptic activity from the scalp electroencephalogram (EEG) [7]. During this intervention, infusion of a constant concentration of propofol was maintained, thus excluding the role of intraoperative anesthetics in the change in EEG activity. Anyway, no postoperative EEG was performed for this patient. The aggressive behavior has completely disappeared.

Case 7 had prompt disappearance of overall disruptive behavior; aggressive bouts now occur only episodically (about once every 2 months), but their duration and intensity is remarkably reduced (from about 9–10 episodes per day to 2–3 episodes per month). This improvement is present at the last follow-up, conducted 2 years after the intervention.

18.4 Discussion

This series shows that patients affected by mental retardation in whom violent and aggressive behavior is associated could consistently benefit from high-frequency stimulation of the pHyp. No patient worsened after surgery, and no patient developed new neurologic symptoms in our series. The patients affected by drug-refractory epileptic syndromes also showed a marked decrease of frequency of epileptic episodes, and in both cases the pharmacologic therapy was consistently reduced. This observation was reported also by Espinosa et al., who used high-frequency stimulation to the pHyp to treat a patient with aggressive behavior and epileptic seizures (personal communication and poster presentation at the meeting of the American Society for Stereotactic and Functional Neurosurgery held in Boston, June 2006). Experimental data are also available on this topic [11].

Besides our series, two other cases treated with posterior hypothalamic DBS have been reported in the literature; Hernando et al. [8] reported the case of a 22-year-old patient with drug-resistant aggression and comorbid mental retardation who presented a significant improvement at a 18 months' follow-up; low-frequency stimulation was used in this case. Kuhn et al. [9] reported the case of a 22-year-old woman with self-mutilating behavior after severe traumatic brain injury. This patient experienced a resolution of symptoms 4 months after beginning DBS.

18.5 Conclusions

In conclusion, the reversibility and the positive effects of pHyp chronic stimulation make this procedure ethically acceptable in mentally retarded patients with violent aggressive behavior. Our knowledge about the mechanisms that underlie pathologic aggressive and impulsive behavior is still incomplete; nonetheless, it has become clear from previous experimental studies that some specific structures play a role in the pathogenetic mechanism. Our group in the first article published on this topic [5] pointed out the role played by structures connected to the posterior hypothalamus (amygdala, dorsomedial thalamus, and orbito-frontal cortex) through loops reverberating within the limbic circuit; in 1988 Sano and Mayanagi [14] hypothesized the causative role of an imbalance between the "ergotropic" and the "trophotropic" circuits in favor of the former, thus justifying the use of a lesion in the "ergotropic" posterior hypothalamus to treat these patients. Kuhn et al. [9] also considered the role of zona incerta cells and their connections with the thalamus, superior colliculus, and pontomesencephalic tegmentum in the regulation of mood and circadian rhythms, given the proximity of this structure to the posterior hypothalamic area.

The possible adjunctive benefits of stimulation may include the control of refractory epilepsy, which sometimes is associated with these complex syndromes. At any rate, the reported methodology is the only neuromodulation procedure available to treat disruptive and aggressive behavior, and it is still the only alternative to classical lesional surgery; furthermore, it should be emphasized that DBS is a reversible treatment that may help patients chronically isolated in mental institutions to be integrate into society.

References

1. Arjona VE. Stereotactic hypothalamotomy in heretic children. Acta Neurochir. 1974;21(Suppl):185–91.
2. Bejjani BP, Houeto JL, Hariz M, Yelnik J, Mesnage V, Bonnet AM, Pidoux B, Dormont D, Cornu P, Agid Y. Aggressive behavior induced by intraoperative stimulation in the triangle of Sano. Neurology. 2002; 12(59):1425–7.
3. Cordella R, Carella F, Leone M, Franzini A, Broggi G, Bussone G, Albanese A. Spontaneous neuronal activity of the posterior hypothalamus in trigeminal autonomic cephalalgias. Neurol Sci. 2007;28:93–5.
4. Franzini A, Ferroli P, Leone M, Broggi G. Stimulation of the posterior hypothalamus for treatment of chronic intractable cluster headaches: first reported series. Neurosurgery. 2003;52:1095–9.
5. Franzini A, Marras C, Ferroli P, Bugiani O, Broggi G. Stimulation of the posterior hypothalamus for

medically intractable impulsive and violent behavior. Stereotact Funct Neurosurg. 2005;83:63–6.
6. Franzini A, Marras C, Tringali G, Leone M, Ferroli P, Bussone G, Bugiani O, Broggi G. Chronic high frequency stimulation of the posteromedial hypothalamus in facial pain syndromes and behaviour disorders. Acta Neurochir. 2007;97(Suppl):399–406.
7. Franzini A, Messina G, Marras C, Villani F, Cordella R, Broggi G. Deep brain stimulation of two unconventional targets in refractory non-resectable epilepsy. Stereotact Funct Neurosurg. 2008;86:373–81.
8. Hernando V, Pastor J, Pedrosa M, Peña E, Sola RG. Low-frequency bilateral hypothalamic stimulation for treatment of drug-resistant aggressiveness in a young man with mental retardation. Stereotact Funct Neurosurg. 2008;86:219–23.
9. Kuhn J, Lenartz D, Mai JK, Huff W, Klosterkoetter J, Sturm V. Disappearance of self-aggressive behavior in a brain-injured patient after deep brain stimulation of the hypothalamus: technical case report. Neurosurgery. 2008;62:E1182.
10. May A, Bahra A, Büchel C, Frackowiak RS, Goadsby PJ. Hypothalamic activation in cluster headache attacks. Lancet. 1998;352:275–8.
11. Nishida N, Huang Z-L, Mikuni N, Miura Y, Urade Y, Hashimoto N. Deep brain stimulation of the posterior hypothalamus activates the histaminergic system to exert antiepileptic effect in rat pentylenetetrazol model. Exp Neurol. 2007;205:132–44.
12. Ramamurthy B. Stereotactic operation in behaviour disorders. Amygdalotomy and hypothalamotomy. Acta Neurochir. 1988;44(Suppl):152–7 (Wien).
13. Sano K. Sedative neurosurgery. Neurol Medicochirurgica. 1962;4:224b–5b.
14. Sano K, Mayanagi Y. Posteromedial hypothalamotomy in the treatment of violent, aggressive behaviour. Acta Neurochir. 1988;44(Suppl):145–51 (Wien).
15. Sano K, Yoshioka M, Ogashiwa M. Stimulation and destruction of the hypothalamus. Neurol Medicochirurgica. 1963;5:169–70.
16. Sano K, Yoshioka M, Ogashiwa M, Ishijima B, Ohye C. Upon stimulation of human hypothalamus. Neurol Med Chir. 1965;7:280.
17. Schvarcz JR, Driollet R, Rios E, Betti O. Stereotactic hypothalamotomy for behaviour disorders. J Neurol Neurosurg Psychiatry. 1972;35:356–9.
18. Tarnecki R, Mempel E, Fonberg E, Lagowska J. Some electrophysiological characteristics of the spontaneous activity of the amygdala and effect of hypothalamic stimulation on the amygdalar units responses. Acta Neurochir. 1976;23(Suppl):135–40.
19. Torelli P, Manzoni GC. Pain and behaviour in cluster headache. A prospective study and review of the literature. Funct Neurol. 2003;18:205–10.

Radiosurgery for Psychiatric Disorders 19

Antônio De Salles and Alessandra A. Gorgulho

19.1 Introduction

Behavioral surgery, previously know as Psychosurgery initiated with lesions disconnecting pathways in the brain. The infamous Frontal Lobotomy proposed by Moniz [1], designed to interrupt the pathways of the frontal lobes evolved to more elegant disconnections with the use of the stereotactic technique by Spiegel and Wicys interrupting the thalamo-connections to the frontal lobe through lesions the anterior thalamus. Indeed, the collaboration of the Austrian Neurologist Spiegel with the Neurosurgeon Wicys in Philadelphia led to the first stereotactic surgery in humans. It was an anterior thalamotomy to modify behavior [2]. The progressive refinement of the understanding of the frontal lobe, know them to control behavior, called for precise lesions in strategic areas, instead of the massive initial lesions in the frontal lobe. Dr. Leksell from Karolinska University in Stockholm, living that era envisioned the necessity of a non invasive way to treat functional diseases of the brain, i.e. realizing precise lesions in specific brain pathways without opening the skull to avoid the unacceptable complications, as psychiatric patients were then being brutally violated by the trans orbital frontal lobectomy [3]. The ideas of radiosurgery matured during the 1950s and 1960s to culminate with the development of the Gamma Knife which was suitable and promptly applied to treat psychiatric diseases, the one chosen then was obsessive-compulsive disorder (OCD) [4].

The evolution of radiosurgery initiated with the idea to focus external beam radiation to concentrate dose to the pathology and spare the peripheral structures appeared in the literature in 1906. It was described by Kohl only 18 years after the discovery of X-rays. During the following years focus radiation progressed with spiral converging beams, pendulum beams and finally rigid hemispheric attached beam directed with stereotactic precision [5]. Leksell attached an X-ray tube to his stereotactic frame and delivered radiosurgery to the first patient submitted to the technique. The trigeminal ganglion was the target for treatment of trigeminal neuralgia. The term "radiosurgery" was coined [6]. This was actually the first application of photon radiosurgery. Radiosurgery was used to make thalamic lesions for cancer pain control, giving the first autopsy generated appearance of the lesions in the gray matter of humans as reported in 1955 [7]. Already in 1983, 26 patients had been submitted to radiosurgery for treatment of malignant obsessive-compulsive disorders (OCD) [4]. In 1985, Dr. Leksell et al. reported for

A. De Salles (✉) · A.A. Gorgulho
Department of Neurosurgery and Department of Radiation Oncology, David Geffen School of Medicine, University of California, 10495 Le Conte Ave, Suite 2120, Los Angeles, CA 90095, USA
e-mail: adesalles@mednet.ucla.edu; afdesalles@yahoo.com

A. De Salles · A.A. Gorgulho
HCor Neuroscience, Sao Paulo, Brazil

B. Sun and A. De Salles (eds.), *Neurosurgical Treatments for Psychiatric Disorders*, DOI 10.1007/978-94-017-9576-0_19
© Shanghai Jiao Tong University Press, Shanghai and Springer Science+Business Media Dordrecht 2015

the first time the appearance of lesions in the internal capsule within 1 month and within 24 hours after gamma capsulotomy (Fig. 19.1). In this report, the right side lesion, the 1 month old lesion was caused by 100 Gy, while the left side, 24 hours old lesion was caused by 120 Gy. At the time, the lesions appeared the same size, although fainter at 24 h, and the patient's symptoms were still unchanged [8]. In 1987, Mindus et al. [9] studied in details the gamma thalamotomy lesions in 6 patients, trying to obtain an uniform response to radiosurgery in the internal capsule.

Since the initial efforts of Radiosurgery, functional diseases and specifically for Psychiatry Neurosurgery became important focus of the technique. This occurred until the development of computerized image capable to demonstrate the morphological targets, i.e. tumors and the remarkable response of arteriovenous malformations to single dose of radiation took the attention of the Neurosurgeons interested in the technique. Radiosurgery evolved during the last 20 years of the last century linked to the explosion of the imaging techniques [10]. While dependent on ventriculography, cysternography and angiography until the late 1970s and early 1980s the applications of radiosurgery were largely limited to the pathologies visualized by these techniques. Behavioral surgery applications, as the other functional applications of radiosurgery, were based on principles of functional neurosurgery localization, for example using the anterior commissure (AC) and posterior commissure (PC) seen by ventriculography to guide targeting. Meckel's cave contrast material injection and cysternography provided visualization of targets such as the trigeminal ganglion in the Mekel's cave and the acoustic neuroma's prominence in the cerebellopontine angle, previously not seen in plain skull radiographs also became focus of the enthusiasts of radiosurgery [11, 12].

19.2 The Inception of the Gamma Knife

Dr. Leksell needing a device capable to treat large number of patients, precise and amenable to the hospital setting recurred to the principle of the cobalt units, then widely used in radiotherapy, to devise the first commercially available, dedicated radiosurgery device. In 1968, Leksell and Larsson developed the first Gamma Knife Unit in Sweden. Larsson was a medical physicist dedicated to develop Gamma Knife and to treat patients with this technique for many decades. The unit was housed in a private setting at the Queen Sophia Hospital (Sophiahemmet) in Stockholm; in 1982 this Unit was transferred to the University of California Los Angeles, being the first Gamma Knife in the USA. This unit was used to treat the first Psychiatric patient with Radiosurgery [8].

The remarkable results obtained with the Gamma Unit treatment of AVMs, starting in 1972 impressed the neurosurgical community, realizing the potential of the technique as a solution for treatment of these formidable lesions. Angiography provided the visualization of arteriovenous malformations (AVMs), making them the classic application of radiosurgery [13].

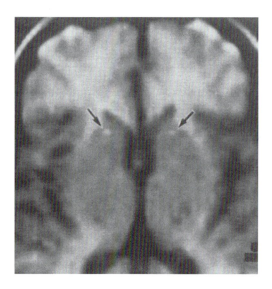

Fig. 19.1 Appearance of lesions in the internal capsule within 1 month and within 24 h after gamma capsulotomy. *Right side lesion*, 1 month old lesion was caused by 100 Gy, while the *left side*, 24 h old lesion was caused by 120 Gy. At the time, the lesions appeared the same size, although fainter at 24 h, and the patient's symptoms were still unchanged [8]

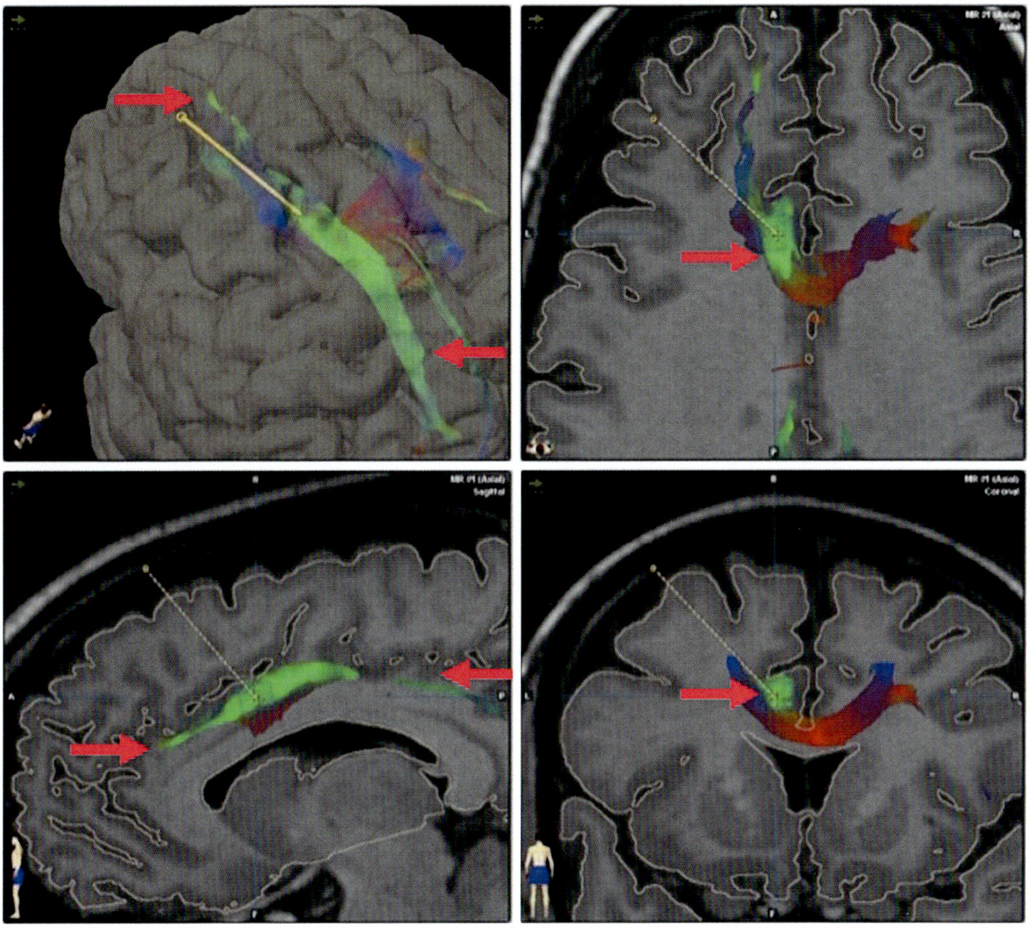

Fig. 19.2 Cingulotomy target sampled with fiber tracking showing spread of fibers mostly to the pre-frontal cortex, high in the frontal lobe **a** 3D rendering and **b** axial MRI representation of the cingulate fasciculus spread to the mid-frontal gyrus cortex. Mostly to towards the prefrontal cortex. **c** Demonstrates the fibers spreading medially in the frontal lobe. **d** Demonstrates precise location of the sampling in the cingulotomy target

Psychosurgery during this period, on the other hand, became highly controlled in the majority of the countries across the world, thanks to the abuse of the trans orbital frontal lobectomy [3]. Therefore losing the center of attention of Neurosurgeons and, specifically of Radiosurgeons that saw in the technique the possibility of treating diseases of easy management and acceptable indications such as AVMs and brain tumors [14]. The technique initially restricted to few institutions and having to provide care for large numbers of patients with structural disease, was not applied in large scale for Psychiatric disorders. Few institutions in the world continue with the work in Psychosurgery, mostly in Spain, USA and Sweden. Careful comparison of radiosurgery with radiofrequency lesions in the brain were carried out at Karolinska, where the main disease treated was OCD with the anterior limb of the internal capsule, the same target was also used for depression during those years [15].

The Gamma Knife evolved to be the only dedicated radiosurgery device for intracranial lesions, competing favorably among neurosurgeons with the various linear accelerator adaptations, when using single dose of radiation,

Table 19.1 Evolution of gamma unit models—technical and economical demands

Gamma Knife U	I. Pioneer: functional neurosurgery (^{60}Co 179 sources)
	II. Initial applications for morphological radiosurgery
Gamma Knife B	I. Initial worldwide demand: devices for large-scale treatment and diversity of histology and applications
	II. Economical pressure: replacement of sources at ±7 years interval (^{60}Co 201 sources) became possible
Gamma Knife C	I. Computer integration allowing initial efforts of robotization
	II. Computerized treatment plan—replacement of Kula planning—expediting the number of patients treated daily
Gamma Knife perfexion	I. Full robotization decreasing possibility of human error
	II. Maximization of collimator interplay for conformality and treatment speed. Replacement of 4 hemispherical helmets of apertures in mm (4, 8, 14, 18) each by one conical helmet with apertures in mm (4, 8, 16) capability, sectors accepting exposure of different number of the ^{60}Co 192 sources available. The GK Perfexion plus brings imaging check capabilities at the time of the treatment

which was dedicated mostly to structural diseases. The appearance of computerized imaging in the 1970s and 1980s amplified the radiosurgery applications, making the demand for dedicated devices for radiosurgery throughout the world [10]. Several models of Gamma Knife represent the evolution of the machine to its state now called commercially Perfexion®. During the evolution of the gamma knife technique lesions in the internal capsule were carried out with searching doses and many times having to adapt to new models, leading to surprises on the size of lesions obtained in the internal capsule, believed to be due to differences in dosimetry between the models of Gamma Knife (Table 19.1).

take advantage of modulation and shaping capabilities [16]. The previous collimation system of the models U, B and C (Table 19.1), which was dependent on four exchangeable helmets with 4 different sizes of apertures (4, 8, 14, 18 mm) was replaced by a single dynamic conic helmet. This new collimation system is capable of movement throughout three different apertures (4, 8, 16 mm), as well as plugging them strategically to modulate and shape the dose distribution, as desired to optimize the intensity conformity and intensity. The cumbersome process of hoisting the collimators every time that size of the isocenter was changed, serving to delay and bring possible errors to the procedure, is now bypassed in the GK Perfexion [17].

19.3 Technical Aspects of Radiosurgery

19.3.1 The Energy and Collimation System

^{60}Cobalt decays to ^{60}Ni leading to a half-life of 5.26 years to the cobalt sources powering the GK. The gamma rays resulting from this decay are collimated to the target to achieve the biological effect. Gamma rays of 1.17 and 1.33 MeV are grouped by three different collimation sizes available in the GK Perfexion to automatically

19.4 Flow of Patient Treatment

The psychiatric patient is treated as outpatients after acquisition of the MRI dedicated for the treatment. They are recommended to come to the Gamma Knife department fasting. The day before the procedure they are advised to wash their heads with an antiseptic shampoo. They are advised of the risks of the procedure and sign the informed consent understanding the implications of the radiation, including immediate, delayed and long-lasting effects, as well as the purpose of the procedure, i.e. slow and long lasting effect of radiation in the brain tissue. Therefore the delayed nature of any effect of the procedure in their disease and advised to continue taking their usual medication.

19.5 Placement of the Stereotactic Frame

They are prepared sterile in the forehead and occipital region with topical anesthetic cream followed by injection of 5 cc of mixed Lidocaine/Marcaine and sodium bicarbonate in each stereotactic frame pin site. The frame is applied strategically with the care of including the anterior limb of the internal capsule, i.e. the central part of the brain, AC and PC, central in the stereotactic space. The compatibility of the stereotactic frame placement with all hardware attachments of the Gamma Knife is checked. Measurements of the head surface are acquired with a plastic stick helmet, as well as the measurements of the stereotactic hardware for input in the Gamma Plan for calculation of beam attenuation. The patient is transferred to the CT scan for the stereotactic image acquisition to be merged to the previously obtained MRI. The contour of the patient's head obtained based on the CT can be used instead of the manual measurements previously obtained to calculate the attenuation of the beams.

19.6 Targeting and Treatment Planning

The target for anterior gamma capsulotomy has been perfected over the years, as well as the dose. Studies are still ongoing to determine whether the most ventral portion of the capsule is most effective or even if there is a lateralization on the brain, which could lead to need of only one side lesion. Now that lesions can be seen, as well as the fibers interrupted by the these lesions can be identified with MRI fiber tracking techniques,

understanding may improve on the effects specific lesion localization with consequent optimization of the results (Fig. 19.2).

The initial targets for capsulotomy as described by Mindus et al. [9] was 10 mm in front of the AC, 8 mm above the inter-commissural line and on average 17 mm lateral to the mid-plane. This target was chosen when the first Gamma Unit was available in Stockholm. It was applied a cross-firing of 179 gamma beams precisely collimated with 3×5 mm beams. On the basis of experience gained from post-mortem observations on patients subjected to gamma thalamotomy for cancer pain, it was used a central irradiation dose of 160 Gy. The treatment planning now available, the Gamma Plan, takes advantage of full computerized system which can optimize the shape of the lesion, even using different sizes of collimators to reach most ventral portions of the internal capsule in an elongated shape, it has been suggested double isocenters of 4 mm (Fig. 19.3).

19.7 Functional Lesion Considerations

19.7.1 Prescribing to a Point

Sharp and well-circumscribed lesion to disconnect pathways or ablate nuclei are the goals of this application. The prescription dose for functional neurosurgery is by convention and by tradition to the isocenter since the initial work of Leksell in psychiatric surgery [9]. This means that 100 % of the dose (=maximal dose) is prescribed to a target point, i.e. prescribed to the isocenter. The radiation prescription dose is the same as the maximal dose, when prescribing to the maximum [18]. The fall off distance, i.e. the volume of tissue receiving at least 50 % of the dose is proportional to the diameter of the aperture. The application of this concept is nicely seen during the targeting of the root entry zone in trigeminal neuralgia with the 4 mm field. The diameter of the 50 % isodose line is 4 mm. The placement of the isocenter while planning

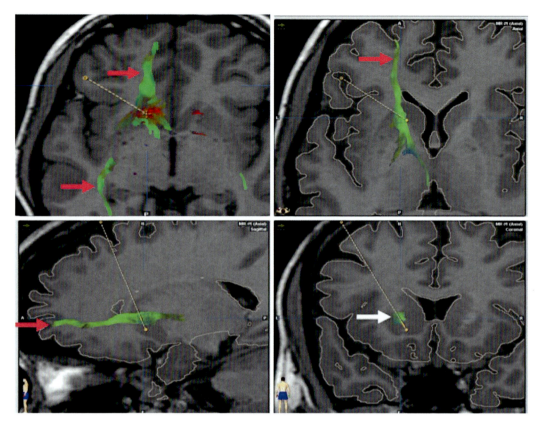

Fig. 19.3 a Demonstrates axial MRI obtained for fiber tracking. Sampling of fibers was obtained at the most ventral portion of the anterior limb of the internal capsule, reaching the shell of the nucleus accumbens, notice the spread of fibers towards the mid frontal lobe, but also towards the temporal and occipital regions through the uncinate fascculum (*arrows*). **b–d** Demonstrate axial, Sagittal and Coronal respectively with sampling in the mid-putaminal point (*white arrows* in **b** and **c**). Notice more restrict spreading of fibers only towards the mid and mesial frontal region (*arrows*)

radiosurgery for trigeminal neuralgia relies on the isodose line to determine the distance of the isocenter to the brainstem. The dose distributions in the case of capsulotomy can be tailored to elongate in the cranial-caudal direction in the internal capsule to achieve the desired disconnection of the flowing fibers in the direction of the frontal basal region (Fig. 19.3).

19.8 Imaging

MRI distortion is a reality and can happen for multiple reasons, since poor calibration of the machine, common in radiological units not linked to stereotactic services, until the presence of metal in the patient's clothes, teeth, hair, etc. Therefore strict care need to be taken when obtained images to input in the Gamma Plan®. The images must be isomorphic and orthogonal, i.e. no gantry tilt when obtaining volumetric scans. Now that image fusion is promptly obtained without the difficulty of the early years [19], acquisition of a stereotactic CT immediately before the procedure, with the patient wearing a well centered stereotactic frame, provides for most reliable stereotactic coordinates with correction of distortions that can hamper the quality of the behavioral Gamma Knife surgery. This

19 Radiosurgery for Psychiatric Disorders

Table 19.2 Minimal quality of imaging and sequences for treatment planning

Functional procedures	T2—volumetric fast spin echo recovery through basal ganglia axial T1 v/a—1 mm tck, n/g, w/c, w/fs, whole brain
Stereotactic CT	Axial a/q, 1 mm tck, n/c and w/c, whole brain

tck thickness, *n/g* no gap, *n/c* no contrast, *w/c* with contrast, *w/fs* with fat saturation, *v/a* volumetric acquisition, *a/q* acquisition

also allows for the convenience of obtaining the MRI days before the procedure to study the patients' brain in detail with functional and morphological images, including fiber tracking to understand which pathways will be interrupted (Table 19.2).

The CT, a faster acquisition image, with fewer issues of claustrophobia, movement issues and possible distortions is the ideal imaging modality to obtain in a psychiatric patient in the day of the procedure. To improve quality of the fusion, a CT post contrast is recommended, using the vascular structures seen on the CT and MRI [20].

19.9 Clinical Applications

Gamma Knife radiosurgery is indicated for all psychiatric disorders already treated with lesion and that the effectiveness is proven. This is however still under study, as much of the literature existent for lesions involving the limbic system date before the advent of computerized imaging. For example, lesions for depression in the cingulum, the limbic leucotomy, subcaudate tractotomy, the anterior thalamotomy [21], all lack of studies with modern scientific methodology correlating the location of the lesions and the clinical effects. More recently, it has been suggested that placing the lesions lower in the internal capsule has led to better control of obsessive symptoms. The body of literature involving Gamma Knife in Psychiatric surgery concentrates on the treatment of OCD having as target the anterior limb of the internal capsule, as early developed by Leksell in collaboration with Talairach in the 1950s [4], further perfected by the studies at Karolinska University, Brown University and University of

Sao Paulo, where sham randomized procedures where performed [22].

19.10 Penetration Worldwide

The patients' appeal for a more comfortable treatment, avoidance of large surgeries and reliability of the treatment and prognosis was met by radiosurgery. Progressively the treatment of the patient does not depend on the manual skills of a person, but on the intellectual and mathematical expertise of a team of specialists dedicated to provide the most reliable and comfortable care for the patient. This development worldwide based on the mushrooming of the computer technology permitted the introduction of robotized medicine and the Gamma Knife is a prototype of this approach, relying exclusively in computer capability to deliver treatment. This promises uniformity of treatment for psychiatric patients suggesting it will have a progressive number of patients undergoing Gamma Knife surgery to relieve their suffering. The indication and the management of the patient are still dependent on the doctor expertise, mostly when the medical therapy is unable to provide the comfort and/or cure. As Gamma Knife provides this immediate population need, it received immediate acceptance in the developed world and marches progressively through the countries in development, as resources become available offering hope for psychiatric patients needing a minimally invasive surgical procedure.

19.11 Obsessive Compulsive Disorder

The target for obsessive-compulsive disorder (OCD) has been in anterior limb of the internal capsule, as determined by the head of the caudate medially and the putamen laterally [8, 23]. It has evolved from the midpoint of the internal capsule as one sees it in the coronal MRI scan to the most inferior portion of the capsule in the proximity of the nucleus accumbens [24]. It became apparent over the years of experience by the groups of Karolinska University and Brown University that as the target was brought ventrally the results improved [15, 25]. Sheehan et al. [24] suggest placement of the 50 % IDL at the most ventral portion of the internal capsule. Recently a randomized trial performed by the Brazilian Group showed that indeed this rational might hold true [26]. Studies are under way to confirm this hypothesis.

The GK capsulotomy calls for a 4-mm collimator aimed to the anterior limb of the internal capsule on each side. It is planned to be located 19–21 mm anterior to the AC on the intercommissural plane. This approximately corresponded to the mid-putaminal point. T1 and T2 weighted MRI demonstrates precisely the mid-putaminal point of the anterior limb of the capsule. The most ventral portion of the 50 % isodoseline reaches the most ventral portion of the internal capsule. Doses in the literature have varied from 140 to 200 Gy [24–26], therefore 70–100 Gy reaches the shell of the accumbens at the base of the IC (Fig. 19.1). Kondziolka et al. [27] showed consistent lesions in the internal capsule using two isocenters of 4 mm, trying to obtain an oval shaped lesion of 48 mm^3 with its most inferior extension in the ventral portion of the internal capsule. The dose used in his study was 140 and 150 Gy.

19.12 Conclusion

Modern Gamma Knife radiosurgery offers easiness of treatment planning and delivery with patient's comfort as an important goal. It is an excellent choice as an instrument of lesion making for patients with Psychiatric diseases, as it is non-invasive, its effect is slow setting allowing for re-adaptation of the patient to its new therapeutic condition, facilitating rehabilitation and permitting the caring physician observe the patient closely to adjust medication in a progressive and sensible work frame.

References

1. Moniz E. How I came to perform prefrontal leucotomy. J Med (Oporto). 1949;14(355):513–5.
2. Gildenberg PL. Spiegel and Wycis—the early years. Stereotact Funct Neurosurg. 2001;77(1–4):11–6.
3. De Salles A. Evolution of radiosurgery. In: De Salles AAF, Agazaryan A, Selch M, Gorgulho AA, Slotman B, editors. Shaped beam radiosurgery. Berlin: Springer; 2011. p. 3–10.
4. Leksell L. Stereotactic radiosurery. J Neurol Neurosurg Psychiatry. 1983;46:797–803.
5. Holly FE. Radiosurgery equipment: physical principles, precision, limitations. In: De Salles AAF, Goetsch SJ, editors. Stereotactic surgery and radiosurgery. Madison: Medical Physics Publishing Corporation; 1993. p. 185–200.
6. Leksell L. The stereotaxic method and radiosurgery of the brain. Acta Chir Scand. 1951;102:316.
7. Leksell L, Herner T, Liden K. Stereotaxic radiosurgery of the brain. Report of a case. Kungl Fysiograf Sallsk Lund Forhandl. 1955;25(17):1–10.
8. Leksell L, Herner T, Leksell D, Persson B, Lindquist C. Visualisation of stereotactic radiolesions by nuclear magnetic resonance. J Neurol Neurosurg Psychiatry. 1985;48(1):19–20.
9. Mindus P, Bergström K, Levander SE, Norén G, Hindmarsh T, Thuomas KA. Magnetic resonance images related to clinical outcome after psychosurgical intervention in severe anxiety disorder. J Neurol Neurosurg Psychiatry. 1987;50 (10):1288–93.
10. De Salles AAF, Gorgulho A, Agazaryan N. Linear accelerator radiosurgery: technical aspects. In: Youmans neurologic surgery, vol. 3. 67th ed. Amsterdam: Elsevier; 2011. pp. 2622–32.
11. Gorgulho AA, Ishida W, De Salles AAF. General imaging modalities: basic principles. In: Lozano AM, Gildenberg PL, Tasker RR, editors. Text book of stereotactic and functional neurosurgery. Berlin: Springer; 2009.
12. De Salles AA, Gorgulho AA, Pereira JL, McLaughlin N. Intracranial stereotactic radiosurgery: concepts and techniques. Neurosurg Clin N Am. 2013;24(4):491–8. doi:10.1016/j.nec.2013.07.001.

13. Steiner L, Leksell L, Greitz T, Forster DMC, Backlund EO. Stereotaxic radiosurgery for cerebral arteriovenous malformations. Report of a case. Acta Chir Scand. 1972;138:459–64.
14. de Lunsford DL, Flickinger J, Lindner G, Maitz A. Stereotactic radiosurgery of the brain using the first United States 201 cobalt-60 source gamma knife. Neurosurgery. 1989;24(2):151–9.
15. Lippitz BE, Mindus P, Meyerson BA, Kihlström L, Lindquist C. Lesion topography and outcome after thermocapsulotomy or gamma knife capsulotomy for obsessive-compulsive disorder: relevance of the right hemisphere. Neurosurgery. 1999;44(3):452–8; discussion 458–60.
16. Bhatnagar JP, Novotny J Jr, Huq MS. Dosimetric characteristics and quality control tests for the collimator sectors of the Leksell Gamma Knife(®) Perfexion(TM). Med Phys. 2012;39(1):231–6.
17. Régis J, Tamura M, Guillot C, Yomo S, Muraciolle X, Nagaje M, Arka Y, Porcheron D. Radiosurgery with the world's first fully robotized Leksell Gamma Knife PerfeXion in clinical use: a 200-patient prospective, randomized, controlled comparison with the Gamma Knife 4C. Neurosurgery. 2009;64(2):346–55.
18. Leksell L. Cerebral radiosurgery. I. Gammathalanotomy in two cases of intractable pain. Acta Chir Scand. 1968;134(8):585–95.
19. De Salles AAF, Asfora WT, Abe M, Kjelberg RN. Transposition of target information from the magnetic resonance and CT-scan images to the conventional X-ray stereotactic space. Appl Neurophys. 1987;50:23–32.
20. Jonker BP. Image fusion pitfalls for cranial radiosurgery. Surg Neurol Int. 2013;4(Suppl 3):S123–8.
21. Hazari H, Christmas D, Matthews K. The clinical utility of different quantitative methods for measuring treatment resistance in major depression. J Affect Disord. 2013;150(2):231–6.

22. Cecconi JP, Lopes AC, Duran FL, Santos LC, Hoexter MQ, Gentil AF, Canteras MM, Castro CC, Norén G, Greenberg BD, Rauch SL, Busatto GF, Miguel EC. Gamma ventral capsulotomy for treatment of resistant obsessive-compulsive disorder: a structural MRI pilot prospective study. Neurosci Lett. 2008;447(2–3):138–42.
23. Leksell L, Backlund EO. Radiosurgical capsulotomy–a closed surgical method for psychiatric surgery. Lakartidningen. 1978;75 (7):546–7 (Swedish. No abstract available).
24. Sheehan JP, Patterson G, Schlesinger D, Xu Z. Gamma Knife surgery anterior capsulotomy for severe and refractory obsessive-compulsive disorder. J Neurosurg. 2013;119:1112–8.
25. Ruck C, Karlsson A, Steele D, et al. Capsulotomy for obsessive-compulsive disorder. Long-term follow-up of 25 patients. Arch Gen Psych. 2008;65(8):914–22.
26. Lopes A, Greenberg B, Noren G, et al. Treatment of resistant obsessive-compulsive disorder with ventral capsular/ventral striatal gamma capsulotomy: a pilot prospective study. J Neuropsych Clin Neurosci. 2009;21(4):381–92.
27. Kondziolka D, Flickinger JC, Hudak R. Results following gamma knife radiosurgical anterior capsulotomies for obsessive compulsive disorder. Neurosurgery. 2011;68(1):28–32; discussion 23-3.

Index

A

Ablation, 55, 60, 62, 64, 90, 106, 111, 114, 125–129, 132, 134, 145, 164, 165, 169, 170, 172, 181, 182, 192

Ablative neurosurgery, 78, 87, 194

Aggressive behavior, 194, 203, 204, 206, 207, 211, 215, 216

Anorexia nervosa, 11, 30, 39–41, 82, 98, 165, 175, 176, 184

Anterior capsulotomy, 55, 59, 61, 62, 87, 107, 109, 115, 126, 180–182, 191–194

Anterior limb of internal capsule, 115

Antipsychotic, 146

Antipsychotic drugs, 146, 203

Autonomy, 78, 79, 83

B

Basal ganglia, 4, 11, 50, 56, 57, 59, 100, 106, 125, 144, 145, 150, 151, 204, 223

Behavioral surgery, 217, 218

Bilateral anterior cingulotomy, 71, 74, 87, 88, 108, 126, 182

Bilateral limbic leukotomy, 89–92

Brain neurotransmitter systems, 203

C

Capsulotomy, 61, 96, 97, 100, 107, 109, 114, 132, 137, 179, 180, 192–194, 200, 205, 221, 222, 224

Caudate nucleus, 4, 5, 41, 56, 57, 59, 106–108, 116, 125, 126, 144, 145, 166, 190, 197, 205, 206

Cerebello-thalamo-cortico-pontine loop, 4

Cingulate cortex, 4, 36, 106

Cingulotomy, 58–61, 87, 96, 98, 107–109, 114, 126, 147–149, 162, 164, 179–182, 191–194, 200, 206, 207, 219

Cognitive-behavior-emotional circuit, 115

Compulsion, 105, 108, 110, 113, 125, 148, 180, 205

Cortical-striatal-thalamic circuit, 106

Corticostriatal–thalamocortical circuitry, 145

D

Deep brain stimulation, 11, 39, 47–50, 55, 60–62, 71, 77, 95, 114, 120, 125, 134, 149, 165, 175, 177, 180, 194, 206

Diffusion spectrum imaging, 21, 22, 24, 27

Diffusion tensor imaging, 2, 21, 26, 35

Dopamine, 1, 3, 12, 37–39, 56, 146, 151, 152, 163, 176, 190

Doppler effect, 127

Drug addiction, 161–165, 167, 168, 170–172, 181

F

Fiber crossing, 24

Functional magnetic resonance imaging, 2, 35–38, 96, 115

G

Gamma capsulotomy, 218, 221

Gamma knife, 55, 59, 108–110, 120, 125, 217–224

H

Hippocampus-amgydala complex, 3, 5, 11

L

Lesions, 42, 48, 53–58, 60–64, 88–91, 93, 96, 97, 106–108, 110, 126, 127, 130, 135, 137, 138, 148, 162, 179, 181, 189, 192, 193, 205, 217–221, 223, 224

Limbic leucotomy, 59, 60, 96, 108, 109, 114, 147–149, 191–193, 207, 223

M

Magnetic resonance imaging, 2, 21, 36, 145, 181, 211

Major depressive disorder, 11, 29, 30, 38, 48, 59, 60, 78, 95, 176

Medial forebrain bundle, 98–100, 164

MRI guided high frequency focused ultrasound, 91

N

Network, 1, 6, 21, 23, 28, 30, 36, 88, 96, 115, 180

Neural circuits, 2, 95, 115, 117, 125, 126, 176–178

Neuroanatomy, 27, 56, 106, 203

Neurobiological circuits, 1

Neuroimaging, 27, 35, 37, 42, 43, 79, 88, 98, 105, 106, 114, 115, 145, 175–177, 189, 191, 194

Neuromodulation, 2, 11, 48, 62, 81, 95, 96, 101, 114, 118, 120, 126, 152, 216

B. Sun and A. De Salles (eds.), *Neurosurgical Treatments for Psychiatric Disorders*,
DOI 10.1007/978-94-017-9576-0
© Shanghai Jiao Tong University Press, Shanghai and Springer Science+Business Media Dordrecht 2015

Nucleus accumbens, 9, 56–58, 71, 98–100, 115, 116, 126, 150, 151, 162, 166, 175, 177, 181, 190, 194, 205, 207, 222

O
Obsession, 105, 108, 110, 113, 125, 135, 148
Obsessive compulsive disorder, 11, 29, 39, 41, 42, 48, 56, 69, 71, 78, 105, 113, 125, 126, 132, 164, 176, 180, 205, 217, 224
Orbital frontal cortex, 40
Orbitofrontal circuit, 57

P
Papez's circuit, 13
Patient selection, 54, 77, 80, 118–120, 132, 150, 182, 183, 191, 194
Physiological dependence, 161
Positron emission tomography, 36, 38, 39, 88, 96, 100, 106, 115, 116, 164, 177
Psychiatric comorbidities, 82, 145, 146, 176, 181
Psychiatric disorder, 1, 2, 4, 10, 22, 27, 29–31, 35, 37, 42, 43, 48, 50, 53, 55, 63, 64, 77–84, 88–91, 97, 106, 110, 114, 118, 125, 144, 165, 175, 176, 178, 180, 182, 184, 191, 203, 205, 219, 223
Psychosurgery, 49, 61, 74, 114, 190, 217, 219

Q
Quality of life, 77–79, 81, 82, 84, 105, 109–111, 117, 144, 152, 169, 172, 175, 185

R
Radiosurgery, 55, 62, 71, 87, 90, 108–111, 125, 129, 185, 204, 205, 217, 218
Refractory psychiatric disorders, 79, 114

Refractory schizophrenia, 191
Region of interest, 28, 29, 35
Replacement therapy, 161

S
Schizoaffective disorder, 60, 204
Serotonin, 69, 72, 190
Serotonin reuptake, 38, 69, 72, 105, 113, 114, 132, 146, 150, 178
Stereotactic surgery, 48, 55, 62, 87, 91, 111, 147, 149, 162, 164, 165, 167, 171, 172, 184, 185, 194, 204, 217
Subcaudate tractotomy, 59, 60, 62, 108, 109, 114, 191–194, 207, 223
Substantia innominata, 3, 5, 6, 8, 10, 59, 108
Surgery, 42, 50, 59, 62, 70, 71, 80–83, 87, 89, 91

T
Thalamotomy, 49, 55, 147, 203, 217, 218, 221, 223
Thermocoagulation, 58, 59, 61, 62, 90, 148, 205
Tourette syndrome, 48, 125, 143, 149–151
Tractography, 6, 22, 23, 25–27, 29, 30, 106, 107, 110
Transcranial magnetic resonance-guided focused ultrasound, 125, 127–130, 132, 133, 135–138
Treatment refractory depression, 71, 87

V
Ventral capsule and ventral striatum, 100, 115, 116, 180
Violent psychosis, 203
Voxel-based morphometric analyses, 2, 23–25, 29

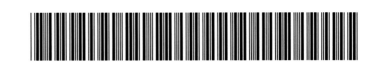

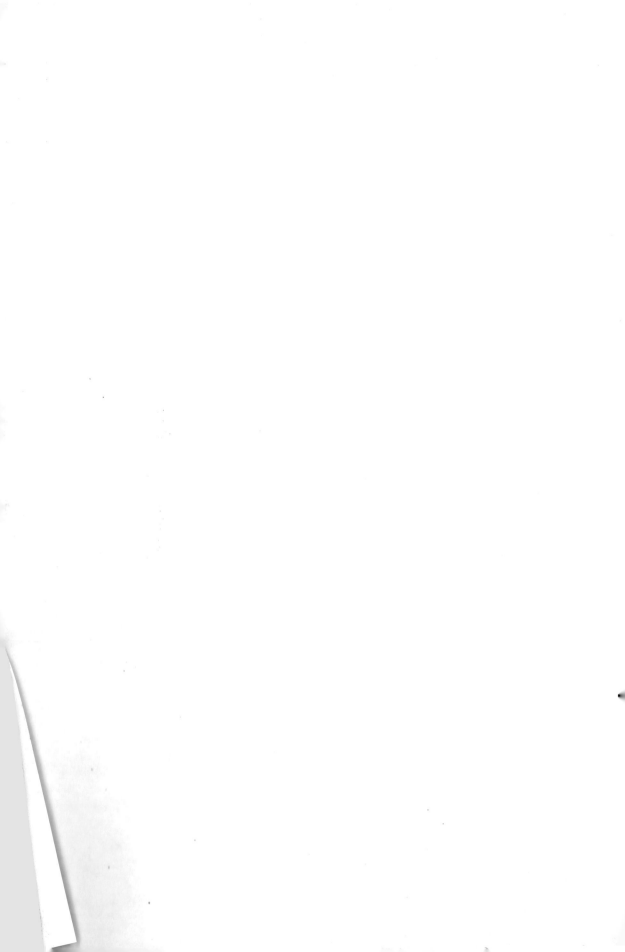